Musculoskeletal Pain Management

Musculoskeletal Pain Management

Editor
Abdul Ghani MBBS MS MRCS
Professor
Department of Orthopedics
Goverment Medical College
Jammu, Jammu & Kashmir, India

Foreword
J Maheshwari

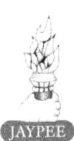

JAYPEE BROTHERS MEDICAL PUBLISHERS
The Health Sciences Publisher
New Delhi | London

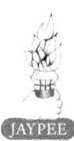

Jaypee Brothers Medical Publishers (P) Ltd

Headquarters
EMCA House
23/23-B, Ansari Road, Daryaganj
New Delhi 110 002, India
Landline: +91-11-23272143
+91-11-23272703, +91-11-23282021
+91-11-23245672
E-mail: jaypee@jaypeebrothers.com

Corporate Office
Jaypee Brothers Medical Publishers (P) Ltd.
4838/24, Ansari Road, Daryaganj
New Delhi 110 002, India
Phone: +91-11-43574357
Fax: +91-11-43574314
E-mail: jaypee@jaypeebrothers.com

Overseas Office
JP Medical Ltd.
83, Victoria Street, London
SW1H 0HW (UK)
Phone: +44-20 3170 8910
E-mail: info@jpmedpub.com

EU GPSR Authorised Representative
Logos Europe, 9 rue Nicolas Poussin
17000, La Rochelle, France
Phone: +33 (0) 6 67 93 73 78
E-mail: Contact@logoseurope.eu

Website: www.jaypeebrothers.com
Website: www.jaypeedigital.com

© 2025, Jaypee Brothers Medical Publishers

The views and opinions expressed in this book are solely those of the original contributor(s)/author(s) and do not necessarily represent those of editor(s) or publisher of the book.

All rights reserved. No part of this publication may be reproduced, stored or transmitted in any form or by any means, electronic, mechanical, photocopying, recording or otherwise, without the prior permission in writing of the publishers.

All brand names and product names used in this book are trade names, service marks, trademarks or registered trademarks of their respective owners. The publisher is not associated with any product or vendor mentioned in this book.

Medical knowledge and practice change constantly. This book is designed to provide accurate, authoritative information about the subject matter in question. However, readers are advised to check the most current information available on procedures included and check information from the manufacturer of each product to be administered, to verify the recommended dose, formula, method and duration of administration, adverse effects and contraindications. It is the responsibility of the practitioner to take all appropriate safety precautions. Neither the publisher nor the author(s)/editor(s) assume any liability for any injury and/or damage to persons or property arising from or related to use of material in this book.

This book is sold on the understanding that the publisher is not engaged in providing professional medical services. If such advice or services are required, the services of a competent medical professional should be sought.

Every effort has been made where necessary to contact holders of copyright to obtain permission to reproduce copyright material. If any have been inadvertently overlooked, the publisher will be pleased to make the necessary arrangements at the first opportunity.

Inquiries for bulk sales may be solicited at: jaypee@jaypeebrothers.com

Musculoskeletal Pain Management / Abdul Ghani

First Edition: **2025**

ISBN: 978-93-5696-953-7

Dedication to

Almighty

and

All

The contributing authors

Contributors

Abhai Singh Bhadwal MBBS
Postgraduate Orthopedics
Resident
Department of Orthopedics
Government Medical College
Jammu, Jammu & Kashmir, India

Abhishek Mahajan MBBS
Postgraduate Orthopedics
Resident
Department of Orthopedics
Government Medical College
Jammu, Jammu & Kashmir, India

Akash Narangyal MBBS Postgraduate Orthopedics
Resident
Department of Orthopedics
Government Medical College
Jammu, Jammu & Kashmir, India

Anchal Gupta MBBS MD(Radiodiagnosis)
Associate Professor
Department of Radiodiagnosis and Imaging
Government Medical College
Jammu, Jammu & Kashmir, India

Anita Kour MBBS MD(Anesthesiology)
Senior Resident
Department of Anesthesia, Critical Care and Pain Medicine
Government Medical College
Jammu, Jammu & Kashmir, India

Anita Vig Kohli MBBS MD(Anesthesiology)
Professor
Department of Anesthesiology, Pain Management and Critical Care
Government Medical College
Jammu, Jammu & Kashmir, India

Ankita Khajuria MBBS
Resident
Department of Orthopedics
Government Medical College
Jammu, Jammu & Kashmir, India

Anjali Mehta MBBS MD
Professor
Department of Anesthesia, Pain Management and Critical Care
Government Medical College
Jammu, Jammu & Kashmir, India

Arti Mahajan MBBS MD
Associate Professor
Department of Anesthesia, Pain Management and Critical Care
Government Medical College
Jammu, Jammu & Kashmir, India

Ashwani Kumar MBBS MD(Anesthesia)
Professor
Department of Anesthesia, Pain Management and Critical Care
Government Medical College
Jammu, Jammu & Kashmir, India

Azhar Ud Din MBBS MS(Orthopedics)
Consultant Orthopedics
Department of Orthopedics
District Hospital
Kargil, UT Ladakh, India

Bias Dev MBBS MS
Associate Professor
Department of Orthopedics
Government Medical College
Jammu, Jammu & Kashmir, India

Deepika Saroj BPT MPT in Sports Physiotherapy
Physiotherapist
Department of Physiotherapy
Government Medical College
Jammu, Jammu & Kashmir, India

Contributors

Deepali Gupta BPT MPT in Sports Physiotherapy
Physiotherapist
Department of Physiotherapy
Government Medical College
Jammu, Jammu & Kashmir, India

Farid Hussain MBBS
MS(Orthopedics)
Assistant Professor
Department of Orthopedics
Government Medical College
Jammu, Jammu & Kashmir, India

Gagandeep Singh Raina MBBS
MS(Orthopedics)
Senior Resident
Department of Orthopedics
Government Medical College
Jammu, Jammu & Kashmir, India

Harsh Chauhan MBBS Postgraduate Orthopedics
Resident
Department of Orthopedics
Government Medical College
Jammu, Jammu & Kashmir, India

Muhammad Haseeb Gani MBBS
MS(Orthopedics)
Senior Consultant
Department of Orthopedics
Paras Hospital
Srinagar, Jammu & Kashmir, India

Heena Saini MBBS MD(Anesthesia)
Assistant Professor
Department of Anesthesia
Government Medical College
Jammu, Jammu & Kashmir, India

Jasmeen Chowdhary MBBS
MD(Anesthesia)
Assistant Professor
Department of Anesthesia, Critical Care and Pain Medicine
Government Medical College
Jammu, Jammu & Kashmir, India

Jawahar Mehmood Khan MBBS
MS(Orthopedics)
Assistant Professor
Department of Orthopedics
Government Medical College
Srinagar, Jammu & Kashmir, India

John Mohd MBBS MS(Orthopedics)
Senior Resident
Deparment of Physical Medicine and Rehabilitation
SKIMS Soura
Srinagar, Jammu & Kashmir, India

Khalid Muzzafar MBBS
MS(Orthopedics) DNB(Orthopedics)
Associate Professor
Department of Orthopedics
Government Medical College
Doda, Jammu & Kashmir, India

Kunal Sharma MBBS MD(Anesthesia)
Assistant Professor
Department of Anesthesia and Critical Care
Government Medical College
Jammu, Jammu & Kashmir, India

Madan Lal Katoch MBBS
MD(Anesthesia)
Professor
Department of Anesthesia, Critical Care and Pain Medicine
Government Medical College
Jammu, Jammu & Kashmir, India

Manish Singh MBBS MS(Orthopedics)
Assistant Professor
Department of Orthopedics
Government Medical College
Jammu, Jammu & Kashmir, India

Mushtaq Ahmed Wani MBBS
MD(Anesthesia)
Associate Professor
Department of Anesthesia, Critical Care and Pain Medicine
Government Medical College
Jammu, Jammu & Kashmir, India

Contributors

Nalini Birpuri MBBS MS(Ophthalmology)
Senior Resident
Department of Ophthalmology
Government Medical College
Jammu, Jammu & Kashmir, India

Nanie Bhadrala MBBS MD(Anesthesia)
Associate Professor
Department of Anesthesia, Critical Care and Pain Medicine
Government Medical College
Jammu, Jammu & Kashmir, India

Neha Sharma MBBS MD(Anesthesia)
Assistant Professor
Department of Anesthesia and Critical Care
Government Medical College
Jammu, Jammu & Kashmir, India

Nitin Choudhary MBBS MS(Orthopedics)
Senior Resident
Department of Orthopedics
Government Medical College
Jammu, Jammu & Kashmir, India

Nusrat Jabeen MBBS MS(Anatomy)
Professor
Department of Anatomy
Government Medical College
Jammu, Jammu & Kashmir, India

Nusrat Kreem Bhat MBBS MD(Pharmacology)
Professor
Department of Pharmacology
Government Medical College
Jammu, Jammu & Kashmir, India

Pankaj Vir Singh MBBS MS(Orthopedics)
Senior Resident
Department of Orthopedics
Government Medical College
Jammu, Jammu & Kashmir, India

Parul Raina MBBS MD(Anesthesia) GFPM(Global Fellowship in Palliative Medicine)
Consultant
Department of Anesthesia
Cytecare Cancer Hospital
Bengaluru, Karnataka, India

Rajesh Mahajan MBBS MD(Anesthesia)
Professor
Department of Anesthesia, Pain Management and Critical Care
Government Medical College
Jammu, Jammu & Kashmir, India

Rashid Anjum MBBS MS DNB MNAMS FIPO
Associate Professor
Department of Orthopedics
AIIMS, Vijaypur
Jammu, Jammu & Kashmir, India

Renu Wakhloo MBBS MD(Anesthesia)
Associate Professor
Department of Anesthesia and Critical Care
Government Medical College
Jammu, Jammu & Kashmir, India

Rifaaqat Ghani MBBS(Pursuing)
Student
Vardhman Mahavir Medical College
New Delhi, India

Sachin Kudyar MBBS MS(Orthopedics)
Senior Resident
Department of Orthopedics
Government Medical College
Jammu, Jammu & Kashmir, India

Sakib Arfee MBBS MS(Orthopedics)
Consultant
Department of Orthopedics
Medcard Multi-speciality Hospital
Amritsar, Punjab, India

Sanjeev Gupta MBBS MS(Orthopedics)
Professor
Department of Orthopedics
Government Medical College
Jammu, Jammu & Kashmir, India

Saransh Bahl MBBS Postgraduate
Orthopedics
Resident
Department of Orthopedics
Government Medical College
Jammu, Jammu & Kashmir, India

Contributors

Shruti Gupta MBBS MD(Anesthesia)
Associate Professor
Department of Anesthesia, Critical Care and Pain Medicine
Government Medical College
Jammu, Jammu & Kashmir, India

Shubham Pandoh MBBS
MS(Orthopedics)
Senior Resident
Department of Orthopedics
Government Medical College
Jammu, Jammu & Kashmir, India

Shubam Surmal MBBS
MS(Orthopedics)
Senior Resident
Department of Orthopedics
Government Medical College
Jammu, Jammu & Kashmir, India

Siddhartha Sharma MS FRCS PhD
Additional Professor
Department of Orthopedics
Postgraduate Institute of Medical Education and Research
Chandigarh, India

Sonakshi Gupta MBBS
MD(Anesthesia)
Senior Resident
Department of Anesthesia and Critical Care
Government Medical College
Jammu, Jammu & Kashmir, India

Sukhil Raina MBBS MS(Orthopedics)
Senior Resident
Department of Orthopedics
Government Medical College
Jammu, Jammu & Kashmir, India

Sumeet Singh Charak MBBS
MS(Orthopedics)
Assistant Professor
Department of Orthopedics
Government Medical College
Jammu, Jammu & Kashmir, India

Sunana Gupta MBBS MD(Anesthesia)
Additional Professor
Department of Anesthesiology
AIIMS Vijaypur
Jammu, Jammu & Kashmir, India

Suraydev Aman Singh MBBS
MS(Orthopedics)
Senior Resident
Department of Orthopedics
Government Medical College
Jammu, Jammu & Kashmir, India

Tanveer Ahmed Bhat MBBS
MS(Orthopedics)
Consultant
Department of Orthopedics
Government Medical College
Jammu, Jammu & Kashmir, India

Updesh Kumar MBBS MD(Anesthesia)
Assistant Professor
Department of Anesthesia, ICU and Pain Medicine
Government Medical College
Jammu, Jammu & Kashmir, India

Yassir Mehmood MBBS Postgraduate Orthopedics
Resident
Department of Orthopedics
Government Medical College
Jammu, Jammu & Kashmir, India

Younis Kamal MBBS MS(Ortho) DNB(Ortho) MNMS(Ortho)
Postdoc Fellowship in Spine Surgery (Ganga Hospital)
Department of Orthopedics and Spine Surgery
Government Medical College
Anantnag, Jammu & Kashmir, India

Zubair Ahmad Lone MBBS
MS(Orthopedics)
Assistant Professor
Department of Orthopedics
Government Medical College
Rajouri, Jammu & Kashmir, India

Foreword

It is a pleasure to write a foreword for this one-of-its-kind title, authored by an orthopedic surgeon.

Surgeons know the importance of pain management in surgery. Recent emphasis has been put on making surgery painless. Unfortunately for too long, surgeons have remained focused on techniques of surgery, and this important aspect of patient care—pain management—has been relegated to our anesthesia team.

Yes, some anesthesia colleagues are highly motivated to embrace newer pain relief techniques, and it is an asset to have such colleagues in your team. But, largely, surgeon–anesthetist communication is rather impersonal as a new anesthetist is on the head-end every day.

Hence, more often than not, ensuring pain management becomes the responsibility of the surgical team. It is in this background that a book dedicated to pain management is a novel thought.

I compliment Ghani for conceptualizing this title and putting effort into giving it the shape of a book. I am sure that it will become a much sought-after title with surgeons and anesthetists.

I wish the book all the success!

J Maheshwari MBBS MS(Orthopedics)
Author of Essential Orthopedics
Knee and Shoulder Clinic
Sitaram Bhartia Hospital
New Delhi, India

Preface

The complexity and diversity of musculoskeletal pain disorders demand a comprehensive approach to its management. It is with this need in mind that I present this book "*Musculoskeletal Pain Management*".

The primary goal of this book is to provide a brief, crisp, and practical guide to treating musculoskeletal pain effectively and scientifically in any situation or condition. This book is based on the latest research and clinical practices in this field and therefore aims to equip healthcare professionals with the latest knowledge and means to address these issues.

Throughout the book, almost all the topics have been explored with various treatment modalities. Also, the wide range of day-to-day challenges faced by clinicians has been covered. Each chapter is designed to offer a blend of insights and practical applications, ensuring that the reader gains a holistic understanding of the subject matter.

One of the unique features of this book is its multidisciplinary approach. It was recognized that musculoskeletal pain often requires the expertise of various healthcare professionals. Therefore, this book has included perspectives from orthopedists, anesthetists, pharmacologists, general practitioners, physiotherapists, pain specialists, and other relevant practitioners. This collaborative approach emphasizes the importance of an integrated treatment strategy in achieving optimal patient outcomes.

This book is intended to be a comprehensive resource for anyone involved in the management of musculoskeletal pain. Whether a seasoned practitioner seeking to update current knowledge or a resident embarking on a medical career, I find the information within these pages enlightening and practical.

Thank you for your interest in this book. I trust that it will serve as a valuable guide in your professional journey. There are deliberate repetitions and overlap of a few important aspects to reinforce the key concepts.

I welcome any feedback or suggestions from readers as we continue to advance our understanding and treatment of musculoskeletal pain. Together, let us strive to alleviate the burden of pain and improve the quality of life for those affected.

Please feel free to share your critical valuable feedback at drghani31@gmail.com.

Sincerely,

Abdul Ghani

Acknowledgments

First and foremost, I would like to express my heartfelt gratitude to the Almighty who has given me the insight and wisdom to write this book.

A big thanks go to all the contributing authors, for coming forth and contributing very proactively. I am also grateful to them for their encouragement, as it was instrumental in bringing this project to fruition. Their insights and feedback have been invaluable.

I am profoundly thankful to my family, whose unwavering support has meant the world to me. I thank my wife Nusrat in particular, for her endless patience and understanding during this process. I thank my son Rifaaqat for his love and for being a constant source of my energy.

A big thank you goes to Dr J Maheshwari, for agreeing to write a foreword for this book.

Special thanks goes to Dr Farid Hussain, whose keen eye and thoughtful suggestions greatly improved the content a lot. His sincere input has been crucial in shaping this book.

I extend my thanks to my colleagues and peers, for the stimulating discussions and for sharing their thoughts and input. Their support has been greatly appreciated.

I am highly obliged to M/s Jaypee Brothers Medical Publishers (P) Ltd., New Delhi, India, especially Mr Ashish Kumar (Senior Business Development Manager), Sheeba Khan (Development Editor), and Priyansh Saxena (Development Editor), for getting this book into real shape.

I would also like to acknowledge the invaluable help and support from Mr Vikram Singh Khullar for shaping this manuscript.

Finally, I thank the readers for their interest in this book. I hope they find it as enlightening and enjoyable to read as it was for me to write.

Writing this book has been a journey of both challenge and discovery, and I am deeply grateful to many people who have supported me along the way.

Once again, I thank all for being a part of this journey.

Kind regards,

Abdul Ghani

Contents

1. Understanding Musculoskeletal Pain ... 1
   Anjali Mehta

2. Anatomy and Physiology of Pain ... 3
   Nusrat Jabeen, Rifaaqat Ghani

3. Assessment of Musculoskeletal Pain ... 6
   Akash Narangyal

4. Management of Acute Musculoskeletal Pain ... 10
   Kunal Sharma

5. Managing Chronic Musculoskeletal Pain ... 15
   Mushtaq Ahmed Wani

6. Transition from Acute to Chronic Pain ... 20
   Anita Kour

7. Pain Flare Management ... 23
   Nitin Choudhary

8. Current Guidelines for Musculoskeletal Pain Management ... 27
   Pankaj Vir Singh

9. Nonsteroidal Anti-inflammatory Drug and Acetaminophen ... 31
   Arti Mahajan

10. Opioids and Opioid-sparing Strategies in the Management of Musculoskeletal Pain ... 40
    Nusrat Kreem Bhat, Farid Hussain

11. Role of Muscle Relaxants in Musculoskeletal Pain Management ... 47
    Nusrat Kreem Bhat, Farid Hussain

12. Adjunct Analgesics ... 52
    Sachin Kudyar

13. Topical Analgesia ... 56
    Farid Hussain, Nusrat Kreem Bhat

14. Pediatric Musculoskeletal Pain ... 63
    Neha Sharma

15. Approach to Back Pain in Children ... 68
Younis Kamal

16. Geriatric Musculoskeletal Pain ... 74
Neha Sharma

17. Management of Musculoskeletal Pain in Pregnant and Lactating Mothers ... 78
Jasmeen Chowdhary

18. Management of Musculoskeletal Pain in Liver Failure ... 86
Nalini Birpuri, Updesh Kumar

19. Management of Musculoskeletal Pain in Renal Failure ... 89
Updesh Kumar, Nalini Birpuri

20. Management of Musculoskeletal Pain in the Phantom Limb ... 94
Renu Wakhloo

21. Management of Neuropathic Pain ... 98
Ashwani Kumar

22. Management of Rheumatoid Arthritis Pain ... 101
Suraydev Aman Singh

23. Management of Acute and Chronic Gouty Pain ... 104
Rashid Anjum

24. Pain Management in Osteoporotic Vertebral Fracture ... 111
Sukhil Raina

25. Pain Management in Ankylosing Spondylitis ... 117
Sakib Arfee

26. Sports Injury ... 121
Neha Sharma, Suraydev Aman Singh

27. Approach to Management of Low Backache in Adults ... 124
Bias Dev

28. Pain Management of Osteoarthritis ... 132
Suraydev Aman Singh

29. Pain Management of Cervical Spondylosis ... 135
Suraydev Aman Singh, Zubair Ahmad Lone, Shubam Surmal

30. Approach to Management of Shoulder Pain ... 139
Gagandeep Singh Raina

31. Management of Tennis Elbow and Golfer's Elbow ... 143
Khalid Muzzafar

32. De Quervain's Disease — 148
Sanjeev Gupta

33. Management of Carpal Tunnel Syndrome — 153
Sakib Arfee

34. Approach to the Management of Knee Pain — 156
Jawahar Mehmood Khan

35. Approach to Heel Pain — 160
Muhammad Haseeb Gani

36. Management of Foot and Ankle Pain — 164
Manish Singh

37. Fibromyalgia — 168
Azhar Ud Din, Saransh Bahl

38. Management of Complex Regional Pain Syndrome — 175
Saransh Bahl

39. Myofascial Syndrome — 181
Saransh Bahl

40. Interventional Techniques for Pain Relief — 185
Sunana Gupta, Rajesh Mahajan

41. Joint Injection Techniques — 190
Siddhartha Sharma, Tanveer Ahmed Bhat

42. Role of Radiology in Managing Musculoskeletal Pain — 199
Anchal Gupta

43. Local Anesthesia in Musculoskeletal Pain Management — 203
Zubair Ahmad Lone, Shubam Surmal

44. Surgical Management of Musculoskeletal Pain — 207
Sumeet Singh Charak

45. Preemptive Analgesia — 210
Yassir Mehmood

46. Intraoperative Measures to Reduce Postoperative Pain — 214
Heena Saini

47. Postoperative Pain Management Strategies — 220
Madan Lal Katoch

48. Enhanced Recovery after Surgery Protocols — 225
Anita Vig Kohli

49.	Role of Steroid in Musculoskeletal Pain Management *Abhai Singh Bhadwal*	232
50.	Role of Physiotherapy in the Management of Musculoskeletal Pain *Deepika Saroj, Deepali Gupta*	238
51.	Role of Integrated Medicine Including Alternative Medicine in Pain Management *Harsh Chauhan*	243
52.	Role of Acupuncture in the Management of Musculoskeletal Pain *Nusrat Jabeen*	247
53.	Musculoskeletal Pain and Mental Health *Ankita Khajuria*	250
54.	Essentials of Regenerative Medicine in Pain Management *Rashid Anjum*	253
55.	Multidisciplinary Approaches to Pain Management *John Mohd, Parul Raina*	257
56.	Palliative Care and End-of-Life Pain Management in Musculoskeletal Pain *Rajesh Mahajan, Sunana Gupta*	260
57.	Preventive Strategies for Musculoskeletal Pain *Abhishek Mahajan*	264
58.	Occupational and Ergonomics Considerations in Musculoskeletal Pain Management *Shubham Pandoh*	268
59.	Pain Education and Patient Empowerment *Sonakshi Gupta*	273
60.	Technology and Innovation in Pain Management *Shruti Gupta*	276
61.	Emerging Trends and Future Directions in Musculoskeletal Pain Management *Nanie Bhadrala*	281

Index — *285*

CHAPTER 1

Understanding Musculoskeletal Pain

Anjali Mehta

■ INTRODUCTION

Musculoskeletal pain is a widespread and often debilitating issue affecting millions globally. It impacts approximately 47% of the population and poses challenges for both patients and healthcare providers alike. This type of pain encompasses a broad range of disorders involving bones, muscles, ligaments, tendons, and other connective tissues.

Pain is a common symptom associated with musculoskeletal disorders, influencing patients' physical and emotional well-being. Managing pain effectively not only aids in the recovery process but also improves overall patient outcomes. Effective pain management is crucial in orthopedics and trauma care as inadequate pain control. Inadequate pain control can hinder wound healing, increase infection risks, and delay patient mobilization, potentially leading to complications like pulmonary embolism and thrombosis.

Musculoskeletal pain can stem from various causes, including acute injuries, chronic conditions, degenerative diseases, and inflammatory processes such as arthritis and fibromyalgia. It can manifest as localized discomfort or widespread pain affecting multiple areas.

Pain management strategies are classified into acute and chronic categories. Acute pain typically arises suddenly from an injury and resolves within weeks with appropriate treatment. Chronic pain persists for longer periods, often beyond 3 months despite intervention, significantly impacting daily life.

The principles of managing musculoskeletal pain involve a comprehensive approach that integrates pharmacological, nonpharmacological, and interventional methods. The goal is not only to alleviate pain but also to enhance functionality and improve quality of life.

Implementing multimodal analgesia regimens has been effective due to their synergistic effects in pain relief. Early administration of oral medications post surgery can shorten hospital stays and reduce healthcare costs, minimizing complications associated with prolonged hospitalization.

A multidisciplinary approach is essential for addressing complex musculoskeletal pain, involving collaboration among various healthcare professionals such as physicians, physical therapists, psychologists, and occupational therapists. This team effort ensures a tailored treatment plan that addresses individual needs comprehensively.

Structured pain management programs incorporating education, physical therapy, psychological support, and medication management have shown promise in improving outcomes for chronic pain sufferers. These programs emphasize patient education, goal setting, and active participation in treatment decisions to achieve better results.

CONCLUSION

Effective musculoskeletal pain management requires a holistic understanding of its causes and symptoms, along with a patient-centered approach that integrates evidence-based treatments. By adopting a comprehensive strategy that considers the diverse aspects of pain and individual patient needs, healthcare providers can significantly enhance the well-being of those affected by musculoskeletal pain. Continued research and innovation in pain management offer hope for more personalized and effective treatments in the future.

BIBLIOGRAPHY

1. Bannwarth B, Kostine M. Targeting the prostaglandin E2 pathway: background for rational design of novel therapeutic strategies in pain management. Curr Opin Rheumatol. 2014;26(2):150-9.
2. Baron R. Mechanisms of disease: neuropathic pain—a clinical perspective. Nat Clin Pract Neurol. 2006;2(2):95-106.
3. Chou R, Turner JA, Devine EB, Hansen RN, Sullivan SD, Blazina I, et al. The effectiveness and risks of long-term opioid therapy for chronic pain: a systematic review for a National Institutes of Health Pathways to Prevention Workshop. Ann Intern Med. 2015;162(4):276-86.
4. Latremoliere A, Woolf CJ. Central sensitization: a generator of pain hypersensitivity by central neural plasticity. J Pain. 2009;10(9):895-926.
5. Woolf CJ, Salter MW. Neuronal plasticity: increasing the gain in pain. Science. 2000;288(5472):1765-9.

CHAPTER 2

Anatomy and Physiology of Pain

Nusrat Jabeen, Rifaaqat Ghani

■ INTRODUCTION

Understanding the anatomy and physiology of pain is crucial for professionals across the medical field. The musculoskeletal system is a foundation of human anatomy, encompassing bones, muscles, tendons, ligaments, and cartilage, forming the essential structural framework of the body.

Musculoskeletal pain refers to pain in the muscles, bones or joints, ligaments, tendons, bursae, and nerves.

■ ANATOMY OF PAIN

Pain perception begins at the periphery, where nociceptors—specialized sensory neurons—detect noxious stimuli. Nociceptors are distributed throughout the skin, joints, and viscera and can be classified into various types based on their response to thermal, mechanical, or chemical stimuli.

- *Peripheral nociceptors*: These primary afferent neurons include A-delta and C fibers. A-delta fibers are myelinated and transmit sharp, well-localized pain quickly, while C fibers are unmyelinated, transmitting dull, diffuse pain more slowly.
- *Spinal cord and dorsal horn*: After nociceptors are activated, the pain signal travels along peripheral nerves to the dorsal horn of the spinal cord. Here, neurotransmitters like glutamate and substance P are released, transmitting the signal to secondary neurons. The dorsal horn integrates and modulates these signals before they ascend to higher brain centers.
- *Ascending pain pathways*: Pain signals ascend via the spinothalamic tract to the thalamus, a crucial relay station. From the thalamus, signals are sent to various cortical regions, including the somatosensory cortex, insula, and anterior cingulate cortex, which are involved in the sensory-discriminative and affective-motivational aspects of pain.

- *Brain regions involved in pain perception*: The perception of pain is a result of the integration of sensory input in various brain regions. The primary somatosensory cortex (S1) is responsible for the localization and intensity of pain, while the insula and anterior cingulate cortex are involved in the emotional response to pain.

PHYSIOLOGY OF PAIN

The physiology of pain encompasses the mechanisms by which pain is detected, transmitted, and modulated.
- *Transduction*: Pain transduction begins when nociceptors convert noxious stimuli into electrical signals. This process involves ion channels and receptors such as TRPV1, which respond to heat and capsaicin, and ASICs, which are activated by acidic conditions.
- *Transmission*: Following transduction, the electrical signal travels along afferent neurons to the spinal cord. Here, neurotransmitters are released into the synaptic cleft, activating secondary neurons. This process is influenced by various factors, including ion channel activity and receptor sensitivity.
- *Modulation*: Pain modulation occurs at multiple levels of the nervous system. In the dorsal horn, inhibitory interneurons release neurotransmitters like gamma-aminobutyric acid (GABA) and glycine, which can dampen pain signals. Descending pathways from the brainstem, involving structures like the periaqueductal gray (PAG) and the rostral ventromedial medulla (RVM), can enhance or inhibit pain through the release of endogenous opioids.
- *Perception*: The final perception of pain is a complex interplay of sensory, cognitive, and emotional factors. Pain perception can be influenced by various factors including attention, expectation, and previous experiences.

Pain can be classified into two types (**Table 1**):
1. *Fast pain* is sharp and acute, mediated by myelinated A-delta fibers and transmitted rapidly, often felt immediately after a stimulus
2. *Slow pain* is dull and aching, mediated by unmyelinated C fibers, transmitted more slowly, and can persist longer.

Musculoskeletal pain is not purely nociceptive; peripheral inflammation and central sensitization processes, as well as neuropathic components, may contribute. The pain of mixed origins may respond to the administration of agents that treat both nociceptive and neuropathic components.

CLINICAL IMPLICATIONS

A thorough understanding of the anatomy and physiology of pain is essential for the development of effective pain management strategies. Recent advancements in molecular biology and neuroimaging have provided deeper insights into pain mechanisms, leading to the development of new therapeutic approaches.

Table 1: Comparison of fast (first) pain and slow (second) pain characteristics.

Pain type	Fast/first pain/epicritic pain	Slow/second pain
Nerve fiber	A-delta	C
Axon	Myelinated	Unmyelinated
Duration	0.1 second	1 second
Velocity	6–30 m/s	0.5–2 m/s
Nature	Acute, sharp, stabbing, pricking	Chronic, dull, aching
Occurrence	In superficial tissues only	Both superficial tissue and deep tissue destruction
Stimuli	Mechanical, thermal	Mechanical, thermal, and chemical
Tract	Neospinothalamic tract	Paleospinothalamic tract
Neurotransmitter	Glutamate	Substance P

- *Pharmacological interventions*: Advances in the understanding of pain pathways have led to the development of new pharmacological treatments targeting specific receptors and ion channels involved in pain transmission and modulation. For instance, drugs targeting the TRPV1 receptor or specific sodium channels like Nav1.7 show promise in pain management.
- *Nonpharmacological interventions*: Techniques such as cognitive-behavioral therapy (CBT), mindfulness, and physical therapy have been shown to modulate pain perception and improve patient outcomes. Neurostimulation techniques like transcutaneous electrical nerve stimulation (TENS) and spinal cord stimulation are also increasingly used in clinical practice.

CONCLUSION

The anatomy and physiology of pain involve a complex network of structures and processes designed to detect, transmit, and modulate pain signals. Advances in scientific research continue to unravel the complexities of pain, offering hope for more effective treatments and improved quality of life for individuals experiencing pain.

BIBLIOGRAPHY

1. Apkarian AV, Bushnell MC, Treede RD, Zubieta JK. Human brain mechanisms of pain perception and regulation in health and disease. Eur J Pain. 2005;9(4):463-84.
2. Basbaum AI, Bautista DM, Scherrer G, Julius D. Cellular and molecular mechanisms of pain. Cell. 2009;139(2):267-84.
3. Braz J, Solorzano C, Wang X, Basbaum AI. Transmitting pain and itch messages: a contemporary view of the spinal cord circuits that generate gate control. Neuron. 2021;108(3):366-81.
4. Caterina MJ, Julius D. The vanilloid receptor: a molecular gateway to the pain pathway. Annu Rev Neurosci. 2001;24:487-517.
5. Denk F, McMahon SB, Tracey I. Pain vulnerability: a neurobiological perspective. Nat Neurosci. 2014;17(2):192-200.

CHAPTER 3

Assessment of Musculoskeletal Pain

Akash Narangyal

■ INTRODUCTION

Proper assessment is crucial for accurate diagnosis and effective management.

■ COMPONENTS OF PAIN ASSESSMENT

Patient History

Detailed patient history is the cornerstone of musculoskeletal pain assessment. It should include:
- *Onset and duration*: Acute versus chronic pain
- *Location*: Specific areas affected
- *Quality of pain*: Sharp, dull, throbbing, burning, etc.
- *Intensity*: Using pain scales like the Numeric Rating Scale (NRS) or Visual Analog Scale (VAS)
- *Aggravating and alleviating factors*: Activities or positions that increase or decrease pain
- *Impact on daily activities*: Functional limitations and quality of life

Physical Examination

A thorough physical examination should include:
- *Inspection*: Look for swelling, deformity, or discoloration.
- *Palpation*: Identify tender points and assess muscle tone.
- *Range of motion (ROM)*: Assess active and passive ROM of affected joints.
- *Strength testing*: Evaluate muscle strength using the Medical Research Council (MRC) scale.
- *Neurological examination*: Assess reflexes, sensation, and motor function to rule out neurological involvement.

Diagnostic Imaging

Imaging studies play a vital role in the assessment of musculoskeletal pain:
- *X-rays*: Useful for detecting fractures, osteoarthritis, and alignment issues
- *Magnetic resonance imaging (MRI):* Provides detailed images of soft tissues, including muscles, ligaments, and intervertebral discs
- *Ultrasound*: Useful for assessing soft-tissue injuries and guiding injections
- *Computed tomography (CT)*: Offers detailed bone images and is useful in complex fractures

Laboratory Tests

Laboratory tests can help identify underlying systemic conditions:
- *Complete blood count (CBC)*: To detect infections or inflammatory conditions
- *Erythrocyte sedimentation rate (ESR) and C-reactive protein (CRP)*: Indicators of inflammation
- *Rheumatoid factor (RF) and anti-cyclic citrullinated peptide (anti-CCP) antibodies*: Used in the diagnosis of rheumatoid arthritis

ADVANCED ASSESSMENT TOOLS

Patient-reported Outcome Measures

Patient-reported outcome measures (PROMs) are essential for understanding the patients' perspective on their pain and its impact on their life. Commonly used PROMs include:
- *Short Form-36 (SF-36)*: Measures the overall health status
- *Oswestry Disability Index (ODI)*: Specific for lower back pain
- *Western Ontario and McMaster Universities Osteoarthritis Index (WOMAC)*: Specific for hip and knee osteoarthritis

Functional Assessment Tools

Functional assessments help quantify the impact of pain on daily activities and physical function:
- *Timed up and go (TUG) test*: Assesses mobility and balance
- *Six-minute walk test (6MWT)*: Measures endurance and functional capacity
- Gait analysis

To assess the severity and monitor the progress, use assessment tools like those given in the following text.

Visual Analog Scale
Key Features of the Visual Analog Scale for Musculoskeletal Pain
One end of the line represents "no pain" (0) and the other end represents "worst pain" (10).

Patients are advised to mark a point on the line from 0 to 10 that corresponds to their pain intensity.

An example of a VAS for musculoskeletal pain is:

No pain   Worst pain
0---10

Patients are advised to place a mark on the line that best represents their current level of pain.

Interpretation is as follows:
- 0 cm: No pain
- 1–3 cm: Mild pain
- 4–6 cm: Moderate pain
- 7–10 cm: Severe pain

Numeric Rating Scale

The NRS is a commonly used method for assessing pain intensity, including musculoskeletal pain.

Patients are asked to choose a number between 0 and 10 that best describes their pain intensity at that moment, e.g., "On a scale of 0 to 10, where 0 stands for no pain and 10 starts for worst pain anyone can imagine."

Advantages:
- Simplicity
- Quick
- Versatility

Example is as follows:

0   1   2   3   4   5   6   7   8   9   10
No pain   Worst imaginable pain

Multidisciplinary Approach

Effective assessment of musculoskeletal pain often requires a multidisciplinary approach involving healthcare professionals from various specialties:
- *Clinicians*: Provide diagnosis and medical management.
- *Physical therapists*: Conduct detailed physical assessments and develop rehabilitation programs.
- *Occupational therapists*: Assess the impact of pain on daily activities and suggest modifications.
- *Psychologists*: Evaluate the psychological aspects of chronic pain and provide cognitive-behavioral therapy (CBT).

CONCLUSION

Comprehensive approach to musculoskeletal pain is a good option for proper diagnosis and treatment of pain. Detailed patient history and proper physical examination should performed. Appropriate radiograph, ultrasound, CT, or MRI scans can be performed during assessment. Sometimes a blood investigation or another laboratory test is also ordered to determine the specific cause and extent of the pain. These methods lead to not only the identification of the pain but also the gradation of the pain. Assessment tools such as PROMs is another way of gathering patient perceptions of their pain and is highly effective. For pain intensity VAS and the NRS can be used.

BIBLIOGRAPHY

1. Deyo RA, Mirza SK, Turner JA, Martin BI. Overtreating chronic back pain: time to back off? J Am Board Fam Med. 2009;22(1):62-8.
2. Henschke N, Maher CG, Refshauge KM, Herbert RD, Cumming RG, Bleasel J, et al. Prognosis in patients with recent onset low back pain in Australian primary care: inception cohort study. BMJ. 2008;337:a171.
3. Roos EM, Lohmander LS. The Knee injury and Osteoarthritis Outcome Score (KOOS): from joint injury to osteoarthritis. Health Qual Life Outcomes. 2003;1:64.
4. Suri P, Rainville J, Kalichman L, Katz JN. Diagnosis and treatment of low back pain: a joint clinical practice guideline from the American College of Physicians and the American Pain Society. Ann Intern Med. 2007;147(7):478-91.
5. Woolf AD, Pfleger B. Burden of major musculoskeletal conditions. Bull World Health Organ. 2003;81(9):646-56.

CHAPTER 4

Management of Acute Musculoskeletal Pain

Kunal Sharma

■ INTRODUCTION

Acute musculoskeletal pain is defined as sudden and severe pain perceived in musculoskeletal tissues that is short-lived and lasts for a few days to a few weeks, depending on the underlying cause and severity of the injury.

Effective management of acute musculoskeletal pain is essential for improving patient outcomes, preventing chronic pain development, and reducing the burden on healthcare systems.

■ PATHOPHYSIOLOGY OF ACUTE MUSCULOSKELETAL PAIN

Understanding the pathophysiology of acute musculoskeletal pain is crucial for its effective management. Acute pain typically results from injury, inflammation, or overuse of musculoskeletal structures.

- *Inflammatory response*: Acute injuries trigger an inflammatory response characterized by the release of cytokines, prostaglandins, and other mediators that sensitize nociceptors and cause pain.
- *Mechanical factors*: Mechanical factors such as muscle strain, ligament sprains, and fractures directly stimulate nociceptors in the affected tissues.
- *Neurogenic factors*: Acute pain can also involve neurogenic inflammation, in which nerve fibers release neuropeptides like substance P, further contributing to pain and inflammation.

■ TREATMENT

Numerous treatment options exist, including nonpharmacological and pharmacological interventions (nonopioid and opioid).

Multimodal Analgesia

Multimodal therapy is the use of two or more approaches that have different modes of action. This may include two or more analgesics that will work additively or synergistically. Multimodal therapy can shorten the hospital stay and lessen the adverse effects of opioids by decreasing individual drug dosage and thereby improving patient outcomes.

Pharmacological Management

Pharmacological interventions are a mainstay in the management of acute musculoskeletal pain. The choice of medication should be based on the severity of pain, patient comorbidities, and potential side effects.

- *Acetaminophen*: This is a first-line option for mild-to-moderate pain, particularly in patients in whom nonsteroidal anti-inflammatory drugs (NSAIDs) are contraindicated.
- *NSAIDs*: These are commonly used due to their anti-inflammatory and analgesic properties. They are effective for mild-to-moderate pain but should be used with caution in patients with gastrointestinal or renal issues.
- *Opioids*: Short-term use of opioids may be necessary for severe pain, but their use should be limited due to the risk of dependence and side effects. It is important to monitor patients closely and prescribe the lowest effective dose.
- *Muscle relaxants*: Muscle relaxants like cyclobenzaprine can be used to alleviate muscle spasms associated with acute musculoskeletal pain.
- *Topical analgesics*: Topical NSAIDs and capsaicin creams can provide localized pain relief with minimal systemic side effects.
- *Role of steroids*: They are used very rarely and briefly only.

Nonpharmacological Management

Nonpharmacological interventions play a crucial role in the holistic management of acute musculoskeletal pain.

- *Rest and activity modification*: Encourage patients to rest the affected area and modify activities to avoid further injury while gradually reintroducing movement as the pain subsides.
- *Physical therapy*: Physical therapy, including exercises, stretching, and manual therapy, can help reduce pain, improve function, and prevent recurrence. Early mobilization is key to recovery.
- *Cold and heat therapy*: Cold therapy can reduce inflammation and numb pain in the acute phase, while heat therapy can relax muscles and improve blood flow during the subacute phase.
- *Cognitive behavioral therapy (CBT)*: CBT techniques can help patients manage pain-related anxiety and develop coping strategies, improving overall pain outcomes.

CHAPTER 4: Management of Acute Musculoskeletal Pain

- *Complementary therapies*: Acupuncture, massage, and chiropractic care may provide additional pain relief for some patients and can be considered adjuncts to conventional treatments.

Interventional Therapy

At times, the pain may be more severe and not respond to noninterventional measures; hence, there is a role for interventions. Various interventions are given in the following text.

Nerve Blocks

Acute pain management often involves the use of nerve blocks, which can provide significant pain relief by interrupting pain signals in specific areas of the body. Nerve blocks can be performed using various techniques, including blind techniques, ultrasound guidance, and fluoroscopic guidance, to increase accuracy and safety.
- *Peripheral nerve blocks*
  - *Upper extremity blocks*: These include interscalene, supraclavicular, infraclavicular, and axillary blocks, which are used for acute pain in the shoulder, arm, or hand.
  - *Lower extremity blocks*: These include femoral, sciatic, popliteal, and ankle blocks, used for acute pain in the hip, thigh, knee, lower leg, ankle, or foot.
- *Truncal blocks*:
  - *Intercostal nerve block*: Used for pain relief following rib fractures
  - *Transversus abdominis plane (TAP) block*: Effective for abdominal pain
  - Rectus sheath block
  - Pectoral (PECS) block
- *Spinal and epidural blocks*:
  - *Spinal anesthesia*: Commonly used for acute pain in the lower abdomen, pelvis, rectum, and lower extremities.
  - *Epidural anesthesia*: Provides effective pain relief for the abdomen, pelvis, and lower extremities.
- Trigger point injections

PATIENT EDUCATION AND SELF-MANAGEMENT

Empowering patients with knowledge and strategies to manage their pain is essential for successful outcomes.
- *Pain education*: Educate patients about the nature of acute musculoskeletal pain, the expected course of recovery, and the importance of adhering to the treatment plan.
- *Self-management techniques*: Teach patients self-management techniques such as pacing activities, relaxation exercises, and proper posture to prevent exacerbations.
- *Follow-up*: Regular follow-up is important to assess progress, adjust treatment plans, and provide ongoing support to patients.

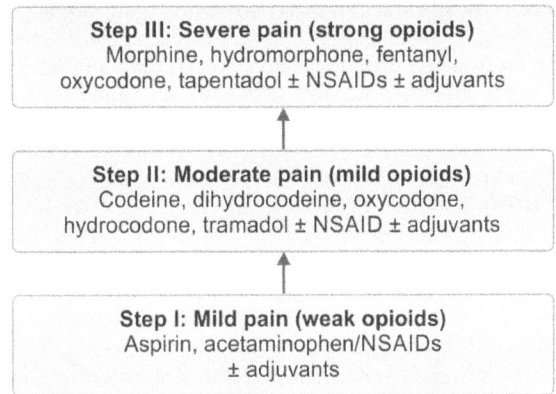

Flowchart 1: WHO pain management ladder.
(NSAIDs: nonsteroidal anti-inflammatory drugs; WHO: World Health Organization)

CLINICAL PRACTICE GUIDELINES

Adherence to evidence-based clinical practice guidelines ensures standardized and effective care for patients with acute musculoskeletal pain.
- *Guidelines*: Refer to guidelines from reputable organizations such as the World Health Organization (WHO) three-step ladder approach **(Flowchart 1)**, the American College of Rheumatology, the American Academy of Orthopaedic Surgeons, and the British Pain Society for comprehensive management strategies.
- Multimodal strategy is the way to go.
- *Multidisciplinary approach*: A multidisciplinary approach involving physicians, physiotherapists, pharmacists, and mental health professionals can enhance patient care and outcomes.

CONCLUSION

Effective management of acute musculoskeletal pain requires a multifaceted and multimodal strategy approach that combines pharmacological and nonpharmacological interventions. By understanding the pathophysiology, conducting thorough assessments, and applying evidence-based treatments, healthcare professionals can significantly improve patient outcomes. Continuous education and a patient-centered approach are essential for the successful management of acute musculoskeletal pain.

BIBLIOGRAPHY

1. Bleakley C, McDonough S, MacAuley D. The use of ice in the treatment of acute soft-tissue injury: a systematic review of randomized controlled trials. Am J Sports Med. 2012;32(1):251-61.
2. Bovill C, Lynch F, Simpson AHRW, Gaston P. NSAIDs in trauma and orthopedic surgery—a review of current practice and information sources. Injury. 2017;48(3):510-7.

3. Chou R, Gordon DB, de Leon-Casasola OA, Rosenberg JM, Bickler S, Brennan T, et al. Management of postoperative pain: a clinical practice guideline from the American Pain Society, the American Society of Regional Anesthesia and Pain Medicine, and the American Society of Anesthesiologists' Committee on Regional Anesthesia, Executive Committee, and Administrative Council. J Pain. 2016;17(2):131-57.
4. Derry S, Wiffen PJ, Kalso EA, Bell RF, Aldington D, Phillips T, et al. Topical analgesics for acute and chronic pain in adults—an overview of Cochrane Reviews. Cochrane Database Syst Rev. 2017;12:CD008609.
5. Ehde DM, Dillworth TM, Turner JA. Cognitive–behavioral therapy for individuals with chronic pain: efficacy, innovations, and directions for research. Am Psychol. 2014;69(2):153-66.
6. Finestone HM, Alfeeli A. Diagnostic imaging in acute musculoskeletal pain disorders. Best Pract Res Clin Rheumatol. 2019;33(1):101418.
7. Foster NE, Hill JC, O'Sullivan P, Hancock M. Stratified models of care. Best Pract Res Clin Rheumatol. 2011;27(5):701-10.

CHAPTER 5

Managing Chronic Musculoskeletal Pain

Mushtaq Ahmed Wani

INTRODUCTION

Chronic musculoskeletal pain (CMP) is a prevalent condition affecting millions worldwide, significantly impacting quality of life and posing a considerable challenge to healthcare systems. It encompasses a wide range of conditions, including osteoarthritis, rheumatoid arthritis, fibromyalgia, and chronic back pain.

PATHOPHYSIOLOGY

Chronic musculoskeletal pain results from a complex interplay of biological, psychological, and social factors. It often involves persistent inflammation, central and peripheral sensitization, and changes in pain processing within the nervous system. Understanding the underlying mechanisms is crucial for effective management.

DIAGNOSIS

Accurate diagnosis involves a detailed patient history, physical examination, and often imaging or laboratory tests. The goal is to identify the underlying cause, assess pain intensity and impact on function, and rule out other conditions.

PHARMACOLOGICAL MANAGEMENT

Pharmacological treatments aim to reduce pain and improve function, although they often need to be combined with other modalities for optimal results.

Nonsteroidal Anti-inflammatory Drugs

Nonsteroidal anti-inflammatory drugs (NSAIDs) are commonly used for their anti-inflammatory and analgesic properties. They are effective in conditions like osteoarthritis and rheumatoid arthritis but can cause gastrointestinal, renal, and cardiovascular side effects with long-term use.

Acetaminophen

Acetaminophen is often recommended for mild-to-moderate pain. It is generally safer than NSAIDs but may be less effective for severe pain or inflammation.

Opioids

Opioids may be prescribed for severe pain unresponsive to other treatments. However, they carry a high risk of dependency, tolerance, and other side effects, making them a less favorable long-term option, especially for chronic pain.

Antidepressants and Anticonvulsants

Medications like tricyclic antidepressants (e.g., amitriptyline) and anticonvulsants (e.g., gabapentin, pregabalin) can be effective in managing neuropathic pain and central sensitization. They are particularly useful in conditions like fibromyalgia.

Topical Agents

Topical NSAIDs and capsaicin creams can provide localized pain relief with fewer systemic side effects. They are beneficial for joint pain in osteoarthritis and localized neuropathic pain.

NONPHARMACOLOGICAL INTERVENTIONS

Nonpharmacological treatments are critical components of a comprehensive pain management plan, addressing the multifaceted nature of chronic pain.

Physical Therapy

Physical therapy aims to improve mobility, strength, and function while reducing pain. Techniques include:
- *Exercise therapy*: Tailored exercise programs to enhance strength, flexibility, and endurance.
- *Manual therapy*: Hands-on techniques to mobilize joints and soft tissues.
- *Modalities*: Use of heat, cold, ultrasound, and electrical stimulation to alleviate pain and promote healing.

Cognitive Behavioral Therapy
Cognitive behavioral therapy helps patients manage pain by changing maladaptive thought patterns and behaviors. It can reduce pain intensity, improve coping strategies, and enhance quality of life.

Mind–Body Techniques
Mind–body practices such as yoga, tai chi, and mindfulness meditation can reduce pain perception and improve psychological well-being. These techniques promote relaxation, reduce stress, and enhance *overall health*.

Occupational Therapy
Occupational therapists assist patients in adapting their work and daily activities to reduce pain and prevent further injury. They may recommend ergonomic adjustments, assistive devices, and strategies for energy conservation.

Acupuncture
Acupuncture is believed to stimulate the body's natural painkillers and has shown efficacy in managing various types of chronic pain.

Lifestyle and Self-management Strategies
Empowering patients to take an active role in managing their pain is essential for long-term success.

Education
Educating patients about their condition, pain mechanisms, and management strategies fosters better understanding and adherence to treatment plans.

Nutrition
A balanced diet rich in anti-inflammatory foods can support overall health and potentially reduce pain. Omega-3 fatty acids, antioxidants, and certain vitamins, especially vitamin D, and minerals play a role in inflammation and pain modulation.

Weight Management
Maintaining a healthy weight reduces stress on the musculoskeletal system, particularly important in conditions like osteoarthritis.

Sleep Hygiene
Chronic pain often disrupts sleep, creating a vicious cycle of pain and sleep disturbance. Good sleep hygiene practices, such as maintaining a regular sleep schedule and creating a restful environment, can improve sleep quality and reduce pain.

Stress Management

Stress exacerbates pain perception and can hinder recovery. Techniques such as deep breathing, progressive muscle relaxation, and biofeedback can help manage stress levels.

INTEGRATIVE AND MULTIDISCIPLINARY APPROACHES

Chronic musculoskeletal pain management often requires a multidisciplinary approach involving various healthcare professionals, including physicians, physical therapists, psychologists, and nutritionists. Integrative pain management centers offer coordinated care that addresses the physical, emotional, and social aspects of chronic pain.

PAIN CLINICS

Specialized pain clinics offer a range of services, including interventional procedures like nerve blocks, radiofrequency ablation, and spinal cord stimulation. These clinics provide access to specialists in pain management who can tailor treatments to individual needs.

REGENERATIVE MEDICINE

Techniques such as platelet-rich plasma (PRP) injections and stem cell therapy show promise in promoting tissue healing and reducing pain in conditions like osteoarthritis.

NEUROMODULATION

Neuromodulation therapies, including spinal cord stimulation and peripheral nerve stimulation, offer new options for patients with refractory chronic pain.

PERSONALIZED MEDICINE

Genetic and biomarker research is paving the way for personalized pain management strategies, allowing treatments to be tailored to an individual's unique pain profile and response to therapies.

CONCLUSION

Managing CMP requires a holistic and patient-centered approach, combining pharmacological treatments with nonpharmacological interventions and lifestyle modifications. By addressing the multifaceted nature of chronic pain, healthcare providers can help patients achieve better pain control, improved function, and enhanced quality of life. Continuing advancements in pain research and the integration of emerging therapies promise to further improve outcomes for individuals living with CMP.

BIBLIOGRAPHY

1. Bannuru RR, Osani MC, Vaysbrot EE, Arden NK, Bennell K, Bierma-Zeinstra SM, et al. OARSI guidelines for the non-surgical management of knee, hip, and polyarticular osteoarthritis. Osteoarthritis Cartilage. 2019;27(11):1578-89.
2. Busse JW, Craigie S, Juurlink DN, Buckley DN, Wang L, Couban R, et al. Guideline for opioid therapy and chronic noncancer pain. CMAJ. 2017;189(18):E659-66.
3. Chou R, Deyo R, Friedly J, Skelly A, Hashimoto R, Weimer M, et al. Noninvasive treatments for low back pain. Rockville, MD: Agency for Healthcare Research and Quality; 2016. Report no. 16-EHC004-EF.
4. Eccleston C, Fisher E, Thomas KH, Hearn L, Derry S, Stannard C, et al. Interventions for the reduction of prescribed opioid use in chronic non-cancer pain. Cochrane Database Syst Rev. 2017;11(11):CD010323.
5. Turk DC, Wilson HD, Cahana A. Treatment of chronic non-cancer pain. Lancet. 2011;377(9784):2226-35.

CHAPTER 6

Transition from Acute to Chronic Pain

Anita Kour

INTRODUCTION

The occurrence of chronic pain following surgery is significantly high. Various theories suggest that the prolonged experience of acute pain, along with long-term changes both within and outside the central nervous system (CNS), leads to chronic pain having a histological and pathological basis. Distinct surgical techniques can result in distinct types of persistent pain following surgery, which is influenced by intricate biochemical and pathophysiological pathways.

FACTORS INVOLVED IN THE CONVERSION OF PAIN FROM ACUTE TO CHRONIC

These factors can be categorized into:
- *Preoperative factors*:
  - *Patient factors*:
    - Psychological factors
      - Preoperative anxiety
      - Depression
      - Unpleasant experience with pain
    - Demographic factors
      - Female sex
      - Younger age
      - Worker's compensation cases
      - Genetic predisposition
    - Social environment
- *Medical factors*:
  - Repeat surgery
  - Pain from surgery that ranges from moderate to severe and lasts longer than a month

- Localized radiation therapy
- Damage to nerves
- Chemotherapy
- *Surgical factors*:
  - *Types of surgery*
    - Certain types of surgeries are more likely to result in chronic pain, e.g., amputation, coronary artery bypass, thoracotomy, and breast surgery.
  - Surgeries lasting > 3 hours
  - Technique and level of experience of the surgeon
  - Prolonged inflammation or pain following surgery
  - Inadequate analgesia after the surgery (crucial and preventable factors).
  - The level of tissue injury determines the degree of nociceptive stimulation.
  - Duration of process of tissue healing.

PREVENTION STRATEGIES TO MITIGATE THE CHANGE IN PAIN FROM ACUTE TO CHRONIC

The principle "prevention is better than cure" is particularly relevant in the context of chronic pain as it is more difficult to treat than acute pain.

There are several physiological shifts that take place during the shift from acute to chronic pain, ranging from the peripheral nervous system to the CNS.

Preventing or reversing these pathophysiological changes could potentially decrease the chances of occurrence of chronic pain.

Timely management of acute pain is crucial for minimizing the chances of development of chronic pain, not only for ethical and humanitarian reasons but also for the overall well-being of patients. Identifying patients at an increased risk for the development of chronic pain early is essential for implementing effective prevention strategies. Risk stratification can greatly lower the likelihood that chronic pain will develop by implementing suitable preventative analgesia that targets different levels of pain pathways.

A multimodal analgesic approach aims to provide synergistic pain control by targeting receptors at different levels of the pain pathway, thereby reducing neuronal excitability.

Preventive strategies to lower the prevalence of persistent pain following surgery include modifying surgical techniques to minimize tissue damage, avoiding nerve damage, and using minimally invasive methods.

Local and regional anesthesia are used to block pain signal transmission and reduce pain sensitivity, potentially reducing central neuroplasticity. The long-term effects of these techniques on chronic pain development are not fully understood, although some studies suggest benefits from epidural analgesia before surgery.

Ensuring adequate postoperative analgesia is the most crucial factor in preventing chronic pain. Multimodal analgesia, involving various pharmacological therapies with different mechanisms of action and delivery routes (enteral, parenteral, epidural, intrathecal) at different time points (preoperative, intraoperative, and postoperative), is essential for optimizing acute pain treatment and preventing chronic pain.

Physical activity or physical therapy is promoted to manage acute pain effectively and prevent its transition to chronic pain. Psychological factors like neuroticism and depression are addressed through a psychosocial approach for patients at an increased risk of developing chronic pain. By adopting these comprehensive strategies, healthcare providers can significantly decrease the prevalence of chronic pain following surgery.

CONCLUSION

Pain, if prevented in a timely manner, reduces the chances of developing chronic pain. Efficient management through the use of multimodal analgesia is key to reducing the incidence of chronic pain.

BIBLIOGRAPHY

1. Harstall C. How prevalent is chronic pain? In: IASP Pain Clinical Updates. Washington, DC: IASP; 2003. pp. XI, 1–4.
2. Ready L. The interface between acute and chronic pain. In: The Management of Pain. New York: Churchill Livingstone; 1998.
3. Schmitt P. Rehabilitation of chronic pain: a multi-disciplinary approach. J Rehabil. 1985;51:72.

CHAPTER 7

Pain Flare Management

Nitin Choudhary

INTRODUCTION

The intensity of chronic musculoskeletal pain may vary over time and there may be times when it is worse than usual. A flare is a period of time when symptoms are more severe than they are on a daily basis. Flares can linger for hours or even days, with little to no warning and no discernible pattern.

The first step in any case of acute flare is to identify whether it is a new pain, flare pain, or a breakthrough pain. While flare pain has been defined as above, new pain refers to a fresh pain in a new location or a new associated symptom like muscle weakness, numbness, and nausea or vomiting. *Breakthrough pain* is defined as sudden and intense increase in pain that occurs even when a person is regularly taking medication to manage chronic pain.

TRIGGERS VERSUS WARNING SYMPTOMS

Triggers

Triggers can be defined as almost anything that leads to exacerbation of pain and results in an episode of pain flare. Various trigger factors include:
- Variation in activity levels
- Elevated stress levels
- Weather variations
- Alteration in sleep quantity or quality
- Difficulties in family or other relationships
- Problems at work or financial difficulties
- Mood swings
- Prolonged periods of static posture or activity
- Recent illnesses such as cold or flu
- Hormonal fluctuations

Certain elements, such as variations in humidity or temperature, are simple to identify but hard to avoid (i.e., outside our control). Two categories can be used to classify other recognizable and preventable factors: Those associated with physical activity (overactivity or underactivity) and those associated with tension, stress, or emotional problems.

Warning Symptoms

Warning symptoms are the symptoms that one feels before having a full-fledged attack of pain flare. Warning symptoms like triggers are specific for each individual; that is, each individual may experience a warning symptom in his or her unique way and intensity.

Identifying both trigger factors and warning symptoms can be important in the management of pain flares as appropriate measures can be taken well in time to prevent an attack or to reduce its intensity.

STRATEGIES FOR MANAGING AND COPING WITH PAIN FLARES

A successful strategy for managing a case of pain flare should include a structured plan that inculcates:

- *Prevention:* It is a well-known fact that "prevention is better than cure." Strategies should be aimed at preventing acute flare-ups by avoiding the avoidable triggers.
- *Learning:* Learning from the previous episode of acute flare-up is important from both the patient's and the doctor's perspective and can guide to better management or even prevention of such acute flare-ups in future.
- *Management of acute flare-ups:* In cases of acute flare-ups, each case should be managed judiciously and the patient should be relieved of his or her distress at the earliest.

Various modes of managing acute pain flare are given in the following text.

Medications

Various classes of opioid and nonopioid medications are routinely used to treat musculoskeletal pain primarily in conjunction with other modalities.

Corticosteroids

Acute pain and acute flare-ups of chronic pain disorders are treated with oral corticosteroids. By suppressing proinflammatory genes and increasing the expression of anti-inflammatory genes, corticosteroids also indirectly lower inflammation. Because long-term uses come with their own set of hazards and consequences, caution must be exercised when using them.

Opioids
Opioids and opioid-like medications are used extensively for managing cases of acute pain flare; however, this class needs to be used cautiously because of various side effects associated with the use of this class of drugs, especially the risk of overdose and addiction.

Antidepressants
The two most popular kinds of antidepressants used to treat chronic neuropathic pain are tricyclic antidepressants (TCAs) and serotonin and norepinephrine reuptake inhibitors (SNRIs). Duloxetine was found to be more effective than venlafaxine in a meta-analysis; however, careful monitoring is advised for adverse effects linked to greater dosages of TCAs.

Topical Medications
Topical medications, especially patches, have been used to manage flares.

Transcutaneous Electric Nerve Stimulation
The activation of large Aβ-fiber afferent neurons by transcutaneous electric nerve stimulation (TENS) stimulation is anticipated to block nociceptive transmission at the dorsal horn of the spinal cord. It has been used to treat acute pain flares in conjunction with medicines.

Interventions
The most commonly used interventions are local steroid injections, epidural injections (in cases of spine pain), sympathetic and ganglionic blocks, trigger point injections, radiofrequency ablation of nerve roots/branches, etc. Although literature is lacking on the efficacy of the above interventions, one can use them judiciously in conjunction with other modalities.

Coping with Acute Pain Flares
Coping with acute pain flares is a multimodal approach; both the patient and the treating physician have to entail a multitude of factors and this has to go alongside other modalities as discussed earlier. The patient's approach and his or her emotional and behavioral attitude toward the pain are mainly comprised of coping strategies and have a significant effect on short-term as well as long-term goals.
- Recognize what is happening and how one is feeling.
- Consume the prescribed drugs but refrain from increasing the dosage over extended periods of time. In order to prevent the long-term requirement for increasing drug dosages, active self-management techniques should be taken into consideration in addition to taking breakthrough medications as directed for the short-term reduction of pain.
- Concentrate on what one can manage.

- Reframe recurring, ineffective thoughts.
- Engage in self-compassion and kindness practices.
- Finding ways to distract oneself
- Expressing and venting thoughts and emotions
- Manage sadness and isolation.
- Keep moving. Recall that you should attempt to move through the suffering.

INCORPORATING PAIN FLARE MANAGEMENT INTO LONG-TERM PAIN MANAGEMENT PLANS

As discussed in the above section, the management plan for acute pain flare includes:

- *Prevention*: Before a flare
- Management of acute episode
- *Learning*: Once the acute phase settles, one has to learn from the experiences and in conjunction with the treating physician devise strategies which can be incorporated into long-term musculoskeletal pain management plans.
- *Find out what did and did not work during the episode*: Both during and after a flare-up, record what helped and did not help ease discomfort or lessen pain. These resources may come in handy later on. Attempt to recognize and stay away from any avoidable triggers as well.
- Stay healthy and keep active.
- Tackling unhelpful repetitive thoughts and managing stress levels

CONCLUSION

In crux, incorporating a pain flare management plan into long-term management involves anticipating triggers, having a toolkit of coping strategies, adjusting medications if necessary, and ensuring ongoing communication with healthcare providers. It is about creating a proactive approach to handle flare-ups while maintaining overall treatment goals.

BIBLIOGRAPHY

1. Carter A. (n.d.). Flare management. Northern Pain Centre. [online] Available from https://www.northernpaincentre.com.au/wellness/managing-chronic-pain-through-challenging-times/flare-management [Last accessed August, 20024].
2. Dey S, Sanders AE, Martinez S, Kopitnik NL, Vrooman BM. (2024). Alternatives to opioids for managing pain. Treasure Island (FL): StatPearls Publishing [Internet].
3. Rodgers-Melnick SN, Trager RJ, Love TE, Dusek JA. Engagement in integrative and nonpharmacologic pain management modalities among adults with chronic pain: analysis of the 2019 National Health Interview Survey. J Pain Res. 2024;17:253-64.
4. Sturgeon JA, Cooley C, Minhas D. Practical approaches for clinicians in chronic pain management: strategies and solutions. Best Pract Res Clin Rheumatol. 2024:101934.

CHAPTER 8

Current Guidelines for Musculoskeletal Pain Management

Pankaj Vir Singh

■ INTRODUCTION

Current guidelines from bodies such as the American College of Physicians (ACP), American Academy of Family Physicians (AAFP), and the Orthopaedic Trauma Association (2018), as well as the World Health Organization (WHO) four-step ladder approach, advocate for a holistic, multimodal strategy that encompasses the biological, psychological, social, and environmental factors influencing pain. These guidelines recommend comprehensive assessment, diagnosis, and management of musculoskeletal conditions, promoting a team-based approach to cater to diverse patient needs and ensure continuous care across various healthcare settings.

■ AMERICAN COLLEGE OF PHYSICIANS AND AMERICAN ACADEMY OF FAMILY PHYSICIANS

These organizations offer clinical recommendations for both non-pharmacological and pharmacological management, balancing evidence on benefits, harms, costs, and patient preferences. Key treatment protocols include:
- Topical nonsteroidal anti-inflammatory drugs (NSAIDs) with or without menthol as the first-line therapy
- Acetaminophen alone or combined with NSAIDs
- NSAIDs alone
- Acupressure and transcutaneous electrical nerve stimulation (TENS)
- Opioids, including tramadol, for pain reduction

ORTHOPAEDIC TRAUMA ASSOCIATION (2018)

This Association provides evidence-based recommendations for pain management, encompassing medication strategies and cognitive and physical approaches, especially for patients on long-term opioids. Recommendations include:
- Multimodal analgesia (MMA) with NSAIDs, acetaminophen, gabapentinoids, and immediate-release opioids
- Use of TENS
- Cryotherapy units
- Periarticular injections as adjuncts
- Mindset strategies such as aromatherapy and music therapy
- Cognitive behavioral therapy

For major musculoskeletal injury procedures (e.g., long bone or complex joint fracture surgeries), the guidelines recommend specific opioid and nonopioid dosages and durations, customized by the treating physician according to patient characteristics, local practices, and state laws.

WORLD HEALTH ORGANIZATION FOUR-STEP LADDER APPROACH FOR MUSCULOSKELETAL PAIN MANAGEMENT

This approach emphasizes integrating nonopioid therapies at every stage to minimize or eliminate the need for stronger opioids. It includes:
- *Step III for severe pain*: Strong opioids (morphine, hydromorphone, fentanyl, oxycodone, tapentadol) ± NSAIDs ± adjuvants
- *Step II for moderate pain*: Mild opioids (codeine, dihydrocodeine, oxycodone, hydrocodone, tramadol) ± NSAIDs ± adjuvants
- *Step I for mild pain*: Weak opioids (aspirin, acetaminophen/NSAIDs) ± adjuvants

A multimodal approach combining drugs with different mechanisms of action is recommended for more effective analgesia with fewer side effects.

SPECIFIC RECOMMENDATIONS BY AMERICAN COLLEGE OF PHYSICIANS AND AMERICAN ACADEMY OF FAMILY PHYSICIANS

- Topical NSAIDs with or without menthol for acute pain from non-low back musculoskeletal injuries (strong recommendation; moderate-certainty evidence).
- Oral NSAIDs or acetaminophen for acute musculoskeletal pain to reduce symptoms and improve physical function (conditional recommendation; moderate-certainty evidence).

CHAPTER 8: Current Guidelines for Musculoskeletal Pain Management

- Acupressure or TENS for patients with acute pain from musculoskeletal injuries (conditional recommendation; low-certainty evidence).
- Opioids, including tramadol, for acute pain from non-low back musculoskeletal injuries (conditional recommendation; low-certainty evidence).

ORTHOPAEDIC TRAUMA ASSOCIATION

- Use MMA with the lowest effective immediate-release dose for the shortest time (strong recommendation; moderate-quality evidence).
- Discuss pain relief, recovery expectations, and patient experiences in all interactions.
- Connect patients with severe pain or significant symptoms to psychosocial interventions (strong recommendation; moderate-quality evidence).
- Consider using TENS and cryotherapy units postoperatively (strong recommendation; low-quality evidence).
- Use the lowest effective opioid dose for the shortest period, avoiding long-acting opioids and benzodiazepines (strong recommendation; high-quality evidence).
- Implement periarticular injections and MMA tailored to patient needs (strong recommendation; moderate-quality evidence).
- Coordinate care for patients on long-term opioids with acute pain services during inpatient care and ensure single-prescriber management (strong recommendation; moderate-quality evidence).

CHALLENGES AND CONTROVERSIES

Developing and implementing guidelines face several challenges, including variability in clinical presentation; lack of communication; overuse of imaging, opioids, and surgery; failure to provide education; and misclassification. Additionally, regenerative medicine shows promise for conditions like osteoarthritis and tendon injuries, but further meta-analyses and randomized controlled trials (RCTs) are needed to incorporate these strategies into guidelines.

CONCLUSION

Current guidelines for musculoskeletal pain management advocate for a patient-centered approach combining pharmacologic and non-pharmacologic treatments. Early intervention with physical therapy, exercise, and cognitive-behavioral strategies, alongside careful use of medications, is crucial. Emphasizing multidisciplinary care and minimizing opioid use while exploring alternative therapies can enhance outcomes and quality of life. Continuous reassessment and individualized treatment are key to effective management and preventing chronic pain.

BIBLIOGRAPHY

1. Hsu JR, Mir H, Wally MK, Seymour RB; Orthopaedic Trauma Association Musculoskeletal Pain Task Force. Clinical practice guidelines for pain management in acute musculoskeletal injury. J Orthop Trauma. 2019;33(5):e158-82.
2. Qaseem A, McLean RM, O'Gurek D, Batur P, Lin K, Kansagara DL, et al. Nonpharmacologic and pharmacologic management of acute pain from non-low back, musculoskeletal injuries in adults: a clinical guideline from the American College of Physicians and American Academy of Family Physicians. Ann Intern Med. 2020;173(9):739-48.
3. Yang J, Bauer BA, WahnerRoedler DL, Chon TY, Xiao L. The modified WHO analgesic ladder: is it appropriate for chronic non-cancer pain. J Pain Res. 2020;13:411-7.

CHAPTER 9

Nonsteroidal Anti-inflammatory Drug and Acetaminophen

Arti Mahajan

■ INTRODUCTION

Nonsteroidal anti-inflammatory drugs (NSAIDs) are a cornerstone in the management of musculoskeletal pain, commonly used for their analgesic, anti-inflammatory, and antipyretic properties. This chapter explores the role of NSAIDs in treating conditions such as osteoarthritis, rheumatoid arthritis, and acute injuries, highlighting their mechanisms of action, efficacy, and safety profile. By inhibiting cyclooxygenase enzymes (COX-1 and COX-2), NSAIDs reduce the production of prostaglandins, which are mediators of pain and inflammation. Understanding the benefits, limitations, and appropriate use of NSAIDs is crucial for optimizing pain management strategies while minimizing potential risks.

■ PHARMACOLOGICAL THERAPY

Commonly used drugs to treat mild-to-moderate pain are:
- Acetaminophen (paracetamol)
- Nonsteroidal anti-inflammatory drugs
  - Nonspecific
  - Cyclooxygenase (COX)-2 inhibitors

Acetaminophen (Paracetamol)

Acetaminophen is a centrally acting nonopioid analgesic. It is the first-line treatment for mild-to-moderate pain because of its relative effectiveness in many pain conditions, high tolerability, and minimum side effects. It has an analgesic and antipyretic activity similar to NSAIDs, but it does not possess significant anti-inflammatory activity. Its molecules do not present the peripheral action on prostaglandin, so it is better tolerated than NSAIDs, especially at the gastrointestinal level, and does not include platelet activity.

CHAPTER 9: Nonsteroidal Anti-inflammatory Drug and Acetaminophen

Paracetamol should be considered in combination with NSAIDs in the management of musculoskeletal pain (MSP) and alone in patients in whom NSAIDs are contraindicated.
- *Route*: PO/IV
- *Dose*: 10–15 mg/kg (average 1 g)
- *Duration*: 6–8 hours

Monitoring the patients who receive acetaminophen regularly and beyond the maximum dosage of 3–4 g/day (in adults) is required.

Paracetamol (also known as acetaminophen) is generally considered safe when used as directed, but it can interact with other medications, leading to potential adverse effects. Some notable drug interactions are as follows:
- *Alcohol*:
  - *Interaction*: Increased risk of liver damage
  - *Mechanism*: Both alcohol and paracetamol are metabolized by the liver, and concurrent use can exacerbate liver toxicity.
- *Warfarin and other anticoagulants*:
  - *Interaction*: Increased risk of bleeding
  - *Mechanism*: Chronic use of paracetamol may enhance the anticoagulant effect of warfarin, although this interaction is generally considered to be minor and occurs primarily with prolonged use.
- *Carbamazepine*:
  - *Interaction*: Reduced effectiveness of paracetamol
  - *Mechanism*: Carbamazepine induces hepatic enzymes that can increase the metabolism of paracetamol, potentially reducing its analgesic effect.
- *Rifampin*:
  - *Interaction*: Reduced effectiveness of paracetamol
  - *Mechanism*: Rifampin induces liver enzymes, which can increase the metabolism of paracetamol.
- *Phenytoin*:
  - *Interaction*: Increased risk of liver toxicity
  - *Mechanism*: Phenytoin can induce liver enzymes, leading to increased formation of toxic metabolites of paracetamol.
- *Isoniazid*:
  - *Interaction*: Increased risk of liver damage
  - *Mechanism*: Isoniazid inhibits the metabolism of paracetamol, increasing the risk of hepatotoxicity.
- *Lamotrigine*:
  - *Interaction*: Reduced effectiveness of lamotrigine
  - *Mechanism*: Paracetamol can increase the clearance of lamotrigine, potentially reducing its effectiveness.
- *Cholestyramine*:
  - *Interaction*: Reduced absorption of paracetamol
  - *Mechanism*: Cholestyramine binds to paracetamol in the gastrointestinal tract, reducing its absorption and effectiveness.

CHAPTER 9: Nonsteroidal Anti-inflammatory Drug and Acetaminophen

- *Metoclopramide and domperidone*:
  - *Interaction*: Increased absorption of paracetamol
  - *Mechanism*: Both drugs increase gastrointestinal motility, potentially leading to faster absorption of paracetamol.
- *Probenecid*:
  - *Interaction*: Increased levels of paracetamol
  - *Mechanism*: Probenecid inhibits the conjugation of paracetamol, which can increase its plasma concentration and prolong its effects.
- *Other hepatotoxic medications (e.g., methotrexate, amiodarone)*:
  - *Interaction*: Increased risk of liver damage
  - *Mechanism*: Concurrent use of other hepatotoxic drugs can exacerbate the risk of liver injury associated with paracetamol.

Paracetamol (acetaminophen) is generally considered safe when used as directed, but there are certain contraindications and situations where its use should be avoided or used with caution. The key contraindications and precautions are as follows:

- *Contraindications*:
  - Hypersensitivity
  - Severe liver disease
  - Severe renal impairment
    - While not an absolute contraindication, caution is advised in patients with severe renal impairment, and dosage adjustments may be necessary.
- *Precautions*:
  - Chronic alcoholism
  - Malnutrition
    - Malnourished individuals may have depleted glutathione stores, which are necessary for the detoxification of paracetamol metabolites, increasing the risk of toxicity.
  - Concurrent use with other medications
    - Caution is needed when paracetamol is used in combination with other hepatotoxic drugs or drugs that interact with its metabolism (e.g., isoniazid, phenytoin).
  - Glucose-6-phosphate dehydrogenase (G6PD) deficiency
    - Individuals with G6PD deficiency may have an increased risk of hemolysis when using paracetamol.
  - Special populations:
    - Elderly:
      - Older adults may be more susceptible to adverse effects due to concurrent illnesses or polypharmacy. Dose adjustments may be necessary based on liver and kidney function.
    - Children:
      - Paracetamol is commonly used in pediatric populations, but dosages must be carefully calculated based on weight to avoid overdose.

Nonsteroidal Anti-inflammatory Drugs

Nonsteroidal anti-inflammatory drugs are a class of medication used for the treatment of pain, fever, and other inflammatory processes.

It has a peripheral action and exerts anti-inflammatory action by inhibiting prostaglandin through the COX pathway. COX is required to convert arachidonic acid into thromboxane, prostaglandin, and prostacyclin. These substances are involved in inflammation, pain, and fever. A more detailed explanation of the mechanism of action of NSAIDs is given in the following text.

There are two main isoforms of the COX enzyme:
1. *COX-1*:
   a. Constitutively expressed in most tissues
   b. Involved in the production of prostaglandins that protect the stomach lining, maintain renal blood flow, and support platelet function.
2. *COX-2*:
   a. Inducible enzyme, usually expressed at sites of inflammation
   b. Produces prostaglandins that mediate inflammation, pain, and fever

Effects of Cyclooxygenase Inhibition
- Anti-inflammatory
- Analgesic
- Antipyretic

Nonspecific Nonsteroidal Anti-inflammatory Drugs (Inhibit both COX-1 and -2)

Commonly used nonspecific NSAIDs include diclofenac, ibuprofen, indomethacin, ketorolac, mefenamic acid, meloxicam, naproxen, and piroxicam.

They are used to treat mild-to-moderate pain, starting from the lowest effective dose and for the shortest possible duration of treatment.

COX-2 selective inhibitors include drugs like celecoxib, rofecoxib, and valdecoxib (the last two were withdrawn from the market in 2004 and 2005, respectively). They are as effective as nonselective NSAIDs for the treatment of mild-to-moderate pain. They exhibit analgesic and anti-inflammatory actions by inhibiting the COX-2 which is present in the inflammatory cells and damaged tissues. However, they are associated with less gastrointestinal side effects.

Selective COX-2 inhibitors should not be prescribed in patients with ischemic heart disease, cerebrovascular disease, and peripheral artery disease and should be prescribed cautiously in patients with hypertension, diabetes mellitus, hyperlipidemia, smokers, and those who are hypersensitive to the drug.

Nonsteroidal anti-inflammatory drugs are contraindicated in patients who are allergic to them, who have undergone coronary artery bypass graft

CHAPTER 9: Nonsteroidal Anti-inflammatory Drug and Acetaminophen

surgery, during the thirdtrimester of pregnancy, and patients with asthma, especially children.

Adverse effects of NSAIDs include *gastric* (it prevents the creation of prostaglandin that protects gastric mucosa), *cardiovascular* [myocardial infarction (MI), thromboembolic event, atrial fibrillation (AF)], *renal* (acute renal dysfunction, fluid and electrolyte disorders), *hematological* (antiplatelet activity), and *anaphylactoid* reactions.

The exact dose of NSAIDs can vary based on the specific medication, the condition being treated, patient factors, and other considerations. The commonly prescribed doses for some widely used NSAIDs are as follows:

- *Ibuprofen*:
  - *Adult dosage*: 400–800 mg orally every 6–8 hours as needed
  - *Maximum daily dosage*: 3,200 mg
- *Naproxen*:
  - *Adult dosage*: 250–500 mg orally every 12 hours as needed
  - *Maximum daily dosage*: 1,000 mg (1,500 mg for the first day of treatment)
- *Diclofenac*:
  - *Adult dosage*: 50 mg orally every 8 hours as needed
  - *Maximum daily dosage*: 150 mg
- *Celecoxib (a COX-2 inhibitor)*:
  - *Adult dosage*: 100–200 mg orally once or twice daily
  - *Maximum daily dosage*: 400 mg
- *Meloxicam*:
  - *Adult dosage*: 7.5–15 mg orally once daily
  - *Maximum daily dosage*: 15 mg
- *Ketorolac*:
  - *Adult dosage*: 10 mg orally every 4–6 hours as needed
  - *Maximum daily dosage*: 40 mg
  - *Note*: Use is typically limited to a maximum of 5 days due to the risk of gastrointestinal and renal side effects.
- *Indomethacin*:
  - *Adult dosage*: 25–50 mg orally two to three times daily
  - *Maximum daily dosage*: 200 mg
- *Aceclofenac*:
  - *Adults*: The usual recommended dose is 100 mg taken twice daily.
  - *Elderly*: Same as adults, but with close monitoring for adverse effects due to increased susceptibility.
  - *Children*: Not recommended for use in children
- *Etoricoxib*:
  - *Dosage*:
    - Osteoarthritis: 30 or 60 mg once daily
    - Rheumatoid arthritis: 60 or 90 mg once daily
    - Ankylosing spondylitis: 60 or 90 mg once daily
    - Acute pain (e.g., gout): 120 mg once daily, limited to a maximum of 8 days

Drug Interaction in Case of Nonsteroidal Anti-inflammatory Drug Usage

Nonsteroidal anti-inflammatory drugs can interact with a variety of other medications, potentially leading to increased risks of adverse effects or decreased effectiveness of treatments. Some common and significant drug interactions with NSAIDs are as follows:

- *Anticoagulants* (e.g., warfarin, heparin, direct oral anticoagulants)
  - *Interaction*: Increased risk of bleeding
  - *Mechanism*: NSAIDs inhibit platelet aggregation and can cause gastrointestinal bleeding, which can be compounded by anticoagulants.
- *Antihypertensive medications* [e.g., angiotensin-converting enzyme (ACE) inhibitors, angiotensin receptor blockers (ARBs), diuretic]
  - *Interaction*: Reduced effectiveness of antihypertensive medications
  - *Mechanism*: NSAIDs can cause sodium and water retention, leading to increased blood pressure.
- *Corticosteroids* (e.g., prednisone)
  - *Interaction*: Increased risk of gastrointestinal ulcers and bleeding
  - *Mechanism*: Both NSAIDs and corticosteroids can cause gastrointestinal irritation and ulceration.
- *Selective serotonin reuptake inhibitors* (SSRIs; e.g., fluoxetine, sertraline)
  - *Interaction*: Increased risk of gastrointestinal bleeding
  - *Mechanism*: SSRIs can inhibit platelet function, and NSAIDs can cause gastrointestinal irritation, leading to a higher risk of bleeding.
- *Lithium*:
  - *Interaction*: Increased lithium levels and potential toxicity
  - *Mechanism*: NSAIDs can reduce renal clearance of lithium.
- *Methotrexate*:
  - *Interaction*: Increased risk of methotrexate toxicity
  - *Mechanism*: NSAIDs can decrease renal clearance of methotrexate.
- *Digoxin*:
  - *Interaction*: Increased digoxin levels
  - *Mechanism*: NSAIDs can reduce renal clearance of digoxin.
- *Cyclosporine*:
  - *Interaction*: Increased risk of nephrotoxicity
  - *Mechanism*: Both NSAIDs and cyclosporine can have nephrotoxic effects.
- *Aspirin*:
  - *Interaction*: Reduced cardioprotective effect of low-dose aspirin; increased risk of gastrointestinal side effects.
  - *Mechanism*: NSAIDs can interfere with the antiplatelet effect of low-dose aspirin.

> **BOX 1** Potential high-risk patients.
> - >60 years of age
> - Previous history of ulceration
> - Concomitant steroid use
> - Systemic disease, e.g., renal impairment, heart failure, carcinomatosis, increased risk of bleeding, e.g., on warfarin
> - Patients on a higher dose of nonsteroidal anti-inflammatory drug

- *Alcohol*:
  - *Interaction*: Increased risk of gastrointestinal bleeding and ulcers
  - *Mechanism*: Both alcohol and NSAIDs can cause gastrointestinal irritation.

It is important to have the information about all the medications the patient is taking and to tailor the treatment to the individual's needs and medical condition. Long-term use of NSAIDs should be monitored due to potential side effects such as gastrointestinal bleeding, cardiovascular risks, and renal impairment.

Various Do's and Don'ts of Nonsteroidal Anti-inflammatory Drug Use
- NSAIDs should be used cautiously in all patients and any alternative analgesics should always be tried first line.
- They should be used initially in normal-risk patients.
- Stop NSAIDs in suspected peptic ulcer.
- Do not initiate NSAIDs during active ulceration.
- If NSAIDs are essential in high-risk patients, add long-term lansoprazole 30 mg OD.
- Patients with more than one risk factor **(Box 1)** can be considered for treatment either with coxib alone or in combination with an established NSAID plus lansoprazole 30 mg OD.

Around 20% of patients prescribed coxibs report dyspeptic symptoms, and these side effects may limit use.

Who Needs Prophylaxis?
- Give prophylaxis against peptic ulcer if the patient has a history of peptic ulcer or bleeding on NSAID.
- Consider prophylaxis in high-risk patients.

MANAGING GASTROINTESTINAL SIDE EFFECTS OF NONSTEROIDAL ANTI-INFLAMMATORY DRUGS

Management of gastrointestinal side effects of nonsteroidal anti-inflammatory drugs is shown in **Flowchart 1**.

CHAPTER 9: Nonsteroidal Anti-inflammatory Drug and Acetaminophen

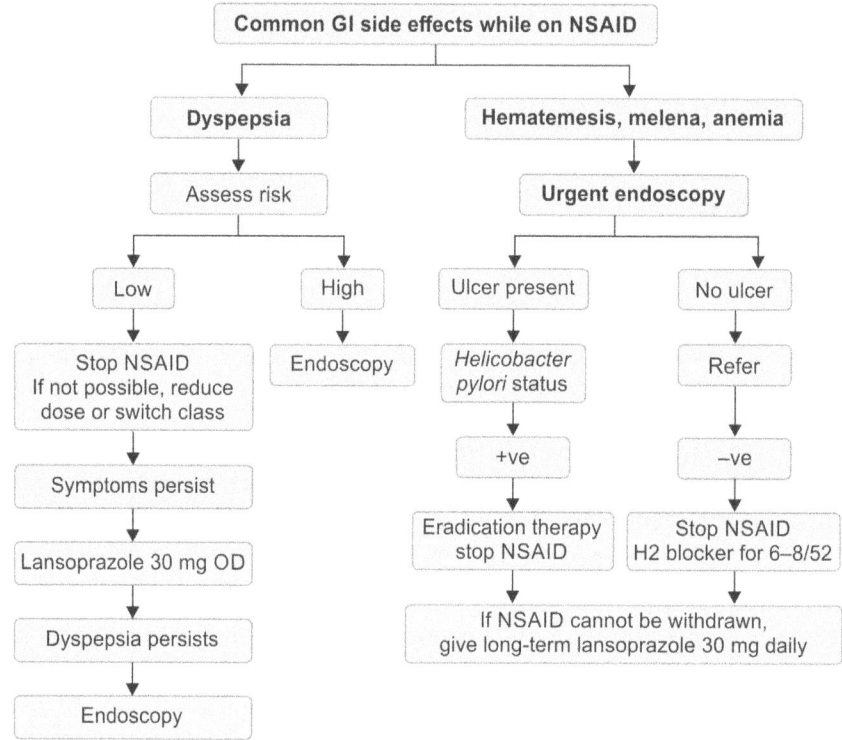

Flowchart 1: Algorithm management of side effects of NSAID.
Note: If gastric ulcer is proven, endoscopy must be repeated after 8–12 weeks of treatment to confirm healing.
(GI: gastrointestinal; NSAID: nonsteroidal anti-inflammatory drug)

CONCLUSION

Nonsteroidal anti-inflammatory drugs play a vital role in managing musculoskeletal pain, providing effective relief for many patients. However, their use must be balanced with considerations of potential side effects, such as gastrointestinal, cardiovascular, and renal risks. Healthcare providers should tailor NSAID therapy to each patient's specific condition, risk factors, and overall health status, incorporating both pharmacologic and non-pharmacologic approaches. As research continues to evolve, a more nuanced understanding of NSAID therapy will help clinicians maximize their benefits while minimizing harm, ultimately improving patient outcomes in musculoskeletal pain management.

BIBLIOGRAPHY

1. Arendt Nielsen L, de Las Peñas CF, Graven Nielsen T. Basic aspects of musculoskeletal pain: from acute to chronic pain. J Man Manipulative Ther. 2011;19(4):186-93.
2. El-Tallawy SN, Nalamasu R, Pergolizzi JV, Gharibo C. Pain management during the COVID-19 pandemic. Pain Ther. 2020;9:453-66.
3. El-Tallawy SN, Nalamasu R, Salem GI LeQuang JAK, Pergolizzi JV, Christo PJ. Management of musculoskeletal pain: an update with emphasis on chronic musculoskeletal pain. Pain Ther. 2021;10:181-209.
4. Schug SA, Palmer GM, Scott DA, Halliwell R, Trinca J. Acute pain management: scientific evidence fourth edition, 2015. Med J Aust. 2016;204(8):315-7.
5. Scottish Intercollegiate Guidelines Network (SIGN). Management of Chronic Pain. Edinburgh: SIGN; 2013. Revised 2019, SIGN publication no. 136. [online] Available from https://www.sign.ac.uk/assets/sign136.pdf [Last accessed August, 2024].
6. World Health Organization. (2019). Musculoskeletal conditions. [online] Available from https://www.who.int/news-room/fact-sheets/detail/musculoskeletal-conditions [Last accessed August, 2024].

CHAPTER 10

Opioids and Opioid-sparing Strategies in the Management of Musculoskeletal Pain

Nusrat Kreem Bhat, Farid Hussain

INTRODUCTION

Opioids are among the most effective medications for moderate-to-severe pain. They increase the pain threshold. They act on " μ", " κ" (kappa) and "δ" (delta) opioid receptors.

Opioids act both presynaptically and postsynaptically to produce an analgesic effect.

Presynaptically, opioids block calcium channels on nociceptive afferent nerves to inhibit the release of neurotransmitters such as substance P and glutamate, which contribute to nociception. Postsynaptically, opioids open potassium channels, which hyperpolarize cell membranes, increasing the required action potential to generate nociceptive transmission. Classification of opioids on the basis of source is given in **Box 1** and on the basis of action being agonist or antagonist is given in **Box 2**.

BOX 1 Classification of opioids.

Natural opium alkaloids
- Morphine
- Codeine

Semisynthetic opiates
- Diacetylmorphine (heroin)
- Pholcodine

Synthetic opioids
- Pethidine (meperidine)
- Fentanyl
- Alfentanil
- Sufentanil
- Remifentanil
- Methadone
- Dextropropoxyphene
- Tramadol
- Tapentadol

CHAPTER 10: Opioids and Opioid-sparing Strategies in the Management...

> **BOX 2** | **Complex action of opioids and opioid antagonists.**
>
> **Agonist–antagonists (κ analgesics)**
> - Nalorphine
> - Pentazocine
> - Butorphanol
> - Nalbuphine
>
> **Pure antagonists**
> - Naloxone
> - Naltrexone
> - Nalmefene
>
> **Partial/weak μ agonist + κ antagonist**
> - Buprenorphine

The various opioids used for the treatment of pain are as follows:
- *Morphine* is considered the classic analgesic among opioids.
- *The various routes of morphine administration* are oral (PO), intravenous (IV), epidural, intramuscular (IM), intrathecal, and sublingual, and morphine can also be used as a suppository. Oral formulations are available in both short and long acting tablets for the treatment of acute and chronic pain.
- The *Food and Drug Administration (FDA)-approved usage of morphine sulfate* for the relief of moderate-to-severe pain when other pain relief medicines are not effective or cannot be used may be acute or chronic.
- The clinical situations in which morphine is indicated are management of palliative/end-of-life care, active cancer treatment, and vaso-occlusive pain during sickle cell crisis. Morphine is widely used off-label for almost any condition that causes pain. In the emergency department, morphine is given for musculoskeletal pain, abdominal pain, chest pain, arthritis, and even headaches when patients fail to respond to first- and second-line agents. Morphine to relieve pain during a myocardial infarction (MI) has been in use since the early 1900s.
- Common unwanted effects of morphine use include constipation, lightheadedness, sedation, dizziness, nausea, vomiting, dry mouth, euphoria, dysphoria, agitation, urinary retention, and biliary tract spasm. Respiratory depression is among the more serious adverse reactions of opiate use that is especially important to monitor in the postoperative patient population. It can also affect the cardiovascular system and reportedly can cause flushing, bradycardia, hypotension, and syncope.
- Respiratory depression caused by morphine is a serious medical condition that requires prompt treatment. The steps typically taken to manage this condition are as follows:
    - *Monitor vital signs*: Check the patient's respiratory rate, oxygen saturation, heart rate, and blood pressure.
    - Assess the patient's level of consciousness and response to stimuli.
    - *Supportive care*:
        - Positioning: Place the patient in a position that maximizes airway patency, such as the recovery position or sitting upright.

- Oxygen therapy: Administer supplemental oxygen to maintain adequate oxygenation.
  ○ Pharmacological intervention
- *Codeine* is similar to morphine, converted in the body to morphine. It is less efficacious and less potent than morphine. It plays a role in treating mild-to-moderate pain. Codeine is often used as a combined medication with acetaminophen or with nonsteroidal anti-inflammatory drugs (NSAIDs) like ibuprofen. It is also used for the treatment of chronic cough and restless leg syndrome.
- *Naloxone*: It is a competitive antagonist over all types of opioids receptors. It is an opioid antagonist that can quickly reverse the effects of opioid overdose, including respiratory depression.

Routes of administration:
  ○ *IV*: It is the preferred route for rapid effect. Initial dose is 0.4–2 mg IV, administered slowly over 30 seconds.
    - If the initial dose is ineffective, it may be repeated every 2–3 minutes up to a total dose of 10 mg.
    - If no response is observed after a total dose of 10 mg, the diagnosis of opioid overdose should be questioned.
    - The dose may need to be titrated based on the patient's response and the severity of the respiratory depression.
  ○ *IM or subcutaneous (SC)*: It is used when IV access is not available. Initial dose is 0.4–2 mg. Repeat doses may be given every 2–3 minutes as needed.
  ○ *Intranasal*: Suitable for emergency situations, along with emergency medical treatment to reverse the life-threatening effects of opiate overdose
    - Dose: 4 mg (one spray) in one nostril
    - A second dose may be administered in the opposite nostril if there is no response after 2–3 minutes.

Naloxone is a life-saving medication in the context of opioid overdose and should be readily available in both medical and community settings where opioid use is prevalent.

In cases where respiratory depression is severe and persistent, a continuous infusion of naloxone may be necessary after an initial bolus dose.

Continuous monitoring: If there is no improvement, repeat doses and be prepared for mechanical ventilation.
- *Oxycodone* is a potent semisynthetic opioid agonist for acute or chronic moderate-to-severe pain when opioid medication is considered suitable for the patient and alternative pain management strategies are inadequate.
- *Pethidine* has one-tenth analgesic potency. It has less spasmodic action on smooth muscles and produces tachycardia due to its antimuscarinic action. It is safer in patients with asthma (less histamine release). The various indications are as analgesic, as preanesthetic medication,

and to also provide analgesia during labor (less neonatal respiratory depression).
- *Fentanyl* is 80–100 times more potent than morphine and has little propensity to release histamine; it is not used orally due to high first-pass metabolism. It has a quick onset of action. Peak analgesia is seen in 5 minutes after IV injection with a duration of action of half an hour. Transdermal fentanyl has become available for use in cancer and the patch should be changed every third day.
- *Methadone* has a slow and persistent action with less sedation and less abuse potential. It is used as a substitute therapy for opioid dependence and 1 mg of methadone is equivalent to 4 mg of morphine.
- *Buprenorphine* is a weak μ agonist and k antagonist. It is 25–50 times more potent than morphine. The route of administration is sublingual; transdermal patches are also available. It has a slower onset and longer duration of action. The uses of buprenorphine are in long-lasting cancer pain, postoperative pain, MI, and treatment of morphine dependence.
- *Pentazocine* has agonistic actions and weak opioid antagonistic activity. The drug elicits dysphoric and psychotomimetic effects and increases in blood pressure and heart rate so it is avoided in patients with MI. It is indicated in moderate-to-severe pain as a preoperative medication and as a supplement to anesthesia.
- *Tramadol* also acts by one additional mechanism, i.e., by norepinephrine and 5-hydroxytryptamine (5-HT) reuptake inhibition. The advantages of tramadol are less respiratory depression, constipation, sedation, urinary retention, and abuse potential. The disadvantages are nausea, vomiting, seizure precipitation (contraindicated in epilepsy), and serotonin syndrome with selective serotonin reuptake inhibitor (SSRI). It is mainly used in labor pain, injury, surgery, and other short-lasting pains. It is as effective as morphine for moderate pain and less effective than morphine for severe pain treatment.
- *Tapentadol* has analgesic action by activating the central noradrenergic pathway. It has certain advantages like less nausea and vomiting than tramadol and the disadvantage is seizure precipitation, so it is contraindicated in epilepsy and serotonin syndrome with SSRI.

Some commonly used opioids are given in **Table 1**.

OPIOID-SPARING STRATEGIES

The aim is to reduce or eliminate the need for opioids by alternative treatment and approaches. It includes a combination of nonpharmacological and pharmacological methods as given in **Table 2**.

Decoy molecules [ribonucleic acid–based therapy and soluble epoxide hydrolase (sEH) inhibitors] are newer drugs that act at the molecular level, and are being developed and undergoing animal trials.

A stepwise approach given by the World Health Organization (WHO) for using opioids in the management of pain is shown in **Flowchart 1**.

Table 1: Some commonly used opioids.

Opioid	Onset of action	Routes	Dose	Side effects	Indications
Morphine	45 minutes	Oral, IV, IM, sublingual, suppository	15–60 mg	Sedation, dizziness, nausea, vomiting, dry mouth, constipation, etc.	Severe pain
Codeine	45 minutes	Oral	30–60 mg	Constipation and nausea	Moderate pain
Oxycodone	5–10 minutes	Oral, IV	5–10 mg	Constipation, fatigue, and dizziness	Severe pain
Hydrocodone with paracetamol	30–60 minutes	Oral	5 mg/300 mg	Nausea, vomiting, constipation, and drowsiness	Moderate pain
Methadone	15–45 minutes	Oral	22.5–10 mg	Constipation, somnolence	Severe pain
Buprenorphine	26–36 hours	Transdermal patch, sublingual tablets, buccal films	5, 10, 20 µg	Nausea, vomiting, headache, constipation	Moderate-to-severe pain
Tramadol	10–15 minutes	Oral and IV	50–100 mg	Nausea, vomiting, constipation	Moderate pain
Fentanyl	5–10 minutes	Sublingual, IV, transdermal patch	100–400 µg	Somnolence, diarrhea, nausea	Severe pain
Pethidine	30 minutes	Oral, IV	50–100 mg	Nausea, vomiting, constipation, drowsiness	Severe pain
Tapentadol	30–60 minutes	Oral (IR, ER)	50–100 mg	Nausea, vomiting, constipation, respiratory depression	Severe pain
Tylenol (codeine + paracetamol)	30–60 minutes	Oral	30–60 mg 300–1,000 mg	Nausea, constipation, abuse potential	Moderate pain

(IM: intramuscular; IV: intravenous)

Table 2: Nonpharmacological and pharmacological alternatives to reduce the use of opioids.

Pharmacological strategies and drugs	Nonpharmacological strategies (physical modalities)	Pain interventions	Lifestyle modifications	Surgical interventions

• NSAIDs and paracetamol
• Antidepressants
  ○ Amitriptyline
  ○ Nortriptyline
  ○ Duloxetine
• Anticonvulsants
  ○ Gabapentin
  ○ Pregabalin
  ○ Carbamazepine
• Lidocaine patches
• Capsaicin patches
• Topical analgesics
• Muscle relaxants
  ○ Cyclobenzaprine
  ○ Baclofen
  ○ Tizanidine
• Corticosteroids
  ○ Dexamethasone
  ○ Prednisolone
• Anxiolytics
• N-Methyl-D-aspartate receptor antagonists
• Ketamine
• Dextromethorphan
• Magnesium
	• Cryotherapy
	• Occupational therapy
	• Acupuncture
	• Heat and cold therapy
	• TENS
	• Therapeutic exercises
	• Regular exercise and weight management
	• Massage therapy
	• Chiropractic care
	• Psychological meditation
	• Stress reduction
	• Cognitive behavioral therapy
	  ○ Relaxation technique
	  ○ Music therapy
	• Ultrasound and electric stimulation
		• Local anesthetics
		  ○ Lidocaine nerve block
		• Botulinum toxin
		• Alpha-2-adrenergic agonists like clonidine, dexmedetomidine
		• Neurolytics like alcohol or phenol
		• Radiofrequency ablation and cryoanalgesia
		• Intra-articular injection of corticosteroid or hyaluronic acid
		• Bone marrow concentrates, injections
		• Regional anesthesia techniques
		  ○ Epidural analgesia
		  ○ Bier block
		• Surgical site local infiltration
		• Liposomal Bupivacaine
			• Education
			  ○ Proper body posture, mechanics, and ergonomics to prevent injury
			• Nutraceuticals, diet, and nutrition
			• Herbal products with anti-inflammatory properties
			• Good sleep
			• Avoid smoking
				• Surgical procedures for primary lesion or pathology
				• Neurological procedures for pain management

(NSAID: nonsteroidal anti-inflammatory drug; TENS: transcutaneous electric nerve stimulation)

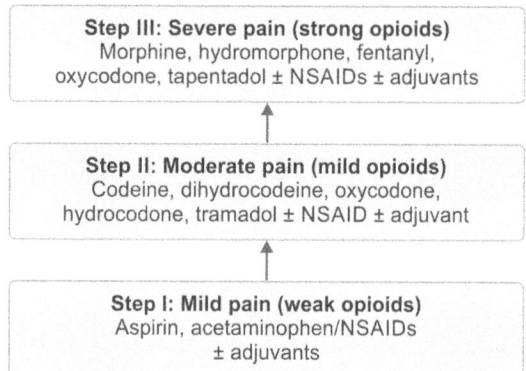

Flowchart 1: WHO pain management ladder.
(NSAIDs: nonsteroidal anti-inflammatory drugs; WHO: World Health Organization)

CONCLUSION

In managing musculoskeletal pain, balancing effective relief with the risks of opioid use is critical. While opioids may still have a role in treating acute or severe cases, the long-term risks of dependence, tolerance, and side effects have driven the need for alternative approaches. Opioid-sparing strategies, including non-opioid medications, physical therapy, and interventional techniques, provide viable pathways to control pain while minimizing harm. By adopting a multidisciplinary approach, healthcare providers can offer safer, more sustainable pain management, ultimately improving patient outcomes and contributing to efforts in reducing opioid misuse.

BIBLIOGRAPHY

1. Anghelescu DL, Guo A, Morgan KJ, Frett M, Prajapati H, Gold R, et al. Pain outcomes after celiac plexus block in children and young adults with cancer. J Adolesc Young Adult Oncol. 2018;7(6):666-72.
2. Christo PJ, Mazloomdoost D. Cancer pain and analgesia. Ann N Acad Sci. 2008;1138: 278-98.
3. Haghjooy-Javanmard S, Ghasemi A, Laher I, Zarrin B, Dana N, Vaseghi G. Influence of morphine on TLR4/NF-kB signalling pathway of MCF-7 cells. Bratisl Lek Listy. 2018;119(4):229-33.
4. Hoy DG, Smith E, Cross M, Sanchez-Riera L, Buchbinder R, Blyth FM, et al. The global burden of other musculoskeletal disorders: estimates from the Global Burden of Disease 2010 study. Ann Rheum Dis. 2014;73:1462-9.
5. Leite Jr JB, de Mello Bastos JM, Samuels RI, Carey RJ, Carrera MP. Reversal of morphine-conditioned behaviour by an anti-dopaminergic post-trial drug treatment during re-consolidation. Behav Brain Res. 2019;359:771-82.
6. Schellack G, Schellack N, Meyer JC. Opioid analgesics—a 2018 update. S Afr Pharm J. 2018;85(1):43.
7. Tripathi KD. Opioid analgesics and antagonists. In: Tripathi KD (Ed). Essentials of Medical Pharmacology, 8th edition. New Delhi: Jaypee Brothers Medical Publishers; 2019. pp. 454-68.

CHAPTER 11

Role of Muscle Relaxants in Musculoskeletal Pain Management

Nusrat Kreem Bhat, Farid Hussain

INTRODUCTION

Musculoskeletal pain often necessitates the use of muscle relaxants which play a crucial role in alleviating discomfort associated with muscle spasms.

TYPES OF MUSCLE RELAXANTS

Muscle relaxants can be broadly classified into two categories:
1. *Antispasmodics:* These are used to alleviate acute muscle spasms and include drugs like:
    - *Cyclobenzaprine*: Effective for short-term relief of muscle spasms
    - *Methocarbamol*: Often used for musculoskeletal pain relief
    - *Carisoprodol*: Prescribed for acute musculoskeletal pain but has potential for abuse
    - *Thiocolchicoside*: A semisynthetic derivative of colchicine, widely used in Europe and other regions for its muscle relaxant properties
2. *Antispastics:* These are primarily used for conditions involving chronic muscle spasticity, such as:
    - *Baclofen*: Commonly used for spasticity related to spinal cord injuries
    - *Tizanidine*: Effective in managing spasticity in multiple sclerosis

INDICATIONS

Muscle relaxants are indicated for:
- Acute musculoskeletal conditions like back pain and neck pain
- Chronic conditions such as fibromyalgia and spasticity due to neurological disorders
- Short-term use to relieve discomfort from acute muscle spasms or injuries

CONTRAINDICATIONS

Contraindications vary depending on the specific muscle relaxant but generally include:
- Hypersensitivity to the drug
- Severe liver or kidney impairment (e.g., tizanidine should be used cautiously in hepatic impairment)
- History of drug abuse or addiction (notably with carisoprodol)
- Concurrent use of monoamine oxidase inhibitors (MAOIs) with certain muscle relaxants like cyclobenzaprine
- *Thiocolchicoside*: Contraindicated in pregnancy and breastfeeding due to potential teratogenic effects

SIDE EFFECTS

Common side effects associated with muscle relaxants include:
- *Sedation*: Drowsiness and dizziness, particularly with drugs like cyclobenzaprine and carisoprodol
- *Dry mouth and blurred vision*: Often seen with antispasmodics
- *Hypotension*: Notable with tizanidine
- *Gastrointestinal disturbances*: Nausea, vomiting, and constipation
- *Thiocolchicoside*: Diarrhea, abdominal pain, and potential for hypotonia (reduced muscle tone)

Severe adverse effects, though rare, may include:
- *Hepatotoxicity*: Especially with tizanidine
- *Dependence and withdrawal*: Primarily associated with carisoprodol
- *Convulsions*: Reported with thiocolchicoside in high doses or prolonged use

DRUG INTERACTIONS

Muscle relaxants can interact with various other medications:
- *Central nervous system depressants*: Concurrent use with alcohol, benzodiazepines, or opioids can enhance sedative effects, increasing the risk of respiratory depression.
- *Antihypertensives*: Tizanidine can potentiate the hypotensive effects.
- *Fluoroquinolone antibiotics*: May increase serum levels of tizanidine, leading to increased side effects
- *Thiocolchicoside*: Potential interaction with other centrally acting drugs, increasing the risk of central nervous system adverse effects

Details regarding dose, metabolism, indications, contraindications, and adverse effects of some medically important antispasmodic and antispastic muscle relaxants are given in **Tables 1 and 2**.

CHAPTER 11: Role of Muscle Relaxants in Musculoskeletal Pain Management

Table 1: Antispastic and antispasmodic skeletal muscle relaxants.

Drugs	Dose	Metabolism	Indications	Contraindications	Adverse effects
Tizanidine	4 mg TDS, can titrate to optimal 2–4 mg TDS, oral route	Liver	• Spasticity reduces in amyotrophic lateral sclerosis • Multiple sclerosis • Spinal injuries	Cautions used in elderly patients	Somnolence, xerostomia, and weakness
Thiocolchicoside (additional anti-inflammatory and analgesic properties)	4–8 mg BD oral, intramuscular, topical gels	Liver	• Acute and chronic muscle spasm including low backache • Sciatica, torticollis, and neurological disorder muscle spasm	• Individual prone to seizures • Teratogenic and decreased fertility in men, children	• Nausea, vomiting, diarrhea • Allergy • Vasovagal reactions, hepatotoxicity in systemic routes
Tolperisone	50–150 mg, oral	Liver	• Multiple sclerosis • Cerebral palsy • Spinal cord injuries • Low back pain • Spondylosis	• Myasthenia gravis • Pregnancy • Lactation	• Dizziness • Headache • Muscle weakness • Arterial hypotension • Dry mouth
Diazepam	2–10 mg, TDS or QID, oral, IM, IV	Liver	• Skeletal muscle spasm • Anxiety • Seizure disorders	• Pregnancy • Glaucoma • Hepatic impairment	• Drowsiness • Fatigue • Hangover effect • Dependence • Cognitive impairment

Table 2: Antispasmodic skeletal muscle relaxants.

Drugs	Dose	Metabolism	Indications	Contraindications	Adverse effects
Carisoprodol	250–350 mg TDS or QID, orally	Liver	Acute painful musculoskeletal disorders associated with muscle spasm	• Pregnancy • Breastfeeding	Dizziness, drowsiness, headache, tremors, seizure, depression dependency
Chlorzoxazone	250–750 mg TDS or QID, orally	Liver	Acute musculoskeletal pain	• Pregnancy • Breastfeeding	Dizziness, malaise, urine discoloration; hepatotoxicity with jaundice may be fatal
Cyclobenzaprine	5 mg 3 times Maximum: 10 mg 3 times daily orally	Liver	Muscle spasm associated with acute musculoskeletal condition	Hepatotoxic, avoided with tramadol, barbiturates, and alcohol	• Dry mouth, fatigue • Constipation, palpitation, cardiac conduction disturbances
Methocarbamol	1,500 mg QID for the first 3 days followed by 750 mg QID by oral route	Liver and kidney	Acute musculoskeletal pain		• Hypotension, syncope • Dizziness, headache, light-headedness
Metaxalone	800 mg 3–4 times daily orally	Liver	Acute musculoskeletal pain	Liver and renal impairment in children, pregnancy, lactation	Central nervous system depression, nausea, vomiting; rare: jaundice, hemolytic anemia
Orphenadrine	100 mg BD, oral and intramuscular	Liver	Acute musculoskeletal pain	Heart failure	Dryness of mouth, constipation

CHAPTER 11: Role of Muscle Relaxants in Musculoskeletal Pain Management

LATEST EVIDENCE AND RECOMMENDATIONS

Recent studies and reviews emphasize the importance of cautious and short-term use of muscle relaxants due to the potential for adverse effects and dependence. A systematic review published in *Journal of Pain Research* (2022) underscores the efficacy of cyclobenzaprine in the short-term management of acute musculoskeletal pain but highlights the need for close monitoring due to sedative effects. Another study in *Current Medical Research and Opinion* (2023) discusses the role of tizanidine in managing spasticity, advocating for its careful use in patients with liver conditions. Additionally, a review in *Journal of Clinical Pharmacy and Therapeutics* (2023) evaluated the safety profile of thiocolchicoside, recommending its use with caution due to the potential for neurological side effects.

CONCLUSION

Muscle relaxants are valuable in the management of musculoskeletal pain, particularly for short-term relief of acute symptoms. Their use should be guided by a thorough understanding of their indications, contraindications, potential side effects, and drug interactions. Clinicians must remain vigilant regarding the risk of dependence and ensure that therapy is tailored to the individual patient's needs, drawing on the latest clinical evidence to inform best practices.

BIBLIOGRAPHY

1. Tizanidine in spasticity management: efficacy and safety considerations. Curr Med Res Opin. 2023.
2. Safety profile and clinical use of thiocolchicoside. J Clin Pharm Ther. 2023.
3. Systematic review of cyclobenzaprine in musculoskeletal pain management. J Pain Res. 2022.

CHAPTER 12

Adjunct Analgesics

Sachin Kudyar

INTRODUCTION

Adjunct analgesics, also called adjuvant analgesics, are drugs that are helpful in managing pain, particularly musculoskeletal pain, but are not mainly meant for pain control. These medications can assist control particular types of pain and improve the effects of basic analgesics. They can also provide extra pain relief. When combined with systemic medications, regional anesthesia, and neuraxial suppression, they significantly contribute to a successful and accelerated recovery following surgery.

Different adjuncts have additive or synergistic effects by targeting distinct pain pathways or receptors. The overview of the various primary adjuncts utilized in multimodal analgesia is given in **Table 1**.

Table 1: Overview of the various primary adjuncts utilized in multimodal analgesia.			
Group	Examples	Reduces opioid requirements	Side effects
Gabapentinoids	Gabapentin, pregabalin	No	Breathlessness, weakness
NMDA receptor antagonists	Ketamine	Yes	Coronary artery disease, liver failure
Alpha-2-adrenergic agonists	Clonidine, dexmedetomidine	Yes	Hypotension, bradycardia
Glucocorticoids	Dexamethasone	Yes	Poorly controlled diabetes
SSRIs	Duloxetine	No	Seizures, uncontrolled hypertension

Note: They have long been a part of pain management.
(NMDA: *N*-methyl-D-aspartate; SSRI: selective serotonin reuptake inhibitors)
Source: Adapted from Bennett and Morison (2022). Adjuncts and multimodal analgesia: A narrative overview. Digestive Medicine Research. [online 5.0]. Available from https://dmr.amegroups.org/article/view/8162/html [Last accessed August, 2024].

CHAPTER 12: Adjunct Analgesics

GABAPENTINOIDS

Pregabalin and gabapentin are examples of gabapentinoids, and both of them are taken orally. Both pregabalin and gabapentin have a half-life of 6 hours; pregabalin reaches its maximal plasma concentration 1 hour after intake, whereas gabapentin takes 4 hours. By blocking calcium channels, these medications lessen the release of excitatory neurotransmitters. Headaches, vertigo, and drowsiness are typical adverse effects. According to a study, pregabalin 300 mg increased sedation but decreased postoperative opioid use in patients undergoing elective hip arthroplasty.

N-METHYL-D-ASPARTATE RECEPTOR ANTAGONISTS

By halting central sensitization, which can result in persistent pain, *N*-methyl-D-aspartate (NMDA) receptor antagonists like magnesium and ketamine aid in the management of pain. Ketamine is used intraoperatively for surgical pain treatment or as "rescue analgesia." It can be injected intramuscularly, sublingually, intravenously, or intranasally. For infusion, the American Society of Regional Anesthesia and Pain Medicine suggests 0.5–1 mg/kg/h and a maximum bolus dose of 0.35 mg/kg. Hypersalivation, bronchodilation, and hallucinations are some of the adverse effects. Patients with elevated intracranial and intraocular pressure, significant liver illness, or coronary artery disease should not take it.

While magnesium similarly functions as an antagonist of NMDA receptors, its analgesic mechanism is uncertain due to its limited blood–brain barrier crossing. The recommended intravenous dosage for this medication is 40–50 mg/kg. Bradycardia, hypotension, and persistent neuromuscular blockade are among its side effects.

ALPHA-2-ADRENERGIC AGONISTS

Clonidine and dexmedetomidine are examples of alpha-2-adrenergic agonists that function by obstructing presynaptic receptors, which lowers noradrenaline release and sympathetic activity. These medications block pain pathways by binding to dorsal horn substantia gelatinosa receptors. Clonidine can be administered intravenously, orally, or by neuraxial injection. Postoperative doses of 50–75 µg are the starting points, and they can be repeated up to three times a day. The dose ranges from 1–2 to 2–4 µg/kg epidurally for intrathecal injection. Both intraoperative and postoperative hypotension are side consequences.

Dexmedetomidine is used only in operating rooms and critical care settings, where it is infused intravenously. Postoperative bradycardia and cardiovascular consequences are examples of side effects.

MEMBRANE STABILIZERS

The amide local anesthetic lidocaine blocks sodium channels to produce its effects. It has analgesic and anti-inflammatory properties when given intravenously. Up to 1.5 mg/kg of loading dosage is administered, and an infusion of up to 1.5 mg/kg/h—a maximum of 120 mg/h—follows. Intravenous lidocaine has a limited therapeutic window and is not approved for use in perioperative analgesia. Therapeutic plasma concentrations fall between 2.5 and 3.5 µg/mL; toxicity develops over 5 µg/mL and manifests as symptoms such as dizziness, numbness in the tongue, and possibly even convulsions. Below 10 µg/mL in plasma, cardiotoxicity is infrequent.

GLUCOCORTICOIDS

Because of its antiemetic qualities, dexamethasone is frequently administered intraoperatively. As a component of a multimodal analgesia regimen, it helps lessen surgical pain by lowering postoperative nausea and vomiting. By inhibiting proinflammatory pathways, it also has anti-inflammatory properties. Most patients can safely receive intravenous dosages of 4-8 mg during surgery. Both the first- and 24-hour postoperative pain scores are improved. Elevated blood sugar levels are one of the side effects; nevertheless, there is no increased risk of wound healing delay or postoperative infection.

SELECTIVE SEROTONIN REUPTAKE INHIBITORS

By raising the levels of serotonin and norepinephrine in the dorsal horn of the spinal cord, duloxetine is used to treat neuropathic and chronic pain. This enhances the suppression of pain by activating different adrenergic and serotonin receptors. It is taken orally, with a maintenance dose of 60 mg once daily after the first 30-60 mg once daily. Breathing difficulties, facial and neck puffiness, and hives are some of the side effects.

COMMONLY USED ADJUNCT ANALGESICS

The following is a list of adjunct analgesics used in the management of musculoskeletal pain, along with information on their uses, dosages, adverse effects, and drug interactions:
- *Antidepressants (e.g., amitriptyline, duloxetine)*:
  - *Indications*: Chronic musculoskeletal pain, neuropathic pain, fibromyalgia
  - *Contraindications*: Recent myocardial infarction, monoamine oxidase (MAO) inhibitor use within 14 days, narrow-angle glaucoma (for tricyclic antidepressants)
  - *Dose*:
    - *Amitriptyline*: Take 10-25 mg by mouth at bedtime; up to 50-100 mg daily can be progressively increased.
    - *Duloxetine*: Take 30 mg at first, and up to 60 mg later.
  - *Side effects*: Sedation, dry mouth, weight gain, constipation, sexual dysfunction

- *Drug interactions*: MAO inhibitors, selective serotonin reuptake inhibitors (SSRIs), and serotonin-norepinephrine reuptake inhibitors (SNRIs; increased risk of serotonin syndrome), anticholinergic drugs (enhanced effects)
- *Anticonvulsants (e.g., gabapentin, pregabalin)*:
    - *Indications*: Neuropathic pain, fibromyalgia
    - *Contraindication*: Hypersensitivity to the drug
    - *Dose*:
        - *Gabapentin*: Begin taking 300 mg of gabapentin daily; gradually increase to 1,800–3,600 mg in separate doses.
        - *Pregabalin*: 75 mg twice a day to start, with a possible increase to 150 mg twice a day
    - *Side effects*: Dizziness, drowsiness, peripheral edema, weight gain
    - *Drug interactions*: Central nervous system (CNS) depressants (enhanced sedation), opioids (increased risk of respiratory depression)

By understanding and appropriately using these adjunct analgesics, healthcare providers can enhance pain management strategies, reduce opioid requirements, and improve patient outcomes.

CONCLUSION

Adjunct analgesia plays a crucial role in optimizing pain management for musculoskeletal conditions. By integrating nonopioid medications, physical therapies, and complementary techniques, clinicians can enhance pain relief, minimize opioid dependence, and improve patient outcomes. The careful selection of adjuncts tailored to individual patient needs is essential for effective, multimodal pain management strategies, reducing side effects while improving quality of life.

BIBLIOGRAPHY

1. Benett V, Morison B. (2022). Adjuncts and multimodal analgesia: a narrative overview. Digestive Medicine Research. [online 5.0] Available from https://dmr.amegroups.org/article/view/8162/html [Last accessed August, 2024].
2. Derry S, Moore RA, Aldington D, Cole P, Wiffen PJ. Adverse events associated with single dose oral gabapentin in acute postoperative pain in adults. J Clin Anesth. 2013;25(3):267-75.
3. Hurley RW, Wu CL. Acute postoperative pain. In: Barash PG, Cullen BF, Stoelting RK (Eds). Clinical Anesthesia, 7th edition. Philadelphia: Lippincott Williams & Wilkins; 2013. pp. 1373-410.
4. Subramaniam K, Subramaniam B, Steinbrook RA. Ketamine as adjuvant analgesic to opioids: a quantitative and qualitative systematic review. Anesth Analg. 2004;99(2):482-95.
5. Vadivelu N, Kai AM, Kodumudi G, Babayan K, Fontes M, Burg MM. The clinical applications of perioperative multimodal analgesia. J Clin Anesth. 2017;40:112-9.

CHAPTER 13

Topical Analgesia

Farid Hussain, Nusrat Kreem Bhat

INTRODUCTION

The systemic use of nonsteroidal anti-inflammatory drugs (NSAIDs) is associated with gastrointestinal, hepatic, renal, and cardiovascular side effects. Therefore, the topical application has a role because it promotes therapeutic concentration in the target tissue with decreased maintenance levels in the plasma to reduce adverse drug reactions.

Topical analgesics (e.g., patches, creams, solutions) represent a growing area of development in pain management because of their relative ease of application, potential for reduced systemic side effects, and lowered risk for end-organ damage.

Topically administered drugs exert peripheral effects near the site of application. They act by depleting and preventing the accumulation of substance P which is a chemomediator of pain impulse from peripheral sensory neurons to the central nervous system (CNS). In addition to reducing the synthesis of prostaglandins and substance P at the pain site, these drugs suppress inflammation by inhibiting leukocyte adhesion and function, reducing platelet aggregation, inhibiting cytokine production, suppressing proteoglycan synthesis in cartilaginous tissue, decreasing cell lysis mediated by the complement system, and inhibiting the formation of free radicals. The pathophysiology of neuropathic pain also has justified the usage of NSAIDs in patients in this condition.

The effectiveness of topical NSAIDs for various musculoskeletal pain syndromes has been proven by several clinical trials and systematic reviews.

Topical medications such as indomethacin, aspirin, and diclofenac have been used for neuropathic pain.

Some benefits and shortcomings of topical routes are given in **Table 1**.

Table 1: Benefits and shortcomings of topical routes.	
Merits of topical routes	**Demerits of topical routes**
<ul><li>Convenient and easy to use</li><li>First-pass metabolism is avoided</li><li>Therapeutic concentration achieved</li><li>Reduced side effects</li><li>Direct access to the target site</li><li>Painless administration</li><li>Greater compliance</li><li>Can be given in unconscious and nauseating patients</li><li>Minimize peak and trough level in blood</li><li>Less cost</li><li>Minimum abuse risk and addiction</li><li>Noninvasive</li><li>Less chances of drug interaction</li></ul>	<ul><li>Skin irritation, allergy, erythema can occur</li><li>Drug potency decreases due to metabolism of drug by skin enzymes</li><li>Interindividual and intraindividual differences in the efficacy</li><li>Efficient dermal penetration needs optimal molecular size which is a difficult task</li><li>Local drug metabolism alters the efficacy</li><li>Less effective in diseases in which absorptive capacity of the skin decreases</li><li>Molecules < 500 Da are absorbed only via skin</li><li>Topical agents must have both aqueous and lipid solubility</li><li>Administration of actual measured dose is difficult</li><li>Little literature is present regarding peer-reviewed, evidence-based formulations, so their efficacy and safety is of limited knowledge</li></ul>

Table 2: Topical agents for the treatment of musculoskeletal pain.	
Formulations	**Active ingredient**
Ointment	Indomethacin
Gel	Piroxicam, diclofenac, felbinac, ketoprofen, indomethacin, ibuprofen, salicylic acid, eltenac
Patch/plaster	Diclofenac, flurbiprofen
Spray P	Indomethacin
Cream	Diclofenac, ibuprofen, benzydamine, salicylic acid
Foam	Ketoprofen, felbinac

Topical analgesics provide a safe and effective therapeutic approach for musculoskeletal pain. The Food and Drug Administration (FDA)–approved topical agents with established safety and efficacy are NSAIDs, capsaicin, lidocaine 2.5% and 5% patches, prilocaine 2.5%, and doxepin.

All these topical formulations are available in the market as a single active ingredient or a combination of different ingredients for musculoskeletal pain. Some formulations of topical NSAIDs with active ingredients are given in **Table 2**.

Some medically important topical analgesic groups along with their drug formulations, mechanism of action, and indications are given in **Table 3**.

Table 3: Formulations, mechanism of action, and indications of some important topical agents.

Group	Drugs	Formulations	Mechanism of action	Indications
NSAIDs	• Diclofenac 10–20% • Ketoprofen 10–20% • Ibuprofen 10% gel • Ketoprofen 2.5% gel • Nimesulide 1% gel • Piroxicam 0.5% gel • Indomethacin gel/spray • Flurbiprofen • Salicylates	• Gel/cream/patch/drops • Foam, spray, ointment	Suppress inflammation by inhibiting COX enzyme	• Acute musculoskeletal pain • Muscle strains • Sprains • Osteoarthritis
Topical anesthetics	• Lidocaine patch 2.5%, 5% • Prilocaine gel	Gels, sprays, adhesive patches	Block activity of sodium-gated channels on sensory afferents	• Postherpetic neuralgia • Painful diabetic neuropathy • Knee osteoarthritis • Burning mouth syndrome
Counter irritants (neuropeptides)	• Capsaicin cream 5%, 8% • Camphor • Menthol • Homeopathic gel (marsh tree + comfrey + poison ivy) • Peppermint oil • Resiniferatoxin (potent capsaicin analogue)	• Cream/patch • OTC camphor balms	• Initially stimulate and then desensitize TRPV1 channels on afferent nerve [transient receptor potential vanilloid-1 receptors (TRPV1)] • By depleting substance P in sensory nerve endings • Menthol blocks calcium channels and also acts via opioid receptors	• Postherpetic neuralgia • Painful diabetic neuropathy • HIV neuropathy • Trigeminal neuralgia • Post-mastectomy pain syndrome • Uremic pruritis • Chronic peripheral polyneuropathy • Surgical neuropathic pain • Rheumatoid arthritis • Psoriasis • Knee osteoarthritis

Continued

Continued

Group	Drugs	Formulations	Mechanism of action	Indications
Tricyclic antidepressant	• Amitriptyline 1–10% in PLO base • Pregabalin • Gabapentin	Cream, ointment, gel		• Neuropathic pain • Complex regional pain syndrome
α-2 agonist	Clonidine	0.1% gel, cream, patch	• Stimulation of α-2-receptor agonist produces antinociception • Blocks NE-induced vasoconstriction	• Painful diabetic neuropathy • Trigeminal neuralgia • Postherpetic neuralgia
Nitric oxide–releasing drugs	• Nitroglycerine patch 5% • Nitrates	• Patch • Capsule soft gel	Release nitric oxide for vasodilation and have anti-inflammatory action	• Shoulder pain • Chronic extensor tendinosis • Painful diabetic neuropathy
NMDA blocking agents	Ketamine (0.5–20%)	Cream, ointment, gel	Downregulation of NMDA receptors	Neuropathic pain
Anticonvulsant	• Carbamazepine (2% in PLO base) • Doxepin • Gabapentin • Phenytoin 5% cream	Ointment, cream, gel	Inhibits the $α_2δ_1$ subunit of voltage-gated Ca^{2+} channels resulting in the reduction of neuropathic pain	Neuropathic pain
Opioids	Morphine in PLO gel solutions	Gel solution	Decrease the release of substance P from peripheral sensory nerve endings	• Chronic arthritis pain • Post-mastectomy pain syndrome • Inflammatory pressure ulcers and erosions • Ca ulcer-related mucositis
GABA agonists	Baclofen 2%, 5%	Cream	Increase K^+ influx and inhibit Ca^{2+} ions	Herniated lumbar disc

Continued

Continued

Group	Drugs	Formulations	Mechanism of action	Indications
Thermotherapy	Hot cloth, hot water bottle, ultrasound, heating pad, hydrocollator packs	Pads, packs, bottles	Produces vasodilation that increases the supply of oxygen and nutrients and the elimination of carbon dioxide and metabolic waste	• Acute low backache • Muscle spasms • Myalgia • Fibromyalgia • Contracture • Bursitis
Medicinal leeches	*Hirudo medicinalis*	Leech saliva	• Anti-inflammatory • Anticoagulation effect	Chronic musculoskeletal pain syndrome

(COX: cyclooxygenase; GABA: gamma-aminobutyric acid; HIV: human immunodeficiency virus; NE: norepinephrine; NMDA: N-methyl-D-aspartate; NSAID: nonsteroidal anti-inflammatory drug; OTC: over-the-counter; PLO: pluronic lecithin organogel)

OTHER FORMS OF TOPICAL ANALGESIA

Topical Herbal Remedies
These include creams, gels, or ointments containing natural ingredients such as capsaicin, menthol, or *Arnica*.

Nonpharmacological Topical Analgesia Options
They have gained attention for their effectiveness in managing pain without the side effects associated with pharmacological treatments. Several methods that can be used are as follows:
- *Cold therapy (cryotherapy)*:
  - Ice packs, cold gel packs, or cooling sprays
  - Effective for acute injuries, postoperative pain, and certain chronic conditions like osteoarthritis
- *Heat therapy*:
  - Heating pads, warm compresses, or heat wraps
  - Commonly used for muscle soreness, chronic muscle pain, and arthritis
- *Transcutaneous electrical nerve stimulation (TENS)*:
  - Proven effective for chronic pain conditions such as back pain, osteoarthritis, and neuropathic pain
- Ultrasound therapy
- Massage therapy
- Acupuncture
- Laser therapy (low-level laser therapy)
- *Hydrotherapy*:
  - Use of water in various forms, including baths, whirlpools, or aquatic exercises
  - Beneficial for musculoskeletal conditions, arthritis, and fibromyalgia
- *Kinesio taping*:
  - *Evidence*: Used for sports injuries, joint pain, and postsurgical recovery
- Compression therapy

The choice of therapy should be based on the type and cause of pain, patient preference, and clinical guidelines.

CONCLUSION

Systemic NSAIDs and opioids are the mainstay of treatment for most acute and chronic musculoskeletal pain conditions. However, concerns regarding the gastric, cardiac, and renal risk from NSAIDs, and issues with opioids, have resulted in increasing demand and attention to nonsystemic topical alternatives. Topical analgesics are great alternatives for pain management and are an essential part of multimodal analgesia with increasing evidence of the efficacy and safety of topical agents in pain control.

Topical agents are simple but effective methods for treating local pain and can play a crucial role in multimodal pain management of musculoskeletal conditions. They can be used alone or in combination with other agents to have a synergistic analgesic effect.

Besides, new drugs are under trials for local use like resiniferatoxin (RTX). This drug could potentially be an efficacious topical capsaicin analog, which is extracted from the resin of the *Euphorbia* cactus.

BIBLIOGRAPHY

1. Bhat C, Rosenberg H, James D. Tropical nonsteroidal anti-inflammatory drugs. CMAJ. 2023;195(36):E1231.
2. Coderre TJ, Fulas OA. Topical drug delivery in the treatment of chronic pain: a review. Chron Pain Manag. 2024;7:152.
3. El-Tallawy SN, Nalamasu R, Salem GI, LeQuang JAK, Pergolizzi JV, Christo PJ. Management of musculoskeletal pain: an update with emphasis on chronic musculoskeletal pain. Pain Ther. 2021;10:181-209.
4. Flores MP, Castro APCR, Nascimento JDS. Topical analgesics. Rev Bras Anestesiol. 2012;62(2):244-52.
5. McCleane G. Topical analgesics. Anesthesiol Clin. 2007;25:825-39.
6. Nosek K, Leppert W, Puchała L, Łoń K. Efficacy and safety of topical morphine: a narrative review. Pharmaceutics. 2022;14:1499.
7. Stanos SP. Topical agents for the management of musculoskeletal pain. J Pain Symptom Manage. 2007;33(3):342-55.

CHAPTER 14

Pediatric Musculoskeletal Pain

Neha Sharma

■ INTRODUCTION

Pediatric musculoskeletal pain is a frequent concern, arising from causes like growth, injury, or infections. Managing this requires a clear understanding of pediatric anatomy, accurate diagnosis, and age-appropriate pain assessment. This chapter outlines key strategies for effective pain management, combining both pharmacological and non-pharmacological treatments.

■ PROBLEM STATEMENT

Musculoskeletal (MSK) pain is a common pediatric problem labeled as a public health disaster with a large prevalence and a significant impact on a child's physical and psychosocial health.

Musculoskeletal pain in children was earlier underreported. An increased prevalence of MSK disorders is now coming to light because of the associated suffering, dependency on family, limitation of activity, and an increased risk of chronic widespread pain in adulthood.

Pain associated with MSK disorders accounts for more than half of all cases of pain reported to physicians by children. It is found to be more common in girls as compared with in boys and children coming from low educational and socioeconomic strata. It peaks at 14 years of age; the probable causation can be that children younger than 14 years do not report symptoms to parents. Even if they do, parents do not take these complaints seriously, dismissing pains as excuses for not participating in sports or going to school.

Musculoskeletal pain in growing children has a major impact on their routine and future lives. Studies have proven that children suffering from MSK disorders suffer long-term impacts in adult life, such as the development of osteoarthritis.

COMMON SITES

Common sites include shoulder joints, lower back, and limbs.

ETIOLOGICAL FACTORS

Improper sitting postures in children are very common. Poorly designed, ergonomically unfavorable school desks with poor back support, or low table height may further exacerbate the problem. This leads to poor back postures and neck or lower back pain.

During sports activities, injury can be a triggering factor. This is seen in both very low and very high physical activity groups.

Other contributing factors are heavy school bags; especially awkward positioning or carrying the bag on one shoulder is known to be a contributing risk factor as compared with the child carrying the bag on both shoulders.

Musculoskeletal disorders are also more common in overweight children as an increase in body mass index (BMI) correlates with a decrease in balance, range of motion, and at times emotional functionality.

Using mobile phones or desktops for a prolonged period, that is, >14 hours per week, may lead to pain in the neck, shoulders, and hands, also known as text neck syndrome.

Overuse sports injuries, which include improper warm-ups and cool-downs, can lead to MSK pain. This is common in football players.

Children who play musical instruments such as violin in improper body posture while practicing for long durations may develop MSK pain.

Musculoskeletal disorders can precipitate bad sleeping habits and vice versa, further compounding the problem.

The child may refuse to participate in sports. Consequently occurring psychosocial personality changes may continue into adulthood.

MANAGEMENT AND PREVENTION

Detailed history and examination and judicious use of investigations are required to establish a clear diagnosis. The most important aspect is not to miss any pathological or serious pathology.

Other important aspects are to treat the basic pathology, along with symptomatic treatment, and to identify and modify any trigger or causative factor like posture.

Psychosocial Therapy and Physical Therapy

Preventive interventions include education which is effective in increasing knowledge as well as awareness regarding MSK discomfort and pain in children. Children should be encouraged to share any discomfort during school or recreational activities with their caretakers.

Exercise must be done under proper guidance using proper protective equipment. There should be experienced physical education teachers monitoring the correct form at schools.

There should be different-sized ergonomically designed desks for differently built children.

The correct dose and type of analgesic for children depends on various factors, including the child's age, weight, the severity of pain, and the specific medication being used. Some commonly used analgesics in pediatric care are given in the following text.

Commonly used analgesics in pediatric patients:
- *Acetaminophen (paracetamol)*:
  - *Use*: Mild-to-moderate pain and fever
  - *Dose*: 10–15 mg/kg per dose
  - *Frequency*: Every 4–6 hours as needed
  - *Maximum daily dose*: Do not exceed 75 mg/kg/day or 4,000 mg/day, whichever is less.
  - *Formulations*: Available in oral suspension, chewable tablets, and rectal suppositories
- *Ibuprofen*:
  - *Use*: Mild-to-moderate pain, inflammation, and fever
  - *Dose*: 5–10 mg/kg per dose
  - *Frequency*: Every 6–8 hours as needed
  - *Maximum daily dose*: Do not exceed 40 mg/kg/day or 2,400 mg/day, whichever is less.
  - *Formulations*: Available in oral suspension, chewable tablets, and tablets
- *Morphine*:
  - *Use*: Moderate-to-severe pain
  - *Dose for oral (immediate-release)*: 0.2–0.5 mg/kg per dose
  - *Frequency*: Every 4 hours as needed
  - *Dose for intravenous (IV)/intramuscular (IM)*: 0.05–0.1 mg/kg per dose
  - *Frequency*: Every 2–4 hours as needed
  - *Maximum dose*: Titrate to response and monitor for side effects.

Considerations for Pediatric Analgesics

- *Weight-based dosing*: Always calculate the dose based on the child's weight in kilograms.
- *Formulation*: Choose a child-friendly formulation, such as liquids for younger children and chewable or dissolvable tablets for older children.

Special Precautions

- *Age and health status*: Consider the child's age, overall health, and any preexisting conditions.
  - *Example calculation for ibuprofen*:
    - For a child weighing 15 kg:
      - Dose range: 5–10 mg/kg
      - Single dose: 15 kg 5 mg/kg = 75 mg to 15 kg 10 mg/kg = 150 mg
      - Administer 75–150 mg per dose every 6–8 hours as needed.

- Example calculation for acetaminophen:
  - For a child weighing 20 kg:
    - Dose range: 10–15 mg/kg
    - Single dose: 20 kg 10 mg/kg = 200 mg to 20 kg 15 mg/kg = 300 mg
    - Administer 200–300 mg per dose every 4–6 hours as needed.

Specific Precautions and Contraindications

Acetaminophen (Paracetamol)
- Use with caution in children with liver disease or those who are malnourished.
- Avoid exceeding the recommended dose to prevent liver toxicity.
- Contraindications:
  - Known hypersensitivity to acetaminophen
  - Severe hepatic impairment or active liver disease

Ibuprofen
- Use with caution in children with a history of gastrointestinal (GI) issues, such as ulcers or gastritis.
- Ensure adequate hydration to prevent kidney damage.
- Avoid in children with dehydration or those taking other nephrotoxic drugs.
- Contraindications:
  - Known hypersensitivity to ibuprofen or other nonsteroidal anti-inflammatory drugs (NSAIDs)
  - History of aspirin-sensitive asthma or other allergic reactions to NSAIDs
  - Severe renal impairment or active GI bleeding or ulceration

Morphine
- Closely monitor for respiratory depression, especially in opioid-naïve children.
- Use with caution in children with compromised respiratory function (e.g., asthma, sleep apnea).
- Consider the risk of dependence and withdrawal with prolonged use.
- Contraindications:
  - Known hypersensitivity to morphine or other opioids
  - Severe respiratory insufficiency, acute asthma attacks, or upper airway obstruction
  - Concurrent use of monoamine oxidase inhibitors (MAOIs) or within 14 days of stopping such treatment

Specific Situations
- Avoid using aspirin in children due to the risk of Reye's syndrome.
- Chronic pain:
  - For chronic pain management, involve a pediatric pain specialist and consider nonpharmacological therapies in addition to medication.

CONCLUSION

Effective management of pediatric musculoskeletal pain relies on accurate diagnosis and a holistic approach. By integrating medications, physical therapy, and psychological support, tailored to the child's needs, healthcare providers can improve outcomes and enhance the child's quality of life.

BIBLIOGRAPHY

1. Merder-Coşkun D, Uzuner A, Keniş-Coşkun Ö, Çelenlioğlu AE, Akman M, Karadağ-Saygı E. Relationship between obesity and musculoskeletal system findings among children and adolescents. Turk J Phys Med Rehabil. 2017;63(3):207-14.
2. Jones GT, Silman AJ, Power C, Macfarlane GJ. Are common symptoms in childhood associated with chronic widespread body pain in adulthood? Results from the 1958 British Birth Cohort Study. Arthritis Rheum. 2007;56:1669-75.

CHAPTER 15

Approach to Back Pain in Children

Younis Kamal

■ INTRODUCTION

Back pain is often overlooked when it occurs in children. However, it is essential to recognize that children can experience back pain too, and understanding its causes, symptoms, and management is crucial for their well-being. The prevalence and impact of back pain in the pediatric population are growing, prompting a need for comprehensive assessment and intervention strategies tailored to their unique needs.

Back pain in children can be multifactorial, ranging from benign musculoskeletal strains to more serious underlying conditions. Unlike adults, who may attribute their discomfort to age-related changes or occupational factors, children's back pain often stems from a different set of circumstances, including rapid growth spurts, sports-related injuries, or structural abnormalities.

The consequences of untreated or improperly managed back pain in children can extend beyond physical discomfort. Chronic back pain can significantly impact a child's quality of life, leading to limitations in daily activities, school performance, and emotional well-being. Additionally, it may herald underlying medical conditions that require prompt attention to prevent further complications.

By gaining insight into the unique challenges posed by pediatric back pain and adopting a proactive approach to its assessment and management, healthcare providers, parents, and educators can collaborate to ensure the holistic well-being of children affected by this condition.

By advocating for early intervention, promoting healthy habits, and fostering a supportive environment, we can mitigate the impact of back pain on the lives of our young ones, enabling them to thrive and flourish unhindered by physical discomfort.

PATTERN OF BACK PAIN IN CHILDREN

Age-related Patterns
- *Infants and toddlers*: Back pain in this age group is rare and often associated with congenital abnormalities, such as spinal dysraphism or developmental disorders.
- *School-aged children*: As children become more active and participate in sports and physical activities, they may experience back pain related to musculoskeletal strains, sports injuries, or poor posture.
- *Adolescents*: Rapid growth spurts during puberty can lead to muscle imbalances, vertebral stress fractures (e.g., spondylolysis), or structural abnormalities like scoliosis, which may manifest as back pain.

Activity-related Patterns
- *Sports-related back pain*: Children involved in athletics, particularly activities requiring repetitive or high-impact movements (e.g., gymnastics, football), are at risk of developing back pain due to overuse injuries, muscle strains, or stress fractures.
- *Postural back pain*: Prolonged sitting, slouching, or carrying heavy backpacks can contribute to postural strain and result in back pain, especially among school-aged children.

Symptom Patterns
- *Acute versus chronic*: Acute back pain may result from sudden injury or strain, while chronic back pain may be indicative of underlying structural or medical conditions.
- *Localized versus radiating*: Back pain may be localized to a specific area of the spine or may radiate to other regions of the body, such as the legs or buttocks, depending on the underlying pathology (e.g., sciatica from a herniated disc).

CONTRIBUTING FACTORS

- *Structural abnormalities*: Conditions like scoliosis, kyphosis, or lordosis can predispose children to back pain due to abnormal spinal curvature or vertebral misalignment.
- *Muscle imbalances*: Weakness or tightness in certain muscle groups, often exacerbated by rapid growth during puberty, can contribute to back pain by altering spinal mechanics and stability.
- *Psychosocial factors*: Stress, anxiety, or emotional distress may exacerbate or contribute to back pain in children, highlighting the importance of addressing the psychological aspects of pain management.

COMMON SIGNS AND SYMPTOMS OF BACK PAIN IN CHILDREN

These include pain, stiffness, tenderness, limited mobility, muscle spasms, postural changes, nighttime discomfort, and activity limitations.

RED FLAGS

- *Pain severity*: Severe or incapacitating
- *Neurological symptoms*: Presence of neurological symptoms such as weakness, numbness, tingling, or loss of bowel or bladder control, suggesting nerve compression or spinal cord involvement
- *Fever*: Back pain accompanied by fever, which may indicate an underlying infection or inflammatory condition
- *Recent trauma*: History of significant trauma or injury preceding the onset of back pain, raising concerns for fractures or spinal cord injury
- *Unexplained weight loss*: Back pain accompanied by unexplained weight loss or loss of appetite, which may indicate a systemic illness or malignancy
- *Night pain*: Persistent back pain that disrupts sleep or worsens at night may be indicative of more serious underlying conditions, such as tumors or infections.

BEHAVIORAL AND PSYCHOLOGICAL SYMPTOMS

These include irritability, school absenteeism, and social withdrawal.

CAUSES OF BACK PAIN IN CHILDREN

- Muscle strain or sprain
- Poor posture
- *Structural abnormalities*: Scoliosis, kyphosis, lordosis
- Sports injuries
- Herniated discs
- *Spondylolysis and spondylolisthesis*:
  - *Spondylolysis*: Stress fracture or defect in the pars interarticularis of the vertebra, often occurring in adolescents engaged in repetitive spinal extension activities (e.g., gymnastics, dancing)

INFECTIONS AND TUMORS

- Rarely, back pain in children may be secondary to infections of the spine (e.g., osteomyelitis, discitis) or tumors (e.g., osteoid osteoma, Ewing sarcoma).

- Infections and tumors typically present with persistent or worsening pain, night pain, fever, or neurological symptoms and require prompt medical evaluation.
- Psychological factors

DIAGNOSIS OF BACK PAIN IN CHILDREN

Diagnosis of back pain in children is based on the following:
- *A detailed history* including history of any pre-existing medical conditions, family history of musculoskeletal disorders or developmental abnormalities, assessment of the activity level, and psychosocial factors
- History should always be followed by a careful and systematic physical examination.
- *Imaging studies*:
  - *X-rays*: Conventional X-rays of the spine can provide valuable information about bony structures, alignment, and the presence of fractures, tumors, or structural abnormalities.
  - *Magnetic resonance imaging (MRI)*: It is more sensitive than X-rays for evaluating soft-tissue structures, such as discs, ligaments, and nerves, and can help identify herniated discs, spinal cord compression, or infections.
  - *Computed tomography (CT) scan*: It may be indicated for assessing bony abnormalities, fractures, or spinal stenosis, especially if MRI is contraindicated or unavailable.
- *Laboratory tests*:
  - *Blood tests*: Laboratory tests, including complete blood count (CBC), erythrocyte sedimentation rate (ESR), and C-reactive protein (CRP), may be ordered to evaluate for signs of infection, inflammation, or systemic diseases.
  - *Genetic testing*: In cases of suspected genetic or developmental abnormalities (e.g., scoliosis), genetic testing or screening may be considered to identify underlying genetic mutations or syndromes.
- *Specialist consultation*:
  - *Orthopedic specialist*: Referral to a pediatric orthopedic specialist may be warranted for further evaluation and management of complex or refractory cases, particularly those involving structural abnormalities or surgical intervention.
  - *Pediatric rheumatologist*: Consultation with a pediatric rheumatologist may be indicated for children with suspected inflammatory or autoimmune conditions affecting the spine (e.g., juvenile idiopathic arthritis).

ROLE OF MINIMAL INVASIVE SURGERY IN CHILDREN WITH BACK PAIN

- Reduced surgical trauma
- Preservation of normal anatomy

- Lower risk of complications
- Improved cosmesis
- Faster recovery and return to activity
- *Application in various spinal conditions*:
  - Minimal invasive surgery (MIS) can be used to treat a wide range of spinal conditions in children, including herniated discs, spinal deformities (e.g., scoliosis), spinal stenosis, and vertebral fractures.
  - The versatility of MIS allows for targeted treatment of specific spinal pathologies while minimizing surgical morbidity and preserving spinal function.
- *Long-term outcomes*:
  - Studies have demonstrated comparable or superior long-term outcomes following MIS compared with those following traditional open surgery in children with various spinal disorders.
  - MIS can achieve effective correction of spinal deformities, relief of nerve compression, and restoration of spinal stability while minimizing the risk of complications and preserving spinal function.

PREVENTIVE MEASURES OF BACK PAIN IN CHILDREN

- Encourage physical activity
- Maintain healthy body weight
- Promote proper posture
- *Ensure proper backpack use*:
  - Advise children to use backpacks that are appropriately sized, lightweight, and worn with both shoulder straps to distribute weight evenly.
  - Teach proper backpack use, including packing heavier items closer to the body and using waist straps for additional support.
- Limit screen time
- Teach safe lifting techniques
- *Provide supportive furniture*:
  - Ensure that furniture such as desks, chairs, and mattresses provide adequate support and promote good posture.
  - Use ergonomic chairs and adjustable desks to promote proper alignment during studying or screen time.
- Address emotional well-being
- *Encourage regular checkups*: Screen for scoliosis and other spinal abnormalities during routine physical examinations, particularly during periods of rapid growth.

CONCLUSION

Addressing back pain in children demands a thorough and cautious approach. While most cases are benign, clinicians must be alert to red flags such as neurological symptoms, systemic signs, or trauma that may suggest serious pathology. A detailed history, focused examination, and selective use of imaging or tests are crucial for accurate diagnosis. Timely intervention and a multidisciplinary approach can help prevent chronic pain and ensure the best outcomes.

BIBLIOGRAPHY

1. American Academy of Pediatrics. Evaluation and management of back pain in children and adolescents. Pediatrics. 2005.
2. Bernstein JA. Pediatric Orthopedic Secrets, 4th edition. Amsterdam: Elsevier; 2020.
3. Lipson LS, Kendall DG. Musculoskeletal Examination and Assessment: A Handbook for Therapists, 5th edition. Amsterdam: Elsevier; 2017.
4. National Institute for Health and Care Excellence (NICE). Low back pain and sciatica in over 16s: assessment and management. NICE Guidelines [NG59]; 2016.
5. Palisano SR, Ratliffe JSC, Orlin M, Clancy JO. Campbell's Physical Therapy for Children. Amsterdam: Elsevier; 2016.
6. Shearer JM, Smith DR, Clark CR. Pediatric back pain: Diagnosis and outcomes in a pediatric population. JAMA. 2019;322(12):1193-201.

CHAPTER 16

Geriatric Musculoskeletal Pain

Neha Sharma

■ INTRODUCTION

Effective pain management in geriatric patients is critical for improving their quality of life. Older adults often face unique challenges, including age-related changes, multiple comorbidities, and the risks of polypharmacy. This chapter explores current best practices for assessing and treating pain in this population, emphasizing tailored, patient-centered approaches. It highlights non-pharmacologic therapies, cautious use of medications, and the importance of balancing pain relief with safety to ensure optimal care for the aging population.

■ PROBLEM STATEMENT

The geriatric population is increasing every day due to ever-increasing longevity. However, this comes with a unique twenty-first-century health problem which is taking care of the elderly and increasing healthcare burden. Fifty percent of the geriatric population complains of aches and pains on and off regularly, out of which around two-thirds use analgesics for the same.

Chronic pain is more common than acute pain and chronic musculoskeletal (MSK) pain is prevalent in one-fourth of elderly people and constitutes the most common nonmalignant disabling condition affecting this age group.

The consequences of people living with pain for long periods include reduced mobility, poor posture, home confinement, and restricted social interaction leading to depression, sleep disturbances, social isolation, and anhedonia. The patient may eventually become bedridden or completely dependent on family. Pressure sores may develop. In extreme cases, even contractures may result because of the disuse of areas where chronic pain is present.

Despite it being a healthcare challenge, MSK pain in the elderly is under-reported. Causes for under-reporting include acceptance of pain and unwillingness to seek help unless functional changes occur. Further, caregivers and family members may accept pain to be a part of the normal consequence of aging and not inquire about it. Family members may be worried about the cost of treatment or difficulty in transporting or investigating elderly people in healthcare facilities, or there may even be reluctance of the elderly to step out of their homes.

ETIOLOGICAL FACTORS

- Degenerative bone, joint, and soft-tissue changes
- Osteoporosis-induced vertebral collapse
- Insufficiency fractures
- Falls and trauma (due to multiple causes which may include neurological disorders, impaired vision, neglect or physical abuse by family members or care providers)
- Other rheumatological disorders such as fibromyalgia
- Malignancy (especially bone metastases)

PRESENTATION

Chronic pain is the most common presentation; however, superimposed acute traumatic events and falls may exacerbate preexisting MSK ailments.

Inability to bear weight, abnormal gait, joint swelling, or deformity may be present.

Neurological symptoms may coexist.

MANAGEMENT AND PREVENTION

Management should be multidisciplinary, involving a team comprising family members, doctors, nurses, physiotherapists, dietitians, and clinical psychologists.

A multidisciplinary approach is most effective as compared with only pharmacotherapy. Pain may be relieved for a short duration by simple analgesics, both opioids and nonopioids. However, a combination of antidepressants, psychosocial therapy, rehabilitation with physiotherapy, and other modalities like the usage of transcutaneous electrical nerve stimulation (TENS) machines or massages may be helpful. Social programs in which the elderly can interact with their peers having similar problems and meditate have shown better results and ensure better compliance.

Government healthcare programs should focus on providing supportive devices like crutches, wheelchairs, good footwear, heating pads, kneecaps, or other devices to the elderly at subsidized rates or free of cost because many of the elderly are financially dependent on other family members.

Early detection and treatment of osteoporosis (silent killer) is of paramount importance, to take care of basic pathology and prevent sequelae like osteoporotic fracture.

Surgical management [total hip replacement (THR), total knee replacement (TKR)] of severely degenerated joints may be indicated to alleviate pain, improve mobility, and improve quality of life.

Programs in which the elderly can be instructed on how to perform safe exercises and stretching may also go a long way in preventing MSK pain. These exercises improve posture and lead to a balanced gait, balanced weight bearing, and overall well-being. The goal of modern healthcare for the elderly should not only be to increase the life span but also to provide a reasonable quality of life.

Using analgesics in elderly patients requires careful consideration due to their increased susceptibility to side effects and potential for drug interactions. Some *special precautions and considerations* are as follows:

- *Start low, go slow*: Begin with the lowest effective dose and titrate slowly to avoid adverse effects.
- *Monitor closely*: Regularly assess for efficacy and side effects, including gastrointestinal, cardiovascular, renal, and central nervous system effects.
- *Polypharmacy*: Be aware of potential drug–drug interactions due to the likelihood of multiple medications.
- *Comorbidities*: Consider the patient's overall health and existing medical conditions, such as cardiovascular disease, renal impairment, and liver dysfunction.

SPECIFIC ANALGESICS

- *Nonsteroidal anti-inflammatory drugs (NSAIDs)*: Risk of gastrointestinal bleeding
    - Use gastroprotective agents like proton-pump inhibitors (PPIs) if NSAIDs are necessary.
    - *Cardiovascular risk*: Increased risk of heart attack and stroke. Use with caution and consider alternatives if the patient has cardiovascular disease.
    - *Renal impairment*: NSAIDs can worsen renal function. Monitor renal parameters regularly.
- *Acetaminophen (paracetamol)*: Preferred first-line agent; generally safer for mild-to-moderate pain
- *Opioids*:
    - *Respiratory depression*: Increased sensitivity to respiratory depressant effects. Use lower doses and monitor closely.
    - *Cognitive impairment and falls*: Higher risk of sedation, dizziness, and confusion leading to falls. Use immediate-release formulations initially and avoid long-acting formulations if possible.
    - *Constipation*: Proactively manage with laxatives or stool softeners due to the high risk of opioid-induced constipation.

CONCLUSION

Analgesic use in elderly patients requires a tailored approach with careful consideration of the risks and benefits. Regular monitoring and a multidisciplinary approach to pain management are essential to ensure safe and effective treatment.

BIBLIOGRAPHY

1. Hwang SW, Kim CW, Jang YJ, Lee CH, Oh MK, Kim KW, et al. Musculoskeletal pain, physical activity, muscle mass, and mortality in older adults: results from the Korean Longitudinal Study on Health and Aging. Medicina (Kaunas). 2024;60(3):462.

CHAPTER 17

Management of Musculoskeletal Pain in Pregnant and Lactating Mothers

Jasmeen Chowdhary

INTRODUCTION

Pregnancy induces significant changes in the musculoskeletal system, leading to strained ligaments, reduced range of motion, and increased muscle tension, often resulting in pain. The growing uterus shifts the body's center of gravity, causing mechanical stress. This typically results in lumbar lordosis, neck flexion, and shoulder drooping. The increased ligamentous laxity in the spine heightens the risk of back injury and contributes to the high prevalence of back pain during pregnancy.

Inadequate treatment of pain can lead to the development of anxiety and depression which can impact on a woman's physical and psychological well-being as well as her ability to provide care for her baby. Proper pain management during pregnancy is crucial to minimize risks to both the mother and the developing fetus.

Nonpharmacological interventions, such as appropriate physical rest, hot and cold compressions, physiotherapy, and acupressure, should be provided before administration of analgesics. All medicines must be assessed for risk versus benefit and be used cautiously to try to minimize harmful effects on the fetus.

EFFECTS OF MEDICATIONS DURING PREGNANCY

The effect of medication on the fetus during pregnancy occurs in three stages:
- *Stage 1 (1–4 weeks)*: Drug produces all-or-none effect. Conceptus either has no anomaly or does not persist.
- *Stage 2 (5–9 weeks)*: It is the stage in which organ formation occurs; therefore, teratogenic effects are more likely to precipitate during this phase.

- *Stage 3 (10 weeks onward)*: Organs grow during this phase and teratogenic effects can occur, but the rate of incidence is lower than in stage 2.

Regardless of drug exposure, all couples have a background risk of 3% of having a baby with serious birth abnormalities, and 15% of pregnancies end in miscarriage. These facts should be emphasized when counseling women on using medications during pregnancy. Analgesics are the most often utilized drug after vitamins, taken by >85% of pregnant women.

A doctor must decide whether to provide medication during pregnancy after taking into account a number of considerations, including:
- Administration route
- The age of the fetus at gestation
- The medication's rate of absorption
- Does the medication pass across the placenta?
- The medication's effective dosage
- The drug's molecular weight
- Possible danger to the mother should the medication not be prescribed

GENERAL PRINCIPLES OF ANALGESIC USE DURING PREGNANCY

- *Justification*: No practice should be adopted unless it offers a positive benefit to a pregnant patient or one likely to become pregnant.
- *Self-assessment before proceeding*:
  - Can the treatment be done without analgesics?
  - Can the treatment be deferred until after delivery?
  - Will delaying the treatment pose a greater risk to the patient?
- *Minimum necessary dose*: If analgesics are required, the dose should be kept to a minimum.
- *10-day rule*: Ideally, delay treatment and pelvic examinations to the 10-day interval after the onset of menstruation.

Prescription drugs ought to be given only when the mother's benefits outweigh the dangers to the developing fetus. The Food and Drug Administration (FDA) of the United States created a five-category drug labeling system in 1979 based on potential teratogenic risks to the fetus, as detailed in **Table 1**.

SAFE USE OF ANALGESICS IN PREGNANCY

When dealing with pain in pregnant patients, class A drugs are safe to use while treating pain in pregnant individuals. Nevertheless, the FDA does not classify painkillers under category A, including opioids, tricyclic antidepressants, local anesthetics, nonsteroidal anti-inflammatory drugs (NSAIDs), and antiepileptics.

Table 1: The FDA's fetal risk classification system.		
FDA classification	**Definition**	**Examples**
Class A	Studies conducted on women under control do not show any danger to the fetus. The likelihood of damage seems low	Multivitamins
Class B	Studies on animals have not shown prenatal harm, but there are no controlled trials on humans, and negative effects in animals have not been verified in females	PO acetaminophen, nalbuphine, lidocaine
Class C	There have been no controlled trials on women or animals, but animal research has revealed teratogenic or embryocidal effects	NSAIDs (sulindac, naproxen), opioids, antidepressants
Class D	There is evidence of positive fetal risk, although the advantages to the mother might outweigh the hazards	NSAIDs (aspirin), steroids, anticonvulsants
Class X	Studies use human experience to illustrate fetal defects or risk. The drugs are contraindicated in pregnant women	Ergotamine, paroxetine, valproic acid

Note: Medications are classified into risk classes A, B, C, D, or X without taking into account the risk to the fetus from breastfeeding, based on the best available scientific or clinical data.
(FDA: Food and Drug Administration; NSAIDs: nonsteroidal anti-inflammatory drugs)

ANALGESICS IN PREGNANCY: RECOMMENDATIONS AND GUIDELINES

First-line Treatment: Acetaminophen (Paracetamol)

- *Use*: For persistent pain requiring medication, acetaminophen (class B when used orally) is recommended as the first-line treatment.
- *Advantages*: It offers effective pain relief similar to NSAIDs without the antiprostaglandin or platelet inhibition effects.
- *Precautions*: Though considered safe, it should be administered cautiously because toxicity can occur when ingested >150 mg/kg over a period of 24 hours.

Nonsteroidal Anti-inflammatory Drugs

- *Usage*: NSAIDs like ibuprofen and diclofenac are relatively contraindicated throughout pregnancy but may be used in the first and second trimesters.
- *Risks*: They raise the possibility of third-trimester uterine artery vasoconstriction and early ductus arteriosus closure.
- *Classification*: These medications are labeled as class C. The FDA advises avoiding NSAIDs during pregnancy unless clinically indicated.

Neuropathic Pain Medications

- *Medications*: Anticonvulsants and antidepressants, such as gabapentin and amitriptyline, are commonly prescribed for neuropathic pain.

- *Risks*: In pregnant women, these drugs can increase the risk of teratogenic effects, including spina bifida, heart defects, or cleft lip.
- *Classification*: Antidepressants fall under class D.

Opioids
- *Usage*: For severe, unrelenting pain, opioids may be prescribed, but precautions should be taken to avoid opioid withdrawal effects in the newborn.
- *Risks*: Opioids are addictive and can quickly cause dependency, leading to a feeling of euphoria.
- *Classification*: Most opioids are labeled as class B, except for codeine (class C).
- *Common opioids*: Include oxycodone, codeine, morphine, tramadol, fentanyl, and buprenorphine

Topical Analgesics
- *Medications*: For the treatment of lower back pain, lidocaine and capsaicin may be applied topically.
- *Classification*: Lidocaine patches (5%) are under class B.

INTERVENTIONAL PAIN MANAGEMENT

For the mother's and the fetus's protection, professional consultation should be advised in cases of acute, uncontrollable discomfort. When medicine and preventive measures are ineffective, other interventional techniques can help with symptoms and functioning.

Epidural Steroids
- *Efficacy*: There is strong evidence supporting the use of epidural steroids for acute radiculopathy due to disc pathology.
- *Imaging*: While image-guided operations are safer, blind, magnetic resonance imaging (MRI)-guided, and ultrasound-guided injections are also options.

Injections Guided by Ultrasound
- *Usage*: Selective nerve root blocks guided by ultrasonography are a better option for treating radicular pain than caudal methods. For sacroiliitis, ultrasound-guided sacroiliac joint injections are advised.

COMMON MUSCULOSKELETAL PAIN DURING PREGNANCY
- *Musculoskeletal pain*:
  - Low back pain
  - Joint pain

- *Rheumatological pain*:
  - Meralgia paresthetica
  - A condition called carpal tunnel syndrome
  - De Quervain's tenosynovitis
- *Neuropathic pain*:
  - Pregnancy-related pelvic pain
  - Intercostal neuralgia

PAIN MANAGEMENT APPROACHES

Nonpharmacological Treatment
- Posture strategies
- Physical intervention
- Use of acupuncture
- Hand treatment
- Hydrotherapy
- Transcutaneous neural stimulation
- Belts for stabilization
- Yoga

Pharmacological Treatment
- Acetaminophen
- NSAIDs
- Opioids
- Anticonvulsants
- Antidepressants
- Transdermal patches

Interventional Treatment
Epidural steroids

PREGNANCY-RELATED LOW BACK PAIN MANAGEMENT

Diagnosing the etiology of backache and differentiating it from other disorders (e.g., prolapsed disc, spondylolisthesis) requires a thorough evaluation.

Postural Methods
- Educate pregnant women on correct posture and ergonomics to avoid stress on the spine.
- Rest on a schedule while keeping your feet elevated to ease painful spasms in your muscles.

Physical Medicine
It includes lumbar pain relief activities such as pelvic tilt, knee pull, curl up, lateral straight leg elevating, and Kegel exercises.

Use of Acupuncture

If acupuncture is given by a qualified and licensed professional, it is usually regarded as safe during pregnancy. However, some acupoints should be avoided since they may cause labor or contractions, especially if the pregnancy is <37 weeks along.

Hand Therapy

A woman's center of mass pushes forward as her pregnancy advances into the second and third trimesters, causing her lumbar lordosis to worsen and causing low back and pelvic girdle pain. When administered by a trained practitioner, manual treatment, which includes massage therapy and chiropractic care such as spinal manipulation, is safe and helpful in treating this discomfort. Osteopathic medicine uses focused muscle and joint mobilization along with soft-tissue massage to reduce pain and promote general function.

Hydrotherapy

Water therapy is exercising in a heated pool where the buoyancy and warmth assist reduce body weight by up to 80% and relax muscles, therefore relieving back pain.

Transcutaneous Electrical Nerve Stimulation

For low back pain during pregnancy, transcutaneous electrical nerve stimulation (TENS) is an additional safe and effective therapy option.

Belts for Pelvic Stabilization

When compared with women who merely exercise or receive general treatment information, women with pelvic girdle pain who wear a pelvic belt have been shown to have reduced impairment and pain severity.

JOINT PAIN

It is advised that pregnant patients with rheumatological disease follow a multidisciplinary treatment approach overseen by a rheumatologist. Options for complementary and alternative medicine can potentially be advantageous.

MERALGIA PARESTHETICA

Typically, treatment for meralgia paresthetica is unnecessary as symptoms usually resolve after delivery. Stretching exercises, local steroid infiltration, local anesthetics, or, in the event that symptoms worsen, a lateral femoral cutaneous nerve block can all provide momentary pain relief.

ABDOMINAL AND PELVIC PAIN

Increased pelvic girdle motion and ligamentous laxity brought on by hormones like relaxin and estrogen are common causes of pelvic pain associated with pregnancy. Work that requires a lot of physical exertion, a history of low back pain, pelvic trauma, or pelvic pain during pregnancy are risk factors. Patient education, ergonomic recommendations, and physical activity suggestions are all part of management. Exercise, acupuncture, massage, water gymnastics, pelvic belts, and acupuncture are examples of nonpharmacological therapy. For pain treatment, acetaminophen is recommended; NSAIDs should be taken with caution and avoided during the third trimester of pregnancy. Pelvic discomfort usually resolves after delivery.

INTERCOSTAL NEURALGIA

Pregnancy-related intercostal neuralgia can be caused by spinal cord lesions, nerve trunk, root, or terminal problems; it is frequently brought on by the uterus's mechanical expansion. Particularly in late gestation, it presents as radiating or searing radicular discomfort. Pain is typically relieved after delivery and is managed with topical lidocaine patches or creams, intercostal nerve blocks, and epidural steroid injections.

ORTHOPEDIC MANAGEMENT FOR LACTATING PATIENTS

- *Pain management*: Select medications compatible with breastfeeding, such as NSAIDs like ibuprofen. Use opioids cautiously and for short durations, as they pass into breast milk in small quantities, rarely causing neonatal toxicity.
- *Physical therapy*: Therapists should ensure exercises and treatments are compatible with breastfeeding, avoiding discomfort or interference with milk production.
- *Orthopedic surgery*: Discuss the implications of breastfeeding before surgery. Temporary interruption may be necessary depending on the procedure and anesthesia, although many surgeries can be performed with minimal impact on breastfeeding with proper planning.
- *Positioning and mobility*: Support devices or pillows can help with comfortable breastfeeding. Mobility and range of motion exercises are essential to prevent complications and support baby care.
- *Monitoring for side effects*: While most antibiotics are safe for breastfeeding infants, monitor for adverse effects like diarrhea, rash, or feeding changes.

Prescribing analgesics to lactating patients should be based on the pain severity, analgesic safety profile, and infant health and age, ensuring careful monitoring to support both pain management and breastfeeding.

CONCLUSION

The management of musculoskeletal pain in pregnancy requires a multidisciplinary approach tailored to the individual. Conservative treatments, such as physical therapy, postural correction, and activity modification, are primary strategies. Pharmacological interventions are limited due to potential fetal risks, emphasizing the importance of non-invasive methods like exercise, manual therapy, and supportive devices. Emerging evidence supports the use of acupuncture, yoga, and mindfulness for pain relief, though more research is needed. Early identification and intervention remain key to improving maternal function and quality of life during pregnancy.

BIBLIOGRAPHY

1. Borg-Stein J, Dugan SA. Musculoskeletal disorders of pregnancy, delivery and postpartum. Phys Med Rehabil Clin N Am. 2007;18(3):459-76.
2. Higuchi H, Takagi S, Zhang K, Furui I, Ozaki M. Effect of lateral tilt angle on the volume of the abdominal aorta and inferior vena cava in pregnant and nonpregnant women determined by magnetic resonance imaging. Anesthesiology. 2015;122:286-93.
3. Kametas NA, McAuliffe F, Krampl E, Chambers J, Nicolaides KH. Maternal cardiac function in twin pregnancy. Obstet Gynecol. 2003;102:806-15.
4. Kerr MG, Scott DB, Samuel E. Studies of the inferior vena cava in late pregnancy. Br Med J. 1964;1:532-3.
5. Kodali B, Chandrasekhar S, Bulich LN, Topulos GP, Datta S. Airway changes during labour and delivery. Anaesthesiology. 2008;108:357-62.
6. McDonnell NJ, Peach MJ, Clavisi OM, Scott KL; ANZCA Trials Group. Difficult and failed intubation in obstetric anaesthesia: an observational study of airway management and complications associated with general anaesthesia for caesarean section. Int J Obstet Anesth. 2009;17:292.
7. Sabino J, Grauer JN. Pregnancy and low back pain. Curr Rev Musculoskelet Med. 2008;1(2):137-41.
8. Smith MW, Marcus PS, Wurtz LD. Orthopaedic issues in pregnancy. Obstet Gynecol Surv. 2008;63:103-11.
9. Taylor DJ, Lind T. Red cell mass during and after normal pregnancy. Br J Obstet Gynaecol. 1979;86:364-70.
10. Thabah M, Ravindran V. Musculoskeletal problems in pregnancy. Rheumatol Int. 2015;35:581-7.

CHAPTER 18

Management of Musculoskeletal Pain in Liver Failure

Nalini Birpuri, Updesh Kumar

INTRODUCTION

Pain is a prevalent and often inadequately managed symptom in patients with cirrhosis. Drug-induced liver injury (DILI) is responsible for approximately 15% of acute liver failure cases. Painkillers in these patients can cause drastic complications such as encephalopathy, renal impairment, and gastrointestinal tract (GIT) hemorrhage, resulting in serious illness and potentially lethal outcomes.

NONPHARMACOLOGICAL APPROACHES

- Physical therapy
- Cognitive restructuring
- *Behavioral self-management techniques*: Including diet, exercise, acupuncture, acupressure, and massage.
- *Heat and cold therapy*: Topical thermal therapy can relieve local muscle spasms, while cryotherapy may reduce inflammation and pain during the acute injury phase.

PHARMACOLOGICAL APPROACHES

- *Reduced liver metabolism*:
  - Advice analgesics with a short duration [immediate release (IR)].
  - Start with small doses and reduce frequency (e.g., every 6–12 hours).
  - Restrict daily acetaminophen to 2 g.
- *Reduced renal excretion*:
  - Decide doses on renal function.
  - No morphine in patients with chronic kidney disease.

- *Risk for predisposing renal impairment and GIT hemorrhage*:
  - Omit nonsteroidal anti-inflammatory drugs (NSAIDs) in patients with chronic liver disease.
- *Risk for predisposing hepatic encephalopathy*:
  - Monitor sedation levels closely.
  - Avoid constipation and use laxatives like lactulose.
- *Potential for abuse*:
  - Consider a "pain agreement" for opioid prescriptions to limit access.

Up to 50% of patients with cirrhosis have concurrent renal disorders, increasing the risk of toxicity due to impaired drug excretion.

IMPORTANT CONSIDERATIONS FOR ANALGESIA IN PATIENTS WITH CIRRHOSIS

- *Acetaminophen*: It is an important cause of acute liver injury and hepatocellular damage. The Food and Drug Administration (FDA) recommends a dose of <2.6 g/day for patients with liver disease. Heavy alcohol users should limit to 1 g/day or less, with regular liver function monitoring.
- *NSAIDs*: These inhibit prostaglandin synthesis, reducing renal perfusion and glomerular filtration rate (GFR) and causing sodium retention. Avoid systemic NSAIDs in patients with chronic liver disease; consider topical NSAIDs if necessary.
- *Opioids*: Metabolized in the liver, opioids have increased bioavailability and prolonged half-lives in chronic liver disease. Short-acting opioids like fentanyl or hydromorphone are preferred in reduced doses and extended intervals. Avoid morphine, meperidine, codeine, oxycodone, and hydrocodone. IR formulations are recommended, with extended-release formulations to be avoided.
  - *Tramadol*: Suitable in low doses for cirrhotic patients. Avoid in seizure disorders and be cautious with selective serotonin reuptake inhibitors (SSRIs) or tricyclic antidepressants (TCAs).
    - Dosage: 25 mg every 8 hours or 50 mg every 12 hours
  - *Morphine*: Metabolized to neurotoxic metabolites with delayed excretion in renal failure
    - Dosage: Start with 5 mg every 6 hours; monitor for side effects.
  - *Hydromorphone*: Potent, with inactive metabolites and a stable plasma half-life
    - Dosage: 1 mg every 6 hours
  - *Fentanyl*: Extremely potent, does not produce toxic metabolites
    - Dosage: 12.5-μg patch every 72 hours, based on total daily short-acting opioid requirements
  - *Meperidine*: Avoid due to the neurotoxic metabolite normeperidine.
  - *Codeine*: Weak analgesic properties, generally to be avoided

- *Hydrocodone*: Ineffective drug metabolism reduces efficacy, often combined with acetaminophen.
  - Dosage: 5 mg every 6 hours
- *Oxycodone*: Highly protein-bound with a prolonged half-life
  - Dosage: 5 mg every 6 hours

ADJUVANTS FOR NEUROPATHIC PAIN

- *TCAs*: Use cautiously in low doses due to increased risk of adverse effects and hepatic encephalopathy. Prefer nortriptyline and desipramine.
  - *Nortriptyline*: 10 mg orally at night
  - *Desipramine*: 10 mg orally at night, with careful sedation monitoring
- *Gabapentinoids*: Not metabolized in the liver but require renal function adjustments
  - *Gabapentin*: 300 mg orally daily, increasing gradually
  - *Pregabalin*: 25–50 mg orally twice daily, increasing gradually
- *Serotonin-norepinephrine reuptake inhibitors (SNRIs)*: Prolonged half-life and reduced clearance in patients with cirrhosis. Use with caution due to potential liver injury.
- *Carbamazepine*: Avoid due to hepatotoxicity risk.
- *Topical anesthetics*: Local lidocaine is effective for localized pain without dosage adjustments.
  - *Lidocaine patches (5%)*: Can be used locally on the involved area for a duration of 12 h/day

CONCLUSION

For patients with cirrhosis and chronic alcohol or substance abuse, start with low doses and adjust carefully. Restrict acetaminophen to ≤2–3 g/day, avoid multiple medications, and observe for side effects.

BIBLIOGRAPHY

1. Chandok N, Watt KDS. Pain management in the cirrhotic patient: the clinical challenge. Mayo Clin Proc. 2010;85:451-8.
2. Heidelbaugh JJ, Bruderly M. Cirrhosis and chronic liver failure: part I. Diagnosis and evaluation. Am Fam Physician. 2006;74(5):756-62.
3. Rogal SS, Winger D, Bielefeldt K, Rollman BL, Szigethy E. Healthcare utilization in chronic liver disease: the importance of pain and prescription opioid use. Liver Int. 2013;33:1497-503.

CHAPTER 19

Management of Musculoskeletal Pain in Renal Failure

Updesh Kumar, Nalini Birpuri

INTRODUCTION

Chronic musculoskeletal pain is common in patients with chronic kidney disease (CKD), especially in patients with end-stage renal disease (ESRD). Individuals with CKD have various musculoskeletal manifestations and account for 60% of the patients with CKD. Musculoskeletal pain in CKD can be either nociceptive or neuropathic. Inflammatory mediators like interleukins, tumor necrosis factor (TNF), prostaglandins, and certain uremic toxins play an important role in the sensitization of peripheral nociceptors and pain receptors in the central nervous system (CNS).

MANAGEMENT OF PAIN IN PATIENTS WITH CHRONIC KIDNEY DISEASE

Multidisciplinary management is required to relieve pain in patients with CKD to improve their quality of life, mental health, and ability to do routine physical activities.

In patients with renal insufficiency [decreased estimated glomerular filtration rate (eGFR) of ≤ 90 mL/min/1.73 m^2], analgesic medicines may last longer in the body leading to toxicity and adverse effects, so drug dosage recommendations in patients with CKD can be made according to the eGFR.

The World Health Organization (WHO) and Centers for Disease Control and Prevention (CDC) guidelines recommend both nonpharmacological and pharmacological interventions for pain management in patients with CKD. Nonpharmacological interventions should be attempted first to manage pain, if applicable, followed by nonopioid drugs instead of opioid drugs.

Pharmacological Management in Patients with Chronic Kidney Disease

The WHO (World Health Organization) step ladder for analgesic pain control has been validated for use in patients with CKD. The ladder follows a three-step approach to pain management as mentioned in **Flowchart 1**. The points given in the following text should be considered while executing pain management in patients with kidney dysfunction. The adjustment of the dosage based on glomerular filtration rate (GFR) becomes central as mentioned in **Table 1**.

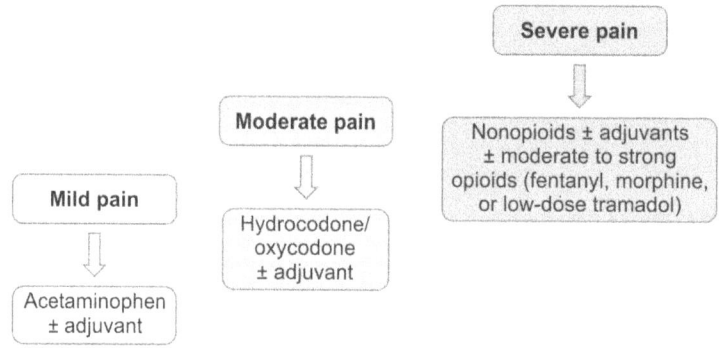

FLOWCHART 1: Pain management in renal patients.

Table 1: Adjusted dosing recommendations based on GFR.					
Dose alteration	>50 mL/min	10–15 mL/min	<10 mL/min		
Morphine	100%	75%	50%		
Fentanyl	100%	75%	50%		
Methadone	100%	100%	50–75%		
Oxycodone	Avoid if GFR <60 mL/min				
Hydrocodone	Not recommended				
TCA	• No dose change requirement • Tolerance of side effect in patient with renal failure is poor				
Duloxetine	Not used if GFR <30 mL/min				
Gabapentin	>80 mL/min	50–79 mL/min	30–49 mL/min	15–29 mL/min	<15 mL/min
	900–3,600 mg/day	600–1,800 mg/day	300–900 mg/day	150–600 mg/day	150–300 mg/day
Pregabalin	>60 mL/min	30–59 mL/min	15–29 mL/min	<15 mL/min	
	600 mg/day	300 mg/day	150 mg/day	75 mg/day	
Acetaminophen	325–650 mg		325–650 mg	325–650 mg	

(GFR: glomerular filtration rate; TCA: tricyclic antidepressant)

Nonsteroidal Anti-inflammatory Drugs
- Nonsteroidal anti-inflammatory drugs (NSAIDs) act by inhibiting the synthesis of prostaglandins in the kidney which leads to reduced GFR, fluid retention, hypertension, and electrolyte disorders.
- NSAIDs causing decreased GFR are indomethacin, naproxen, diclofenac, ibuprofen, and aspirin.
- NSAIDs are best avoided in patients with CKD whose eGFR <60 mL/min/1.73 m² (stage 3).
- Selective cyclooxygenase-2 (COX-2) inhibitors like celecoxib and etoricoxib are also contraindicated in renal failure like the traditional NSAIDs.
- Paracetamol (PCM) (acetaminophen) is safe to use in renal failure. It can be given in therapeutic doses (up to 3–4 g/day).

When it is a must to use NSAIDs (due to the lack of effective alternatives), short-acting NSAIDs are preferred over long-acting agents to avoid prolonged NSAID-induced intraglomerular hemodynamic compromise.

Opioids
- When opioids are required for pain control in patients with CKD, informed consent should be obtained regarding risks and benefits.
- Risk of drug abuse, misuse, or addiction should be assessed before prescribing opioids.
- The optimal dose of opioids is one that either causes a reduction in pain by 30% on the pain rating scale or improves the functional status.

Morphine
- Morphine produces active metabolite morphine-6-glucuronide which gets accumulated in renal failure causing CNS and respiratory depression.
- The dose should be reduced and frequency should be decreased depending on the renal function status. When safer opioids are available, morphine could be avoided.

Hydromorphone
Hydromorphone is more potent than morphine and is generally well tolerated in patients with decreased renal function; still, it should be prescribed with caution in patients with CKD.

Tramadol
- Synthetic opioid
- 30% of the drug and 60% of the metabolites are excreted by the kidneys.
- The risk of toxicity in renal failure is less.
- Easily dialyzable by hemodialysis
- Used with caution in advanced CKD/ESRD as it increases the risk of hypoglycemia and lowers the seizure threshold

Fentanyl
Fentanyl is safe to use in renal failure as it does not produce any active metabolite.

Buprenorphine and Methadone
They are safe for management of moderate to severe pain in patients with CKD.

Oxycodone
Metabolite is excreted through the kidneys. It is not recommended in CKD.

Hydrocodone
It accumulates in renal failure. It is not recommended in CKD.

Adjuvants
Adjuvant drugs are commonly used for the management of musculoskeletal pain having a neuropathic component. Commonly used adjuvants are gabapentin, pregabalin, tricyclic antidepressants (TCAs), and selective serotonin reuptake inhibitors (SSRIs). The dose must be reduced in patients because of the risk of sedation and unwanted adverse effects.

A stepwise approach should be adopted for patients with acute neuropathic pain. When prompt pain relief is required, opioid analgesics may be used alone or in combination with one of the first-line drugs. If first-line drugs alone or in combination fail, consider referral to a pain specialist or multidisciplinary pain center.

Topical Agents
Topical agents (such as topical NSAIDs, lidocaine patch, and capsaicin patch) have been found useful in treating localized pain. They are beneficial in both acute and chronic pain. They have minimal systemic absorption and are safe for use in patients with CKD.

Skeletal Muscle Relaxants
All skeletal muscle relaxants are known to cause sedation, muscle weakness, and dizziness. Thus, they should be avoided in CKD and ESRD.

Regional Blocks
Some regional techniques like epidural steroids and local anesthetic injections have been found useful for short-term pain relief of chronic cervical, lumbar, and osteoarthritic pain symptoms. Therefore, they should be used if and when required. This will lead to less demand for systemic analgesia.

Nonpharmacological Management in Patients with Chronic Kidney Disease

Chronic musculoskeletal pain is the result of multiple biological, psychological, and social factors; therefore, the patient should be offered the use of various nonpharmacological treatment modalities as well.

Thus, in 2016, the National Center for Complementary and Integrative Health (NCCIH) created several treatment modalities.

These include:
- Mind-body interventions
- Diet and lifestyle modifications
- Herbal remedies, manual healing
- Bioelectromagnetics
- Dry needling
- Thermal and cryotherapy
- Neurostimulation like transcutaneous electrical nerve stimulation (TENS), acupuncture, acupressure

Wherever possible, their use should be encouraged because of lesser side effects and hence will decrease the requirement of painkillers.

CONCLUSION

Managing musculoskeletal pain in renal failure patients requires a careful, multidisciplinary approach. Treatment must balance effective pain relief with the unique challenges posed by impaired kidney function, including altered drug metabolism and potential side effects. Non-pharmacologic methods, such as physical therapy and lifestyle interventions, play a key role alongside cautious medication use. A tailored, patient-centered strategy that includes collaboration among healthcare professionals can improve both pain management and quality of life for these patients.

BIBLIOGRAPHY

1. Cohen SD, Patel SS, Khetpal P, Peterson RA, Kimmel PL. Pain, sleep disturbance, and quality of life in patients with chronic kidney disease. Clin J Am Soc Nephrol. 2007;2(5):919-25.
2. Davison SN, Koncicki H, Brennan F. Pain in chronic kidney disease: a scoping review. Semin Dial. 2014;27(2):188-204.
3. Dowell D, Haegerich TM, Chou R. CDC guideline for prescribing opioids for chronic pain—United States, 2016. JAMA. 2016;315(15):1624-45.
4. Kay J, Bardin T. Osteoarticular disorders of renal origin: disease-related and iatrogenic. Best Pract Res Clin Rheumatol. 2000;14(2):285-305.
5. Koncicki HM, Unruh M, Schell JO. Pain management in CKD: a guide for nephrology providers. Am J Kidney Dis. 2017;69(3):451-60.
6. Lim C, Ong K. Various musculoskeletal manifestations of chronic renal insufficiency. Clin Radiol. 2013;68(7):e397-411.
7. National Center for Complementary and Integrative Health. (2016). 2016 Strategic Plan: exploring the science of complementary and integrative health. [online] Available from https://nccih.nih.gov/sites/nccam.nih.gov/files/NCCIH_2016_Strategic_Pla.
8. Pham PC, Khaing K, Sievers TM, Pham PM, Miller JM, Pham SV, et al. 2017 update on pain management in patients with chronic kidney disease. Clin Kidney J. 2017;10(5):688-97.
9. Roy PJ, Weltman M. Pain management in patients with chronic kidney disease and end-stage kidney disease. Curr Opin Nephrol Hypertens. 2020;29(6):671-80.

CHAPTER 20

Management of Musculoskeletal Pain in the Phantom Limb

Renu Wakhloo

■ INTRODUCTION

Phantom limb pain (PLP) is the sensation of pain in an amputated limb. The phenomenon was first documented by Ambroise Paré (1510-1590), a French military surgeon. Historically, the high prevalence and underlying pathophysiology of PLP were not fully appreciated, often being misattributed to psychological factors. Despite continuous research, PLP is still poorly understood due to its complexity and the severe distress it causes.

A systematic review and meta-analysis reveal that approximately 64% of amputees experience PLP, categorizing it as one of the most challenging chronic pain syndromes to manage. It is critical to distinguish PLP from residual limb pain (RLP), which occurs in the remaining stump and can be due to nerve entrapment, ischemia, skin problems, or an infection. While RLP generally subsides with wound healing, it can coexist with PLP in about 50% of cases.

■ CHARACTERISTICS OF PHANTOM LIMB PAIN

Phantom limb pain is typically intermittent, ranging from seconds to minutes, although it can persist for hours or, rarely, indefinitely. It is often described as crushing, pricking, burning, tingling, or shooting pain, primarily localized to the distal part of the phantom limb. The onset usually occurs immediately after amputation but can also begin weeks or months later. The severity and frequency of PLP generally decrease over time, potentially resolving within several weeks to 2 years, although it may continue intermittently throughout life.

Understanding the mechanisms behind PLP is critical to designing effective therapies. Both the peripheral nervous system (PNS) and the central nervous system (CNS) are involved in PLP, which influences therapy options.

MECHANISTIC THEORIES OF PHANTOM LIMB PAIN

Peripheral Nervous System versus Central Nervous System

While amputation has a direct impact on the PNS, changes in sensory and motor signals affect the CNS as well. The cell bodies for PNS somatic axons are located in the dorsal root ganglia (DRG). Following amputation, these axons become disconnected from their targets, leading to inflammation and neuroma formation in the residual limb. These damaged axons generate spontaneous activity, which is transmitted to the spinal cord, increasing N-methyl-D-aspartate (NMDA) activity in the dorsal horn and contributing to neuropathic pain in PLP.

The cortical remapping theory (CRT) is the CNS theory that is most often accepted. According to this theory, areas of the cortex representing the amputated limb are overtaken by neighboring regions in the somatosensory and motor cortices, resulting in maladaptive cortical reorganization closely associated with pain.

RISK FACTORS FOR PHANTOM LIMB PAIN

- Female sex
- Psychological factors such as anxiety, depression, and stress
- Preamputation pain, which increases the likelihood of PLP

TREATMENT APPROACHES

Managing PLP requires a multidisciplinary approach involving orthopedic surgeons, anesthetists, physiotherapists, and rehabilitation specialists. Early intervention with multimodal pain management strategies can help prevent chronic pain development.

PHARMACOTHERAPY

- *Epidural analgesia*: Ropivacaine with adjuvants like ketamine, opioids, or calcitonin, along with patient-controlled analgesia, can reduce PLP during the perioperative period. Prolonged postoperative perineural infusion of local anesthetics via catheters has shown benefits, suggesting the role of local anesthetic blockade in preventing nervous system reorganization.
- *Nonsteroidal anti-inflammatory drugs (NSAIDs) and acetaminophen*: Commonly used to manage PLP, these drugs reduce nociceptive pain at both peripheral and central levels.
- *Opioids*: These may alleviate PLP by reducing cortical reorganization. They should be used alongside antidepressants or neuromodulating agents like gabapentin and pregabalin but with caution due to the risk of tolerance and dependence. Tramadol has shown positive results.

- *Antidepressants*: Amitriptyline, a tricyclic antidepressant, is preferred. Selective serotonin reuptake inhibitors (SSRIs) like duloxetine and milnacipran have shown some efficacy, although their anticholinergic side effects can be problematic for elderly patients.
- *NMDA receptor antagonists*: Drugs like ketamine and dextromethorphan can benefit pain syndromes but are limited by their side effects for long-term use.

SUPPORTIVE NONPHARMACOLOGICAL TREATMENTS

- *Transcutaneous electrical nerve stimulation (TENS)*: Low-frequency and high-intensity TENS is effective for PLP with moderate evidence supporting its use.
- *Transcranial magnetic stimulation*: While results are inconclusive, it may help some patients.
- *Mirror therapy*: This cost-effective, noninvasive treatment involves moving the intact limb in front of a mirror to create a visual representation of the missing limb, reducing pain through visual feedback.
- *Spinal cord stimulation (SCS)*: This therapy, which is frequently successful for PLP, uses an implanted gadget to stimulate the spinal cord's dorsal columns.
- *Virtual reality (VR) and augmented reality training*: Using visual-proprioceptive feedback from VR headsets to visualize the missing limbs has shown momentary pain reduction, warranting further studies.
- *Sympathetic blocks*: A stellate ganglion block can be helpful in resistant cases.
- *Prosthetics*: Functional prostheses offer increased visual feedback during activities, normalizing cortical representation of amputated limbs and aiding in rehabilitation.

Recent surgical techniques like targeted nerve implantation or traction neurectomy aim to prevent neuroma formation. Proper muscle-to-bone attachment is vital for joint movement during rehabilitation.

CONCLUSION

Phantom limb pain remains a complex and challenging condition to treat. The current literature does not support a single superior technique. Small sample sizes and brief follow-up times are the main limitations of most studies. The best therapy for PLP will require the creation of new strategies as well as technological and methodological advancements in the current therapies.

BIBLIOGRAPHY

1. Hanyu-Deutmeyer AA, Cascella M, Varacallo M. Phantom Limb Pain. In: StatPearls. StatPearls Publishing, Treasure Island (FL); 2023. PMID: 28846343.
2. Limakatso K, Bedwell GJ, Madden VJ, Parkern R. The prevalence and risk factors for phantom limb pain in people with amputations: a systematic review and meta-analysis. PLoS One. 2020;15(10):e0240431.
3. Rothgangel A, Braun S, Smeets R, Beurskens A. Feasibility of a traditional and tile treatment approach to mirror therapy in patients with phantom limb pain; a process evaluation performed alongside a randomised controlled trial. Clin Rehabil. 2019;33(10):1649-60.
4. Vaso A, Adahan HM, Gjika A, Zahaj S, Zhurda T, Vyshka G, et al. Peripheral nervous system: origin of phantom limb pain. Pain. 2014;155(7);1384-91.
5. Wittkopf PG, Lloyd DM, Coe O, Yacoobali S, Billington J. The effect of interactive virtual reality on pain perception: a systematic review of clinical studies. Disabil Rehab. 2020;42(26):3722-33.

CHAPTER 21

Management of Neuropathic Pain

Ashwani Kumar

INTRODUCTION

Neuropathic pain, arising from damage or dysfunction in the nervous system, presents a unique challenge in clinical practice. It is characterized by persistent, often severe pain that does not conform to typical nociceptive pain patterns. Understanding its pathophysiology, accurate diagnosis, and effective management strategies is crucial for improving patient outcomes.

Neuropathic pain in musculoskeletal conditions can arise from various causes. Some common causes are as follows:
- *Nerve compression or entrapment*:
  - Herniated disc
  - Carpal tunnel syndrome
  - Thoracic outlet syndrome
- *Nerve damage*:
  - Trauma or injury, surgical procedures
- *Degenerative diseases*:
  - *Osteoarthritis*: Can lead to bone spurs that compress or irritate nearby nerves
  - *Spinal stenosis*: Narrowing of the spinal canal can compress the spinal cord or nerves.
- *Inflammatory conditions*:
  - *Rheumatoid arthritis*: Inflammation can cause nerve compression or damage.
  - Diabetic neuropathy
- *Infections*:
  - Shingles (herpes zoster)
- Tumors
- *Systemic diseases*:
  - Diabetes, multiple sclerosis

- Nutritional deficiencies; B12 deficiency
- *Toxic exposures*:
  - Chemotherapy-induced neuropathy, alcohol abuse

CLINICAL ASSESSMENT

Accurate diagnosis is pivotal for effective management. Neuropathic pain is typically diagnosed based on a detailed patient history and clinical examination, supplemented by specific diagnostic tools such as the Douleur Neuropathique 4 (DN4) questionnaire and the Leeds Assessment of Neuropathic Symptoms and Signs (LANSS) scale. Common symptoms include burning, shooting, or stabbing pain, often accompanied by sensory abnormalities like allodynia and hyperalgesia.

MANAGEMENT

First-line Medications

Antidepressants

Tricyclic antidepressants (TCAs) such as amitriptyline and serotonin-norepinephrine reuptake inhibitors (SNRIs) such as duloxetine are first-line treatments. These agents modulate pain pathways by enhancing descending inhibitory control and modulating serotonin and norepinephrine reuptake.

Anticonvulsants

Gabapentinoids, including gabapentin and pregabalin, are widely used due to their efficacy in reducing neuropathic pain. They work by binding to the $\alpha_2\delta$ subunit of voltage-gated calcium channels, reducing excitatory neurotransmitter release.

Second-line Medications

Opioids

While opioids can be effective, their use is generally reserved for refractory cases due to the risk of tolerance, dependence, and side effects. Tramadol, a weak opioid with additional serotonergic and noradrenergic activity, may be considered as a second-line option.

Topical Agents

Topical agents such as lidocaine patches and capsaicin cream offer localized pain relief with minimal systemic side effects.

Interventional Management

For patients unresponsive to pharmacotherapy, interventional techniques can be considered. Epidural steroid injections, nerve blocks, and spinal cord stimulation (SCS) are among the options. SCS, in particular, has shown promise in reducing pain and improving quality of life in patients with refractory neuropathic pain by modulating pain signals at the spinal level.

Nonpharmacological Management

Physical Therapy
Physical therapy plays a crucial role in managing neuropathic pain, focusing on improving mobility and reducing pain through exercises, manual therapy, and modalities like transcutaneous electrical nerve stimulation (TENS).

Psychological Therapies
Cognitive-behavioral therapy (CBT) and mindfulness-based stress reduction (MBSR) are effective adjuncts, addressing the psychological aspects of chronic pain and helping patients develop coping strategies.

Emerging Therapies
Emerging therapies include monoclonal antibodies targeting nerve growth factor (NGF) and gene therapy approaches aimed at modulating pain pathways at the genetic level.

CONCLUSION

Managing neuropathic pain requires a comprehensive, multimodal approach tailored to the individual patient. Combining pharmacological treatments with interventional and nonpharmacological strategies enhances efficacy and improves patient outcomes. Ongoing research and emerging therapies hold promise for more effective management in the future.

BIBLIOGRAPHY

1. Bouhassira D, Attal N, Fermanian J, Alchaar H, Gautron M, Masquelier E, et al. Development and validation of the Neuropathic Pain Symptom Inventory. Pain. 2004;108(3):248-57.
2. Costigan M, Scholz J, Woolf CJ. Neuropathic pain: a maladaptive response of the nervous system to damage. Annu Rev Neurosci. 2009;32:1-32.
3. Finnerup NB, Sindrup SH, Jensen TS. The evidence for pharmacological treatment of neuropathic pain. Pain. 2010;150(3):573-81.
4. Moore RA, Straube S, Wiffen PJ, Derry S, McQuay HJ. Pregabalin for acute and chronic pain in adults. Cochrane Database Syst Rev. 2009;(3):CD007076.
5. Saarto T, Wiffen PJ. Antidepressants for neuropathic pain. Cochrane Database Syst Rev. 2007;(4):CD005454.
6. Smith BH, Torrance N. Epidemiology of neuropathic pain and its impact on quality of life. Curr Pain Headache Rep. 2012;16(3):191-8.
7. Mantyh PW. The neurobiology of skeletal pain. Eur J Neurosci. 2014;39(3):508-19.

CHAPTER 22

Management of Rheumatoid Arthritis Pain

Suraydev Aman Singh

■ INTRODUCTION

The management of rheumatoid arthritis (RA) aims to control inflammation which in turn relieves pain and stiffness, overall improving the quality of life. Although disease-modifying antirheumatic drugs (DMARDs) remain the mainstay of treatment, nonsteroidal anti-inflammatory drugs (NSAIDs), glucocorticoids, topical capsaicin, opioids, and neuromodulators are key elements for optimal pain management.

■ PHARMACOLOGICAL MANAGEMENT

The treatment recommendations by the American College of Rheumatology (ACR) and European League Against Rheumatism (EULAR) comprise two perspectives.

Symptomatic management of pain associated with RA is achieved by NSAIDs and corticosteroids and sometimes weak opioids may be used for short-term pain relief, while disease-modifying management, i.e., DMARDs, is going to show its effect.

Disease-modifying Antirheumatic Drugs

Disease-modifying antirheumatic drugs are the mainstay pharmacological agents that actually suppress autoimmune activity to promote disease remission and hence delay or prevent joint degeneration. The latest recommendations suggest that treatment with DMARDs should be initiated as soon as possible as early implementation leads to better results, especially given that DMARDs are slow-acting drugs with a delayed onset between 6 weeks and 6 months. Most people tolerate the drug well; however, common side effects include feeling sick, loss of appetite, diarrhea, hair loss, and liver dysfunction.

Nonsteroidal Anti-inflammatory Drugs

Nonsteroidal anti-inflammatory drugs remain an important adjunctive therapy to control inflammation and hence pain in RA. Recent guidelines from the ACR, EULAR and National Institute for Health and Care Excellence (NICE) also emphasize their role in symptom relief, with careful consideration of potential risks associated with their long-term use.

Corticosteroids

Corticosteroids are often prescribed for short-term pain relief while waiting for DMARD response, intending to gradually taper off the medication. They may be recommended as adjunctive therapy in RA that persists despite using DMARDs. At times, to manage flare-ups and severe pain, intra-articular or periarticular steroid injection may be required, although it should not be repeated frequently.

Neuromodulators

Patients with RA manifest a generalized increase in pain perception. Although neuromodulators are not recommended as first-line drugs, they are useful to manage sleep-related symptoms associated with pain. These include the anticonvulsant agents (gabapentin, pregabalin), tricyclic antidepressant (TCA), and serotonin–norepinephrine reuptake inhibitors (SNRIs).

NONPHARMACOLOGICAL THERAPIES

Scientific evidence recommends cold and heat therapy, massage, bracing, thermotherapy, acupuncture, transcutaneous electrical nerve stimulation, and occupational therapy as complementary modalities in nonpharmacological pain management. However, nonpharmacological approaches should be combined with pharmacological treatments to maximize therapeutic success.

SURGERY

Joint surgery is reserved for severe stages of RA to reduce pain and restore joint function. Various procedures include synovectomy, arthroscopy, osteotomy, arthrodesis, and total joint replacement.

CONCLUSION

Effective management of RA pain requires a combination of pharmacological and nonpharmacological approaches. While DMARDs remain central to controlling disease progression and inflammation, NSAIDs, corticosteroids, and neuromodulators play a significant role in addressing symptomatic pain. Nonpharmacological treatments, such as physical therapies and occupational therapy, further complement these strategies, offering holistic relief. In advanced cases, surgical intervention may be necessary to restore joint function and reduce pain, highlighting the importance of a tailored, multifaceted approach to RA management.

BIBLIOGRAPHY

1. Fraenkel L, Bathon JM, England BR, St Clair EW, Arayssi T, Carandang K et al. The American College of Rheumatology's updated treatment guideline for rheumatoid arthritis. Rheumatologist. 2024;12(2):15-22.
2. Smolen JS, Landewé RBM, Bergstra SA, Kerschbaumer A, Sepriano A, Aletaha D, et al. EULAR recommendations for the management of rheumatoid arthritis with synthetic and biological disease-modifying antirheumatic drugs: 2023 update. Ann Rheum Dis. 2024;83(1):3-19.
3. Brown P, Pratt AG, Hyrich KL. Therapeutic advances in rheumatoid arthritis. BMJ. 2024;384:e070856.
4. Fujii T, Murata K, Onizawa H, Onishi A, Tanaka M, Murakami K, et al. Management and treatment outcomes of rheumatoid arthritis in the era of biologic and targeted synthetic therapies: evaluation of 10-year data from the KURAMA cohort. Arthritis Res Ther. 2024;26:30.

CHAPTER 23

Management of Acute and Chronic Gouty Pain

Rashid Anjum

■ INTRODUCTION

Gouty arthritis, caused by urate crystal buildup in joints, leads to intense pain and inflammation. This chapter outlines effective pain management strategies, focusing on medications like nonsteroidal anti-inflammatory drugs (NSAIDs), corticosteroids, and colchicine, along with lifestyle and dietary changes. It provides a concise guide for both acute and long-term management of gout pain to improve patient outcomes.

■ MANAGEMENT OF ACUTE GOUT PAIN

The treatment of gout aims to achieve two primary objectives: Relieving the pain and inflammation of acute gout attacks and managing the condition long term by reducing serum urate (sUA) levels to prevent future episodes. Managing acute pain and inflammation can be challenging due to the presence of comorbidities such as diabetes mellitus (DM), chronic kidney disease (CKD), hypertension, and cardiovascular disease (CVD), which often accompany gout.

Pharmacological Treatment

The American College of Rheumatology (ACR) recently issued updated guidelines for managing gout, including recommendations for treating acute gout. The guidelines propose three first-line therapies but provide minimal direction on how to choose between them.

Nonsteroidal Anti-inflammatory Drugs

Commonly used NSAIDs include indomethacin, naproxen, and ibuprofen. They are most effective when initiated early in the attack.

Considerations: Use with caution in patients with renal impairment, peptic ulcer disease, or cardiovascular risk factors.

Colchicine

Usage: High doses are effective but often cause gastrointestinal (GI) side effects. Low-dose regimens (e.g., 1.2 mg followed by 0.6 mg 1 hour later) are recommended to minimize adverse effects.

Considerations: Use with caution in patients with renal or hepatic impairment.

Corticosteroids

Usage: Options include oral prednisone or intra-articular corticosteroid injections for patients unable to take NSAIDs or colchicine.

Considerations: Long-term use is associated with significant side effects; thus, corticosteroids are typically used for short-term management and are prescribed not too frequently and not for long-term use.

Interleukin-1 Inhibitors

Mechanism: Interleukin-1 (IL-1) inhibitors, such as anakinra, block the activity of IL-1, a key cytokine in gout inflammation.

Usage: Considered for patients with severe or refractory gout attacks not responding to standard treatments

Nonsteroidal anti-inflammatory drugs or cyclooxygenase-2 (COX-2) inhibitors should be taken as prescribed at the starting dose and should be continued until the gout episode has completely subsided. Although every NSAID in the market is thought to be beneficial, only naproxen, indomethacin, and sulindac are authorized for the treatment of acute gout. There are insufficient data to conclude that one NSAID is better than another; there is no discernible variation in their efficacy. There is insufficient data to conclude that selective COX-2 inhibitors, such as celecoxib, work just as well as nonselective NSAIDs but may have fewer side effects overall, especially in the GI tract (6% vs. 16% for GI events). Colchicine has been used for a long time as a prophylactic treatment for acute gout attacks and is endorsed for treating acute episodes. Recent studies suggest that an initial dose of 1.2 mg of colchicine followed by a single 0.6-mg dose 1 hour later is as effective as the traditional regimen of 1.2 mg followed by 0.6 mg every hour for up to 6 hours but with fewer adverse effects **(Flowchart 1)**.

Nonpharmacological Treatment

- *Rest and elevation*: Resting the affected joint and elevating it can help reduce swelling and pain.
- *Ice packs*: Applying ice packs to the inflamed joint can provide symptomatic relief by reducing swelling and numbing the area.
- *Hydration*: Increasing fluid intake helps prevent urate crystal formation by promoting uric acid excretion.

CHAPTER 23: Management of Acute and Chronic Gouty Pain

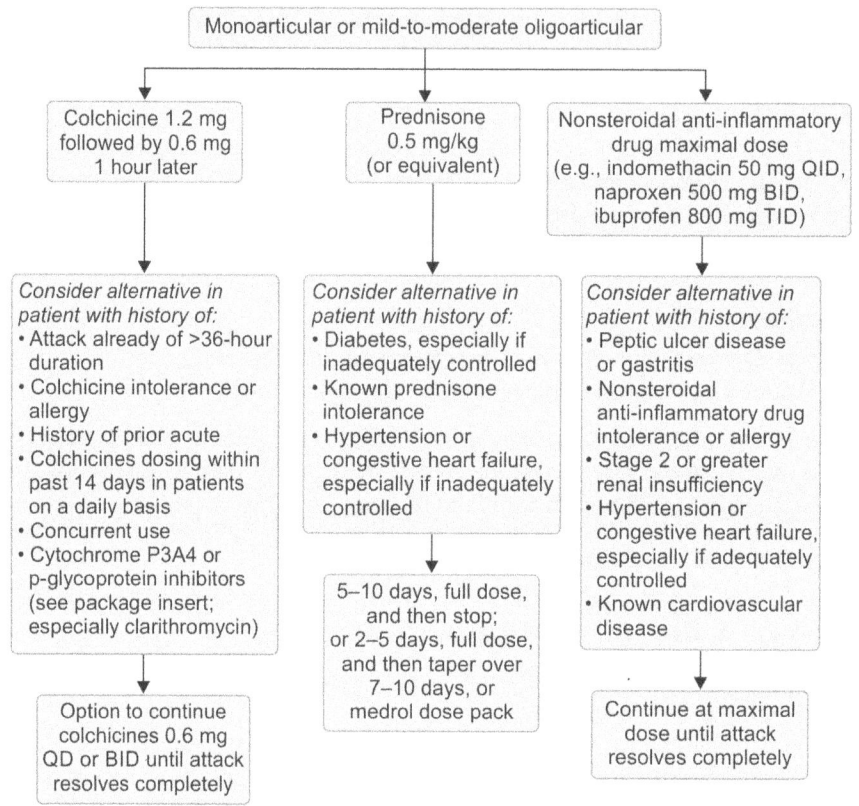

Flowchart 1: Algorithmic management of an acute attack of gout.

MANAGEMENT OF CHRONIC GOUT PAIN

Pharmacological Treatment
- *Urate-lowering therapy (ULT)*:
  - *Allopurinol*: It is a xanthine oxidase inhibitor that reduces uric acid production. Starting at a low dose (e.g., 100 mg daily) and titrating up are recommended to avoid hypersensitivity reactions.
  - *Febuxostat*: It is another xanthine oxidase inhibitor, useful for patients intolerant to allopurinol. Regular liver function tests are necessary due to potential hepatic side effects.
  - *Probenecid*: It is a uricosuric agent that increases renal excretion of uric acid. It is less commonly used due to potential nephrolithiasis.
- *Anti-inflammatory prophylaxis*:
  - Low-dose colchicine or NSAIDs are often prescribed during the initial months of ULT to prevent gout flares.

Nonpharmacological Treatment
- *Lifestyle modifications*:
  - *Diet*: Reducing intake of purine-rich foods (e.g., red meat, seafood), alcohol (especially beer) and fructose-rich beverages can help lower uric acid levels.
  - *Weight management*: Maintaining a healthy weight reduces the risk of hyperuricemia and gout flares.
- *Patient education*: Educating patients about gout triggers, the importance of medication adherence, and lifestyle changes is crucial for long-term management.
- *Regular monitoring*: Regular follow-up visits to monitor serum uric acid levels and adjust therapy as needed to help prevent flares and complications.

Advanced and Adjunctive Therapies
- *Biological agents*: For patients with severe, refractory gout, biological agents like pegloticase (a pegylated uricase enzyme that breaks down uric acid) can be considered. These agents are usually reserved for cases where standard treatments fail.
- *Surgical interventions*: In cases of chronic tophaceous gout causing significant joint deformity or dysfunction or painful/infected tophi, surgical removal of tophi or joint replacement may be necessary.

CONTINUATION OF URATE-LOWERING THERAPY DURING ACUTE GOUT ATTACKS

During the treatment of acute gout attacks, it is essential to maintain ULT initiated before the attack. Evidence suggests that ongoing ULT does not cause adverse effects during attacks. Discontinuing treatment may lead to increased serum uric acid levels, potentially triggering attacks in other joints by destabilizing crystals that are still present. Current recommendations even propose initiating ULT during an attack, contrary to the traditional practice of deferring it until the attack resolves. In a randomized trial comparing patients starting allopurinol 300 mg during an attack with those receiving a placebo (while all patients received anti-inflammatory treatment for the acute attack), no difference in pain outcomes was observed. Regardless of the timing chosen for initiation, lowering and maintaining serum uric acid levels < 6.0 mg/dL remain the primary approach for minimizing the long-term risk of gout attacks.

COMORBIDITIES

Managing acute gout with comorbidities presents a multifaceted challenge, demanding meticulous consideration of various factors. In

CKD, in which approximately 20% of patients with gout have an estimated glomerular filtration rate (eGFR) < 30 mL/min, NSAIDs warrant cautious use, particularly at higher doses. Colchicine emerges as a safer option for stage 3 CKD (eGFR ≥ 60 mL/min), although its use necessitates careful monitoring in severe CKD cases. Alternatively, glucocorticoids or second-line agents like adrenocorticotropic hormone (ACTH) or IL-1 inhibitors may be considered. Hypertension complicates treatment decisions, with NSAIDs and glucocorticoids to be avoided in cases of poorly controlled hypertension, while colchicine stands out as a preferred option in the absence of significant renal impairment. In the context of diabetes and hyperlipidemia, glucocorticoids are best avoided due to their adverse effects on glucose and lipid levels, making colchicine or NSAIDs potentially more suitable alternatives. CVD adds another layer of complexity, with COX-2 inhibitors and NSAIDs posing increased cardiovascular risks, necessitating limited use in patients with a history of myocardial infarction (MI), heart failure, or stroke. In contrast, colchicine shows promise in lowering MI risk, while IL-1 inhibitors present as viable options. Lastly, considerations for hepatic impairment and GI bleeding dictate caution, with NSAIDs to be avoided in cirrhosis due to bleeding risk, and colchicine use warranted with careful monitoring in severe liver impairment. GI bleeding risks necessitate the avoidance of NSAIDs, and the use of proton-pump inhibitors is considered if needed.

Treatment of Asymptomatic Hyperuricemia

Treatment is a matter of debate. A summary of the current recommendations is as follows:
- *General approach*:
  - Lifestyle modifications
  - Regular monitoring of serum uric acid levels and metabolic parameters is recommended.
- *Pharmacological treatment*:
  - *No routine uric acid-lowering therapy*: Most guidelines, including those from the ACR and the European League Against Rheumatism (EULAR), do not recommend routine pharmacological treatment for asymptomatic hyperuricemia.
  - *Consideration in specific populations*: Treatment may be considered in patients with very high serum uric acid levels (e.g., >13 mg/dL in men and >10 mg/dL in women) due to the increased risk of uric acid nephropathy or other complications. Additionally, patients with comorbid conditions such as CKD, CVD, or those at a high risk of gout may be considered for treatment on a case-by-case basis.
- *Emerging evidence*:
  - *Cardiovascular and renal risk*: Some studies suggest that asymptomatic hyperuricemia may be associated with increased cardiovascular

and renal risks. However, definitive evidence supporting the benefit of uric acid-lowering therapy in reducing these risks in asymptomatic patients is lacking.
- *Current guidelines*:
  - *ACR and EULAR*: They advise against ULT in the absence of symptoms. They recommend addressing associated comorbidities and risk factors.
  - *Japanese guidelines*: These guidelines suggest a more proactive approach, in which ULT might be considered in certain high-risk populations, although this approach is more aggressive than that of Western guidelines.
- *Individualized care*:
  - *Risk assessment*: Individual risk assessment is crucial. Physicians should consider patient-specific factors such as uric acid levels, renal function, presence of comorbidities, and risk factors for gout or urate nephropathy.

In summary, the consensus in the current professional literature is that routine pharmacological treatment for asymptomatic hyperuricemia is not recommended. Instead, lifestyle modifications and monitoring are emphasized. Pharmacological treatment may be considered in specific high-risk populations, but this approach is tailored on a case-by-case basis.

CONCLUSION

Effective management of gout pain requires a multifaceted approach, combining pharmacological and nonpharmacological strategies. Acute gout attacks demand prompt treatment with NSAIDs, colchicine, or corticosteroids to alleviate pain and inflammation. Chronic gout management focuses on ULT, lifestyle modifications, and patient education to prevent flares and joint damage. Advanced therapies may be necessary for refractory cases. A comprehensive and personalized treatment plan can significantly improve the quality of life for patients with gout, reducing the burden of this debilitating condition.

BIBLIOGRAPHY

1. Bursill D, Taylor WJ, Terkeltaub R, Abhishek A, So AK, Vargas-Santos AB, et al. Gout, Hyperuricaemia and Crystal-Associated Disease Network (G-CAN) consensus statement regarding labels and definitions of disease states of gout. Ann Rheum Dis. 2019;78(11):1592-600.
2. Bursill D, Taylor WJ, Terkeltaub R, Kuwabara M, Merriman TR, Grainger R, et al. Gout, Hyperuricemia, and Crystal-Associated Disease Network consensus statement regarding labels and definitions for disease elements in gout. Arthritis Care Res (Hoboken). 2019;71(3):427-34.
3. Coburn BW, Mikuls TR. Treatment options for acute gout. Fed Pract. 2016;33(1):35-40.

4. Esser N, Paquot N, Scheen AJ. Anti-inflammatory agents to treat or prevent type 2 diabetes, metabolic syndrome and cardiovascular disease. Expert Opinion Investing Drugs. 2015;24(3):283-307.
5. Khanna D, Khanna PP, Fitzgerald JD, Singh MK, Bae S, Neogi T, et al. 2012 American College of Rheumatology guidelines for the management of gout. Part 2: therapy and antiinflammatory prophylaxis of acute gouty arthritis. Arthritis Care Res (Hoboken). 2012;64(10):1447-61.
6. Zhu Y, Pandya BJ, Choi HK. Comorbidities of gout and hyperuricemia in the US general population: NHANES 2007-2008. Am J Med. 2012;125(7):679-87.e1.
7. Zhu Y, Pandya BJ, Choi HK. Prevalence of gout and hyperuricemia in the US general population: the National Health and Nutrition Examination Survey 2007-2008. Arthritis Rheum. 2011;63(10):3136-41.

CHAPTER 24

Pain Management in Osteoporotic Vertebral Fracture

Sukhil Raina

INTRODUCTION

With the prevalence of osteoporotic fractures on the rise, including vertebral, hip, and wrist fractures, they pose significant challenges due to associated pain and impaired quality of life. Effective pain management not only alleviates suffering but also enhances patient recovery, functional ability, and overall well-being. It has got a crucial role in optimizing outcomes for individuals with osteoporotic fractures. Managing pain in osteoporotic fractures involves a multifaceted approach that aims to alleviate discomfort, promote healing, and improve the patient's overall quality of life.

ASSESSMENT OF PATIENTS WITH OSTEOPOROTIC FRACTURES

Clinical Evaluation
- Identification of fracture location, severity, and associated complications through physical examination and diagnostic imaging
- Assessment of neurological deficits is of paramount importance. Assessment should also include osteoporotic risk factors such as age, sex, family history, previous fractures, glucocorticoid use, smoking, alcohol intake, and low body weight.
- Utilization of validated scales such as the Visual Analog Scale (VAS) and Fracture Risk Assessment Tool (FRAX) is also important for management.

Imaging

- *Vertebral fracture assessment (VFA)*: Performed using X-rays and CT scan (where indicated) imaging to identify vertebral fractures
- Dual-energy X-ray absorptiometry (DXA) is the gold standard for diagnosing osteoporosis and assessing fracture risk. Its indications include:
  - Diagnosis of osteoporosis
  - Monitoring treatment
  - *Risk assessment*:
    - Using bone mineral density (BMD) measurements to estimate the 10-year probability of fractures via tools like FRAX
  - *Screening*:
    - Women aged 65 years and older and men aged 70 years and older, regardless of risk factors
    - Younger postmenopausal women and men aged 50–69 years with clinical risk factors for fracture

Magnetic Resonance Imaging

Magnetic resonance imaging (MRI) is not routinely used for the initial diagnosis of osteoporosis but has specific indications in the context of osteoporotic fractures and osteoporosis pain:

- *Assessment of vertebral fractures*:
  - *Differentiating acute from chronic vertebral fractures*: MRI can show bone edema indicating a recent fracture.
  - Evaluating the integrity of the spinal cord and nerve roots in cases of vertebral compression fractures
- *Detection of nonvertebral fractures*:
  - Diagnosing fractures in complex anatomical regions where X-rays or CT scans are inconclusive
  - Assessing occult fractures, particularly in the hip or pelvis, where patients present with persistent pain but normal X-rays
- *Evaluation of bone marrow*:
  - Identifying marrow pathologies that could contribute to osteoporosis, such as malignancies (e.g., multiple myeloma) or infections (e.g., osteomyelitis)
- *Pain assessment*:
  - Investigating persistent or unexplained pain that may be related to bone lesions, nerve compression, or other soft-tissue abnormalities
  - Useful in cases where pain persists despite normal X-ray findings, helping to identify stress fractures or other subtle pathologies

Laboratory Tests

Serum calcium, phosphate, 25-hydroxyvitamin D, and markers of bone turnover (e.g., C-terminal telopeptide, bone-specific alkaline phosphatase) help in ruling out secondary causes of osteoporosis.

MANAGEMENT OF OSTEOPOROTIC FRACTURES

Management of Pain

Acute Pain

- *Initial bed rest*: It should be as brief as possible as prolonged bed rest exhibits increased comorbidities due to immobilization.
- *Orthotics*: For the treatment of L4 and L5 fractures, lumbosacral orthoses are sufficient. Mid-thoracic to mid-lumbar fractures can be treated with thoracolumbar orthoses.
- *Analgesics*: Nonsteroidal anti-inflammatory drugs (NSAIDs) and acetaminophen are the first-line drugs for mild-to-moderate pain. Opioids may be necessary for severe pain but should be used cautiously.
- *Calcitonin*:
  - It may provide analgesic benefits in acute vertebral fractures, although its use is limited by side effects.
  - It is used in the form of nasal spray or injection.
  - It is generally recommended for short-term use, typically for a duration of up to 4 weeks.
  - Long-term use of calcitonin beyond this period is generally not advised due to potential risks, including hypocalcemia and drug tolerance.

Chronic Pain

Pharmacological Approaches

- *NSAIDs and acetaminophen*:
  - *Antidepressants*: Tricyclic antidepressants and selective serotonin-norepinephrine reuptake inhibitors (SNRIs) for neuropathic pain
  - *Anticonvulsants*: Gabapentin and pregabalin for neuropathic pain management

Nonpharmacological Approaches

- *Physical therapy and rehabilitation*: Emphasize strengthening, stretching, and low-impact aerobic exercises
- Tailored exercise programs to improve balance, strength, and mobility. Weight-bearing and muscle-strengthening exercises are crucial.
- *Fall prevention*: Modifying the home environment, using assistive devices, and reviewing medications to minimize fall risk
- *Lifestyle modifications*: Smoking cessation, moderation of alcohol intake, and ensuring a diet rich in calcium and vitamin D
- *Transcutaneous electrical nerve stimulation (TENS)*:
  - Acupuncture and acupressure

Interventional Procedures

- Local anesthetic injections
- Nerve blocks
- Radiofrequency ablation

- Vertebroplasty and kyphoplasty
- Internal fixation

Surgical Management

Indications for surgery in osteoporotic fractures are:
- Severe pain and disability
- Instability of the fracture
- Neurovascular compromise
- Nonunion or delayed union

MANAGEMENT OF OSTEOPOROSIS

- *Calcium and vitamin D*: Essential for bone health; supplementation is recommended to ensure adequate levels.
- *Bisphosphonates*:
  - *Oral bisphosphonates*: Alendronate, risedronate, and ibandronate
  - *Intravenous bisphosphonates*: Zoledronic acid, ibandronate
  - *Indications*: First-line therapy for most patients with osteoporosis. Particularly useful for patients with a history of fractures or those at a high risk for fractures.
  - *Considerations*: Oral bisphosphonates require strict adherence to dosing instructions to prevent gastrointestinal side effects. Intravenous bisphosphonates may be preferred for patients with gastrointestinal issues or poor adherence to oral therapy.
- *Denosumab*:
  - *Indications*: Alternative to bisphosphonates, especially for patients with renal impairment or those intolerant to bisphosphonates. Administered as a subcutaneous injection every 6 months.
  - *Considerations*: Effective in increasing bone density and reducing fracture risk. Requires ongoing treatment, as discontinuation can lead to rapid bone loss and increased fracture risk.
- *Teriparatide*:
  - *Indications*: Severe osteoporosis, particularly in patients with multiple vertebral fractures or very low bone density. Administered as a daily subcutaneous injection for up to 2 years.
  - *Considerations*: Reserved for patients at a very high risk of fractures. After 2 years of therapy, patients typically transition to an antiresorptive agent (e.g., bisphosphonates or denosumab) to maintain bone density gains.

DECISION-MAKING CRITERIA

- *Severity of osteoporosis and fracture risk*:
  - Patients with mild-to-moderate osteoporosis and fewer fracture risks may start with oral bisphosphonates.
  - Patients with severe osteoporosis or multiple fractures may benefit more from injectable therapies like teriparatide or zoledronic acid.

- *Patient adherence and preferences*:
  - Oral bisphosphonates require strict adherence to dosing schedules and instructions. Patients who may struggle with adherence might benefit from injectable options.
  - Denosumab and zoledronic acid offer less frequent dosing, which can improve adherence.
- *Comorbidities and contraindications*:
  - *Renal function*: Bisphosphonates are contraindicated in patients with severe renal impairment (creatinine clearance <35 mL/min). Denosumab is safer in renal impairment but requires monitoring for hypocalcemia.
  - *Gastrointestinal issues*: Patients with esophageal disorders, gastrointestinal intolerance, or those who have difficulty complying with oral dosing requirements may benefit from intravenous bisphosphonates or subcutaneous denosumab.
  - *History of fractures*: Teriparatide is particularly beneficial for patients with multiple vertebral fractures and extremely low BMD.
- *Previous treatment history*:
  - Patients previously treated with bisphosphonates might benefit from switching to denosumab or teriparatide if their fracture risk remains high or BMD improvement is inadequate.
  - Transition strategies should be considered to maintain or enhance treatment efficacy.

The decision to prescribe a specific osteoporosis treatment involves a comprehensive assessment of the patient's overall health, severity of osteoporosis, fracture risk, comorbid conditions, and treatment preferences. A personalized approach ensures optimal outcomes in reducing fracture risk and enhancing bone health.

The choice between oral or injectable medications and the specific class of drugs depends on several factors, including the severity of the disease, patient comorbidities, preferences, and previous treatment history.

EMERGING THERAPIES

- *Romosozumab*: A monoclonal antibody that inhibits sclerostin, increasing bone formation and decreasing resorption. It has recently been approved for osteoporosis treatment.
- *Stem cell therapy*: Experimental approaches are being investigated to enhance bone regeneration and healing.

MULTIDISCIPLINARY APPROACH TO PAIN MANAGEMENT

- Collaboration between orthopedics, pain specialists, physiotherapists, and psychologists
- Importance of patient education and self-management strategies

- *Psychological support*: Cognitive-behavioral therapy (CBT) to address pain-related anxiety and depression
- Palliative care considerations for advanced cases

CONCLUSION

The management of osteoporotic fractures and associated pain requires a multidisciplinary approach involving pharmacological and nonpharmacological strategies. Adherence to the latest clinical guidelines and evidence-based practices ensures optimal patient outcomes. Early diagnosis, appropriate therapeutic interventions, and preventive measures are key to reducing the burden of osteoporotic fractures and improving patients' quality of life.

BIBLIOGRAPHY

1. Compston J, Cooper A, Cooper C, Davies C, Francis R, Kanis JA, Marsh D, McCloskey EV et al. Diagnosis and management of osteoporosis in postmenopausal women and older men in the UK: National Osteoporosis Guideline Group (NOGG) update 2017. Maturitas. 2017;101:1-16.
2. Cosman F, de Beur SJ, LeBoff MS, Lewiecki EM, Tanner B, Randall S, et al. Clinician's guide to prevention and treatment of osteoporosis. Osteoporos Int. 2014;25(10):2359-81.
3. Kanis JA, McCloskey EV, Johansson H, Cooper C, Rizzoli R, Reginster JY, et al. European guidance for the diagnosis and management of osteoporosis in postmenopausal women. Osteoporos Int. 2013;24(1):23-57.
4. Lems WF, Raterman HG. Critical issues and current challenges in osteoporosis and fracture prevention. An overview of unmet needs. Ther Adv Musculoskelet Dis. 2017;9(12):299-316.
5. Watts NB, Bilezikian JP, Camacho PM, Clarke BL, Harris ST, Hurley DL, et al. American Association of Clinical Endocrinologists and American College of Endocrinology clinical practice guidelines for the diagnosis and treatment of postmenopausal osteoporosis—2016. Endocr Pract. 2016;22(Suppl 4):1-42.

CHAPTER 25

Pain Management in Ankylosing Spondylitis

Sakib Arfee

INTRODUCTION

Ankylosing spondylitis (AS) is diagnosed using *modified New York criteria*. AS diagnosis can be delayed up to 5–6 years and in females the average time of diagnosis can be >10 years. Diagnosis is based on clinical criteria, radiological findings [e.g., sacroiliitis on X-rays or magnetic resonance imaging (MRI)], and presence of human leukocyte antigen B27 (HLA-B27).

CLINICAL CRITERIA

- Low back pain persisting for ≥3 months, reduced by exercise and not relieved by rest
- Limited motion in the lumbar spine in coronal and sagittal planes
- Limited chest expansion compared with normal values for age and sex
- *Radiological criterion*: Grades 3–4 unilateral or grades 2–4 bilateral sacroiliitis
- *Definite AS*: The radiological criterion and ≥1 of clinical criteria are fulfilled.
- *Probable AS*: Three clinical criteria are fulfilled or the radiological criterion alone is fulfilled.

The above-mentioned criteria are adapted from van der Linden S, Valkenburg HA, Cats A. Evaluation of diagnostic criteria for AS. A proposal for modification of the New York criteria. Arthritis Rheum. 1984;27(4):361-8.

MECHANISM OF PAIN IN ANKYLOSING SPONDYLITIS

- *Inflammatory pain:* Chronic enthesitis leads to structural damage and subsequent chronic pain which improves with activity and worsens with rest and inactivity.

- *Mechanical pain:* Certain structural changes in AS lead to the fusion of the spine and various joints, hence altering the biomechanics and resulting in muscle strain, increased joint stress, and altered posture. This change in biomechanics leads to persistent pain in AS.

RADIOLOGICAL AND LABORATORY TESTS

X-rays, MRI, and computed tomography (CT) scans are very crucial for diagnosing AS and for assessment of structural damage. Recent studies report that MRI can diagnose sacroiliitis on average 7.7 years earlier than X-ray imaging. Laboratory tests, e.g., inflammatory markers like erythrocyte sedimentation rate (ESR) and C-reactive protein (CRP), also help in the evaluation of disease activity.

PAIN MANAGEMENT

Nonpharmacological Pain Management

Physical Therapy

Patient education and supervised physical therapy including regular exercises are very effective in relaxing stiff joints and alleviating pain in AS. Physical therapy is a cornerstone of AS management. Recent evidence supports the fact that regular physical activity in AS prevents cardiovascular complications.

Occupational Therapy

Occupational therapy focuses primarily on helping patients with AS to manage and maintain activities of daily living. The therapist helps to reduce spinal and joint strain by providing ergonomic advice, adaptive devices, and various other techniques.

Heat and Cold Therapy

Applying heat using heat pads, warm baths, etc., can relax muscles and reduce stiffness, and cold therapy with ice packs reduces inflammation.

Massage, yoga, and stretching exercises can also provide symptomatic relief and improve overall well-being. Lifestyle modifications and maintaining a good diet and nutrition to keep the body weight within normal limits ultimately reduce stress on joints and the spine.

Pharmacological Pain Management

Nonsteroidal Anti-inflammatory Drugs

Nonsteroidal anti-inflammatory drugs (NSAIDs) are the first-line drugs for the management of pain in AS. Prostaglandin E receptor (PTGER4) is associated with AS and its activation leads to bone resorption. NSAIDs result in inhibition of PGER4 and hence reduce the resorption. It has been well established that regular intake of NSAIDs is associated with better clinical outcomes in terms of progression of disease in comparison to the patients who take them on an SOS basis. NSAIDs reduce inflammation and provide symptomatic relief. Commonly used NSAIDs are naproxen, ibuprofen, and diclofenac. Gastrointestinal, renal, and cardiovascular system (CVS) monitoring is recommended for their long-term use.

Other Medications
Additional analgesics such as acetaminophen and opioids can be used when NSAIDs and biologicals are not giving the expected results. However, with opioids, dependency is the major concern.

Glucocorticoids
Although local glucocorticoid injection can be considered for skeletal muscle inflammation such as enthesitis, systematic administration of steroids is generally not recommended.

Disease-modifying Antirheumatic Drugs
Although the administration of disease-modifying antirheumatic drugs (DMARDs) (e.g., sulfasalazine and methotrexate) is not recommended for axial diseases such as back pain, sulfasalazine is worth considering for the treatment of peripheral arthritis.

Biologicals and Biosimilars
Biological agents are a key treatment option for AS, especially for patients who do not respond adequately to conventional therapies. The current indications for using biological agents in AS based on the latest professional evidence are as follows:
- Inadequate response to NSAIDs
- *Disease activity*: Persistent high disease activity despite treatment with NSAIDs is a primary indication for biological agents. This is typically measured by the Bath Ankylosing Spondylitis Disease Activity Index (BASDAI) score, with a BASDAI score of 4 or higher being a common threshold for initiating biological therapy.
- *Peripheral arthritis*: Biological agents are indicated for patients with AS who also have peripheral arthritis, particularly if they have not responded to conventional DMARDs.
- Extra-articular manifestation
- *Structural damage*: This is particularly relevant if there is a radiographic progression over time.
- *Comorbidities*: Patients with certain comorbid conditions that contraindicate the use of NSAIDs or DMARDs may be candidates for biological therapy.

Types of Biological Agents
- *Tumor necrosis factor (TNF) inhibitors*: The most commonly used biological agents in AS. Examples include:
  - Etanercept
  - Infliximab

- Adalimumab
- Golimumab
- Certolizumab pegol
- *Interleukin-17 (IL-17) inhibitors*: IL-17 inhibitors are an alternative for patients who do not respond to or cannot tolerate TNF inhibitors. Examples include:
  - Secukinumab
  - Ixekizumab

Surgical Management of Pain

Surgical interventions like joint replacement and spine osteotomy along with decompression surgeries can be considered for patients with severe refractory pain and significant functional impairment. These surgeries correct deformities, alleviate pain, and restore functions.

Advances in Pain Management

Janus kinase (JAK) inhibitors and new biologicals show promising results in clinical trials of AS even in refractory cases. Neuromodulation and virtual reality therapy are also being investigated to manage AS.

Finally, AS pain management requires a multifaceted approach including nonpharmacological, pharmacological, and surgical strategies, and orthopedic doctors play a very crucial role in this holistic pain management approach.

CONCLUSION

Managing musculoskeletal pain in renal failure patients requires a careful, multidisciplinary approach. Treatment must balance effective pain relief with the unique challenges posed by impaired kidney function, including altered drug metabolism and potential side effects. Non-pharmacologic methods, such as physical therapy and lifestyle interventions, play a key role alongside cautious medication use. A tailored, patient-centered strategy that includes collaboration among healthcare professionals can improve both pain management and quality of life for these patients.

BIBLIOGRAPHY

1. Braun J, de Keyser F, Brandt J, Mielants H, Sieper J, Veys E. New treatment options in spondyloarthropathies: increasing evidence for significant efficacy of anti-tumour necrosis factor therapy. Curr Opin Rheumatol. 2001;13:245-9.
2. Khan MA. Update on spondyloarthropathies. Ann Intern Med. 2002;136:896-907.
3. van Royen BJ, Dijkmans BAC. Ankylosing Spondylitis: Diagnosis and Management. New York: Taylor & Francis; 2006.
4. Zochling J, Maxwell L, Beardmore J, Boonen A. TNF-alpha inhibitors for ankylosing spondylitis. Cochrane Database Systemic Rev. 2005;3:CD005468.
5. Zochling J, van der Heijde D, Burgos-Vargas R, Collantes E, Davis Jr JC, Dijkmans B, et al. ASAS/EULAR recommendations for the management of ankylosing spondylitis. Ann Rheum Dis. 2006;65:442-52.

CHAPTER 26

Sports Injury

Neha Sharma, Suraydev Aman Singh

■ INTRODUCTION

Pain management in sports injuries is a critical component of recovery, allowing athletes to regain function and return to their sport as quickly as possible. Sports injuries, such as sprains, strains, fractures, and contusions, can lead to acute or chronic pain, affecting both physical performance and overall well-being. Effective pain management strategies aim to reduce discomfort, control inflammation, and promote healing, often using a combination of pharmacological treatments, like nonsteroidal anti-inflammatory drugs (NSAIDs), injectables and nonpharmacological approaches, such as rest, physical therapy, and rehabilitation.

■ DEFINITION

The International Olympic Committee (IOC) defines a sports injury as a new or recurring musculoskeletal complaint that arises during competition or training and requires medical attention. The approach to pain management in sports injuries varies between acute traumatic injuries and chronic pain conditions.

■ ACUTE PAIN

Acute sports injuries have become more prevalent due to the high demands of athletic performance and increased participation in sports by older adults. The management of acute sports injuries begins with nonpharmacological methods, progressing to pharmacological treatments if needed.

Minor injuries can often be managed at home using the RICE protocol:
- *Rest*: Immobilize the injured area to facilitate healing.
- *Ice*: Apply ice to reduce swelling and pain.

- *Compression*: Wrap the injury to support it, but ensure that it does not impair blood circulation.
- *Elevation*: Keep the injured area elevated above the heart level to reduce swelling and pain.

Pharmacological options for noninvasive treatment include:
- NSAIDs, both topical and systemic, which can be nonselective or selective cyclooxygenase-2 (COX-2) inhibitors
- Non-narcotic analgesics and skeletal muscle relaxants
- Narcotic analgesics for severe pain with a high risk of bleeding

Mini-invasive pharmacological approaches include intralesional injections of local anesthetics, corticosteroids, and hyaluronic acid (HA) (viscosupplements). Effective pain management in athletes should aim to reduce pain while minimizing downtime from activity. Other modalities include physical therapy techniques such as traction, bracing, electrical and ultrasonic stimulation, and therapeutic exercises. A tailored, multidisciplinary approach involving temporary activity cessation, pain management, physical therapy, and rehabilitation is recommended for managing sports-related musculoskeletal injuries.

CHRONIC PAIN

Managing chronic pain begins with nonpharmacological strategies, such as optimizing sleep and nutrition and addressing contributing factors from activities, psychosocial elements, or biological issues. Pharmacological treatments for chronic pain include:
- NSAIDs and non-narcotic analgesics on an "as-needed" basis
- Antidepressants, including tricyclic amines (amitriptyline, nortriptyline) and serotonin–norepinephrine reuptake inhibitors (SNRIs) (duloxetine)
- Anticonvulsants such as pregabalin and gabapentin

PHARMACOLOGICAL MANAGEMENT

- *Paracetamol*: It is commonly used for mild-to-moderate pain, alone or in combination with other treatments. Safe up to 3-4 g/day.
- *NSAIDs*: These are widely prescribed for sports injuries. Concerns exist regarding their anti-inflammatory effects potentially hindering tissue healing. Ketorolac, a potent NSAID is commonly used for short term pain management of moderate to severe pain but due to its significant side effects that includes gastrointestinal bleeding, renal impairment and cardiovascular events, it's use is typically recommended for short term use (not more than 5 days). Topical NSAIDs like diclofenac and ketoprofen are recommended before systemic NSAIDs.
- *Opioids*: These are reserved for severe pain and high-risk bleeding, with initial prescriptions not exceeding 5 days to prevent dependence or

addiction. Intravenous morphine is recommended for major trauma in adults in hospital or prehospital settings without affecting coagulation.
- *Topical analgesics*: These are suitable for mild sprains and strains, often containing substances like methyl salicylate, eucalyptus, menthol, capsicum, and camphor. They should not be applied to broken skin to avoid irritation and dermatitis.

INTRALESIONAL INJECTABLES

Intralesional injectables are used in both acute and chronic sports-related injuries. These mini-invasive procedures include:
- *Local anesthetic injections*: Ensure early return to activity
- *Corticosteroid injections*: Effective for chronic pain, but not fully supported for acute injuries due to potential interference with tissue healing
- *HA injections*: Effective and safe for treating joint pain in athletes, with evidence suggesting that they may reduce recovery time

REHABILITATION

Rehabilitation is crucial alongside pharmacological treatments to manage acute and chronic musculoskeletal pain, prevent deconditioning, and enhance physical performance. It should be initiated early, even in acute trauma stages, to optimize physical function and quality of life on returning to activity.

CONCLUSION

A well-rounded, individualized and multidisciplinary management plan that includes brief abstinence from activity, pain management, physical therapy and rehabilitation helps athletes avoid complications, reduces the risk of chronic pain, and facilitates a quicker and safer recover ultimately enhancing long-term performance and well-being.

BIBLIOGRAPHY

1. Buelt A, Narducci DM. Osteoarthritis management: updated guidelines from the American College of Rheumatology and Arthritis Foundation. Am Fam Physician. 2021;103(2):120-1.
2. McAlindon TE, Bannuru RR, Sullivan MC, Arden NK, Berenbaum F, Bierma-Zeinstra SM, et al. OARSI guidelines for the non-surgical management of knee osteoarthritis. Osteoarthritis Cartilage. 2014;22:363-88.
3. National Clinical Guideline Centre. Osteoarthritis: Care and Management in Adults. London, UK: National Institute for Health and Care Excellence; 2014.

CHAPTER 27

Approach to Management of Low Backache in Adults

Bias Dev

INTRODUCTION

Low back pain (LBP) is a leading cause of disability and poses a significant economic burden due to healthcare costs and loss of productivity. This ailment of mankind is the second most common after common cold and is a symptom originating out of several conditions from different organs needing proper evaluation. Effective management of LBP involves a multifaceted approach that includes accurate diagnosis, appropriate treatment, and preventive strategies.

For ease of understanding, the causes of low backache are grouped as spondylogenic (those originating from the spine) and nonspondylogenic (those having their source of pain in organs other than the spine).

SPONDYLOGENIC CAUSES

In the spine, the causes could be the pathologies of soft tissue, osseous components, or both. The degenerative disc disease passes through different stages, pathologies of the contents of the spinal canal, and acute or chronic trauma causing acute fractures or vertebral fractures in osteoporotic patients, respectively. Infective, inflammatory, instability, and tumorous (benign, primary malignant, and secondary) are the common pathologies presenting in patients with backache, and each of them will have different clinical presentations needing a history in detail, clinical examination, and supporting laboratory and radiological investigations.

The acute prolapsed intervertebral disc invariably is associated with an event like lifting, bending, and turning of the back. It may be associated with leg pain which increases with any activity increasing the pressure like coughing and sneezing. The radicular symptoms are dermatomal in presentation, and specific levels can be identified with clinical assessment.

Disc degeneration results in pain that is aggravated by activities in a position for a long period which may be partially relieved by changing position. When the origin of pain is from a prolapsed disc, the pain may become worse by sitting, bending, lifting, and straining, and there can be associated radicular pain as well as sensory and motor symptoms. Pain from facets will be more on extension of the back.

Tubercular infections are more common than other pyogenic infections and will have an insidious onset with constitutional symptoms of loss of weight, loss of appetite, and low-grade fever. Often, these patients may have deformity over the back and neurological deficits and swellings (cold abscess). The pyogenic infections will have a short history and will be associated with high-grade fever. *Salmonella* and *Brucella* infections also need to be kept in mind while suspecting infective pathologies. The pain in such patients is usually worse at night and at rest. History of infection elsewhere, immunocompromise, diabetes, and poor nutritional status are often associated with infections of the spine.

Exposure to some kind of trauma will be present in case of vertebral fractures in normal healthy individuals, whereas the osteoporotic patients may or may not relate the pain to any significant trauma. In osteoporotic patients, a ride on an uneven road may be sufficient to cause a pathological fracture which may present as a low backache. Multiple myeloma and osteoclastic secondaries are other common causes of pathological vertebral fractures.

Ankylosing spondylitis starts by the third decade of life and the patient presents with morning stiffness of the back. Bilateral sacroiliac joint involvement is the earliest and most common presentation. As the disease progresses, the whole spine may get stiff along with the involvement of the hips and shoulder and pulmonary compromise. Facet joint involvement and subsequent instability of the atlantoaxial joint and subaxial subluxations in rheumatoid arthritis of long duration. In inflammatory conditions, there will be morning pain along with stiffness which gradually wanes off as the day passes. It is associated with a gradual increase in stiffness. Other joints may have simultaneous stiffness and pain. Other extraspinal manifestations may be present as inflammatory bowel disease. Spondyloarthropathies have a strong genetic association.

The vertebra is the most common site to have secondaries from primary tumors of the thyroid, breast, lungs, liver, ovaries, and prostate. The majority of these secondaries is osteoclastic. The osteoblastic secondaries are from the prostate. The space-occupying lesions in the spinal canal can be extradural, intradural, extramedullary, and intramedullary, and the lesions could be benign or malignant growths, tuberculomas, or internal gibbus formed secondary to a vertebral body collapse. The pathologies outside the dura are slow to present, whereas the pathologies beneath the dura are rapidly progressive and the intramedullary pathologies are invariably associated with rapidly progressive neurological deficit. A patient with malignant tumors has night or rest pain if there is vertebral destruction. The pain may increase with activity as well and will be associated with constitutional symptoms.

NONSPONDYLOTIC CAUSES

The contents of the abdominal cavity, pelvis, retroperitoneal structures, thoracic cavity, and brain can be sources of the pain in the back. In these nonspondylotic causes, whenever there is a backache, symptoms related to the primary organ have to be present along with back pain. Unlike in spondylogenic pain, non-spondylogenic is not affected by activity and does not relieved by rest. Aortic aneurysm may present boring, deep-seated lumbar pain unrelated to activity. The claudication of peripheral disease may mimic neurogenic claudication of lumbar canal stenosis where the patient will need to sit to relieve the symptoms in comparison with vascular claudication where symptoms will decrease with standing still for some time. Neuropathies and myopathies also need to be ruled out, especially when low backache is associated with loss of sensation and weakness. The pathologies of the hip joint and sacroiliac joint can also present as low back and thigh pain and can mimic pathologies of the spine.

PSYCHOSOMATIC BACK PAIN

Patients with these pains are overtly strained and tense. The significant finding is tense, firm, and tender muscles. There is no nerve root involvement.

PSYCHOGENIC BACK PAIN

Patients with psychogenic pain are emotionally ill. These patients have a preceding history of emotional trouble. In the patient's history, emotional components can be reached out and the patient is convinced that he or she is ill. The important finding in such patients will be the paucity of findings on physical examination.

MECHANICAL BACKACHE

Despite having so many causes of backache, the most common backache does not have any particular structural cause. Mechanical pain is usually more common in females especial in their third decade of life and also in females with pendulous abdomen, obesity and with anemia. There is no structural abnormality evident on radiographs and, generally, they respond well to exercises and nutritional supplements. These patients have a characteristic history of morning pain on coming out of bed which lasts for some time. This is sharp pain of muscle spasm which gets relieved with activity. A dull aching pain of fatigue reappears after a pain-free duration which gets relieved only with rest. Patients with mechanical backache do not have any other symptom related to leg pain or any constitutional symptom.

LEG PAIN

Leg pain is often commonly associated with back pain and different conditions that can produce leg pain are:
- *Intraspinal conditions*:
  - Proximal to disc, conus, and cauda equina lesions (e.g., neurofibroma, ependymoma)
  - At the disc level, herniated nucleus pulposus, central and lateral stenosis
  - Infections (vertebral osteomyelitis, discitis) and inflammation (arachnoiditis)
  - Neoplasms (benign or malignant causing root irritation)
- *Extraspinal causes*:
  - Peripheral vascular disease, gynecological disorders
  - Hip pathologies like avascular necrosis and osteoarthritis of the hip and sacroiliac joint diseases
  - Peripheral nerve diseases like neuropathies, conditions causing pressure over the sciatic nerve like piriformis syndrome, inadvertent injection in the vicinity of the sciatic nerve or tumor, as well as herpes zoster

RED FLAG SITUATIONS

Some conditions are considered red flag situations as they will warrant urgent care. Identifying red flag conditions is to rule out serious underlying conditions that require immediate attention. These include:
- *Unexplained weight loss*: May indicate malignancy
- *Fever and chills*: Possible signs of infection
- *Neurological deficits*: Weakness, numbness, or bowel/bladder dysfunction, which could suggest cauda equina syndrome
- *History of trauma*: Consider fractures or structural damage.
- *Age*: LBP in patients younger than 20 years or older than 60 years

ALERTS AS PER AGE

Certain conditions are associated with age in infancy and adolescence, and vertebral osteomyelitis, osteoid osteoma in adolescents, spondylolysis, and Scheuermann disease are to be considered. In young and middle age group, disc degeneration and spondyloarthropathies need to be suspected. In older adults, an individual having no history of pain if presents with backache of sudden onset needs to be suspected of having a tumor. The most common tumor would be metastasis. Infections and osteoporotic fractures are other causes of back pain in this age group.

ASSESSMENT AND DIAGNOSIS

The initial step in managing is a thorough clinical evaluation. This includes taking a proper history especially concerning pain, its onset, duration, radiation, and aggravating and relieving factors. There has to be emphasis on looking for any of the red flags.

A comprehensive physical examination should include: Inspecting posture and gait and looking for any visible deformities. On palpation, identify tender points and muscle spasms. Assess flexibility, range of motion, and pain on movement followed by neurological examination and check for motor strength, sensory deficits, and reflexes.

Special Tests

Straight leg raise (SLR): For lumbar radiculopathy and for nerve tension. A quick examination of hip joint should be done by performing simple clinical signs like FABER (Flexion, Abduction and External Rotation; Patrick's) test to differentiate hip pathology from spinal issues.

Laboratory Tests

In cases with suspected infection, malignancy, or inflammatory conditions, complete blood count (CBC) to detect infection or anemia, erythrocyte sedimentation rate (ESR), and C-reactive protein (CRP) are markers of inflammation.

Specific Tests

For conditions like ankylosing spondylitis, human leukocyte antigen B27 (HLA-B27) needs to undertaken. If the tissue/pus is available from cold abscess, then it needs to be subjected to GeneXpert/cartridge-based nucleic acid amplification test (CBNAAT) and for culture.

Imaging and Diagnostic Tests

Imaging should be reserved for cases where red flags are present or conservative treatment has failed. Appropriate imaging modalities include:
- *X-ray*: Useful for detecting fractures, severe degenerative changes, or structural abnormalities and instabilities
- *Magnetic resonance imaging (MRI)*: Preferred for evaluating soft-tissue structures, such as intervertebral discs, spinal cord, and nerves
- *Computed tomography (CT) scan*: An alternative to MRI, especially when MRI is contraindicated. CT is a good tool to reach out to cervicodorsal and occipitocervical areas where normal radiographs do not give adequate information.

MANAGEMENT

Nonpharmacological Interventions
- *Education and reassurance*:
  - *Patient education*: Informing patients about the benign nature of most low backache cases and encouraging them to maintain a positive outlook. Patients are advised to stay active and avoid prolonged bed rest, which can delay recovery.
- *Physical therapy*:
  - *Exercise programs*: Supervised exercises focusing on strengthening, flexibility, and aerobic conditioning. Evidence supports structured exercise regimens in reducing pain and improving function.
- *Behavioral therapy*:
  - *Cognitive-behavioral therapy (CBT)*: Effective in managing chronic pain by altering pain perceptions and improving coping strategies
  - *Mindfulness-based stress reduction (MBSR)*: Techniques to manage pain and improve quality of life

Pharmacological Treatment
- *First-line medications*:
  - *Nonsteroidal anti-inflammatory drugs (NSAIDs)*: Effective for pain relief and inflammation reduction. Consideration of patient-specific contraindications is necessary.
- *Second-line medications*:
  - *Muscle relaxants*: For short-term relief in acute settings
  - *Opioids*: Limited use in severe pain unresponsive to other treatments, with caution to avoid dependence
- *Adjuvant medications*:
  - *Antidepressants*: Such as tricyclic antidepressants (TCAs) and serotonin–norepinephrine reuptake inhibitors (SNRIs) for chronic pain management
  - *Anticonvulsants*: Such as gabapentin and pregabalin for neuropathic pain

Interventional Procedures
For patients with persistent pain despite conservative measures, interventional procedures may be considered:
- *Epidural steroid injections*:
  - Useful for radicular pain, providing short-term relief by reducing inflammation around nerve roots
- *Selective nerve root blocks*:
  - Selective nerve root blocks address radicular pain by delivering drugs at the root–disc interface. Approximately 50% of patients with radicular pain can have good pain relief through it.

- *Facet joint injections and medial branch blocks*:
  - Diagnostic and therapeutic interventions for facet joint pain

Surgical Options

Surgery is reserved for cases with specific indications such as severe neurological deficits, cauda equina syndrome, or structural abnormalities unresponsive to conservative treatment:
- *Discectomy*: For herniated discs causing radicular pain or neurological deficits. Discectomy is commonly done through fenestration which does not create any instability and thus the patient can be mobilized out of bed as and when he/she is comfortable.
- *Laminotomies/extended fenestration/laminectomies/with or without fusion*: These procedures can be undertaken for spinal stenosis, for relieving pressure on the spinal cord or nerves, and in case there is instability, the unstable segments have to be fused through posterior as well as anterior instrumentation.

Multidisciplinary Approach for Managing Back Pain

Chronic LBP often requires a multidisciplinary approach involving various healthcare professionals like pain specialists, psychologists, occupational therapists, physiotherapists, and surgeons.

LATEST EVIDENCE AND RECOMMENDATIONS

Recent guidelines and studies highlight several key points in the management of back pain:
- *Early mobilization*:
  - Encouraging patients to stay active and avoid bed rest, which can exacerbate pain and prolong recovery
- *Mind-body interventions*:
  - Incorporating techniques such as mindfulness and yoga, which have shown benefits in managing chronic LBP
- *Personalized treatment plans*:
  - Tailoring interventions based on individual patient profiles, considering comorbidities, preferences, and responses to previous treatments

CONCLUSION

Managing LBP effectively requires a comprehensive, evidence-based approach that integrates patient education, appropriate use of pharmacological and nonpharmacological treatments, and consideration of psychological and social factors. Early identification of serious conditions, personalized treatment plans, and a multidisciplinary approach are essential for improving patient outcomes and quality of life. In endemic areas, patients need to be screened to rule out infective processes to pick up caries spine at the earliest. Despite many causes of backache, mechanical backache is still the most common which has to be diagnosed with a history and responds well to treatment.

BIBLIOGRAPHY

1. Chou R, Deyo R, Friedly J, Skelly A, Weimer M, Fu R, et al. Nonpharmacologic therapies for low back pain: a systematic review for an American College of Physicians clinical practice guideline. Ann Intern Med. 2016;166(7):493-505.
2. Foster NE, Anema JR, Cherkin D, Chou R, Cohen SP, Gross DP, et al. Prevention and treatment of low back pain: evidence, challenges, and promising directions. Lancet. 2018;391(10137):2368-83.
3. Oliveira CB, Maher CG, Pinto RZ, Traeger AC, Lin CC, Chenot JF, et al. Clinical practice guidelines for the management of non-specific low back pain in primary care: an updated overview. Eur Spine J. 2018;27(11):2791-803.
4. Qaseem A, Wilt TJ, McLean RM, Forciea MA. Noninvasive treatments for acute, subacute, and chronic low back pain: a clinical practice guideline from the American College of Physicians. Ann Intern Med. 2017;166(7):514-30.

CHAPTER 28

Pain Management of Osteoarthritis

Suraydev Aman Singh

■ INTRODUCTION

Management of osteoarthritis (OA) pain often requires a multimodal approach; however, it can be broadly categorized into the following:
- Nonpharmacological
- Pharmacological
- Intra-articular injections
- Surgery

■ NONPHARMACOLOGICAL

Exercise and Self-management Programs

The recent guidelines from the American College of Rheumatology and Arthritis Foundation (ACR/AF) recommend exercises, comprising muscle strengthening around joints and general aerobic conditioning and self-management activities, such as using activity trackers, cognitive–behavioral therapy, and goal setting, as first-line treatment for OA.

Weight Loss

It is estimated that even a slight (5%) reduction of body weight in obese patients provides a notable improvement in pain, presumably by reducing biomechanical stress on weight-bearing joints.

Thermotherapy

Cryotherapy causes vasoconstriction of blood vessels and blockade of nerve impulses, thereby alleviating pain. Alternatively, heat therapy helps by relaxing muscles and increasing blood circulation to the applied area. Thermotherapy is easily implemented and a relatively safe recommendation as an adjunctive therapy. The ACR/AF guidelines recommend thermotherapy for symptomatic management as a part of a holistic approach along with other modalities with modest benefits in pain relief and function from both hot and cold therapies.

Foot Orthoses and Bracing

Laterally wedged insoles can be considered in the treatment of medial knee OA because of their potential to reduce the knee adduction moment and hence offloading medial knee. Similarly, knee bracing by unloading of medial compartment and also through general biomechanical and neuromuscular effects leads to improved proprioception and joint stability, and is often recommended by ACR/AF and Osteoarthritis Research Society International (OARSI) guidelines as adjunctive treatment.

PHARMACOLOGICAL

Pharmacological therapies include:
- Acetaminophen
- Nonsteroidal anti-inflammatory drugs (NSAIDs)
- Opioids
- Chondroprotective agents
- Topical capsaicin
- Flexiseq gel
- Centrally acting drugs [such as antidepressants, and particularly serotonin-norepinephrine reuptake inhibitors (SNRIs)]

Topical Capsaicin and Flexiseq

Capsaicin acting via selective depression of type C nociceptive fibers has been well tolerated and hence recommended for adjunctive pain management in OA. On the other hand, Flexiseq gel contains phospholipid vesicles that provide lubrication to minimize friction between cartilage and can be used along with other topical agents.

Chondroprotective Agents

Glucosamine and chondroitin are two of the most popular dietary supplements marketed for the effective improvement of joint health and hence presumably improve the symptoms of OA.

These may be beneficial for some individuals with mild-to-moderate OA. However, the evidence on their efficacy is mixed; hence, the recent guidelines do not strongly endorse these agents for symptomatic management of OA.

INTRA-ARTICULAR INJECTIONS

Intra-articular Corticosteroids

Rarely used for rapid and significant short-term pain control due to their anti-inflammatory effect, recent guidelines from OARSI and ACR/AF conditionally recommend intra-articular corticosteroids (IACs) after considering the due risk/benefit with their effectiveness varying up to 26 weeks. However, they are indicated only where the patient is not fit or willing for surgery or at times to manage severe flare of OA.

Intra-articular Hyaluronic Acid

Hyaluronic acid, a polysaccharide found naturally in synovial fluid, promotes shock absorption and lubrication. The reduced concentration of hyaluronic acid results in low-viscosity synovial fluid in patients with OA and hence increased cartilage loading. Recent literature recommends hyaluronic acid as an effective alternative to corticosteroids, due to its better safety profile and longer duration of action. However, there is no conclusive evidence to support its use.

SURGERY

Patients whose function and mobility remain compromised despite maximal medical therapy should be considered for surgical intervention. Joint replacement surgery is performed to produce a painless, mobile joint; compartment unloading osteotomies should be considered for severe diseases significantly affecting the quality of life of patients.

CONCLUSION

Effective pain management in osteoarthritis requires a comprehensive approach that combines pharmacological treatments, lifestyle modifications, and non-pharmacological interventions.

Understanding the underlying mechanisms of pain in osteoarthritis helps guide treatment decisions tailored to each patient. A multimodal approach, including medications, physical therapy, weight management, and patient education, is essential for improving quality of life and reducing disability. Collaboration between healthcare providers and patients is crucial for long term success in managing pain and enhancing function in osteoarthritis.

BIBLIOGRAPHY

1. Bannuru RR, Osani MC, Vaysbrot EE, Arden NK, Bennell K, Bierma-Zeinstra SMA, et al. OARSI guidelines for the non-surgical management of knee, hip, and polyarticular osteoarthritis. Osteoarthritis Cartilage. 2019;27(11):1578-89.
2. Conaghan PG, Porcheret M, Kingsbury SR, Gammon A, Soni A, Hurley M, et al. Impact and therapy of osteoarthritis: the Arthritis Care OA Nation 2012 survey. Clin Rheumatol. 2013;32(8):1124-30.
3. Felson DT, Neogi T. Osteoarthritis: is it a disease of cartilage or of bone? Arthritis Rheumatol. 2023;75(3):521-8.
4. Hunter DJ, Bierma-Zeinstra S. Osteoarthritis. Lancet. 2023;392(10155):1745-59.
5. Kolasinski SL, Neogi T, Hochberg MC, Oatis C, Guyatt G, Block J, et al. 2019 American College of Rheumatology/Arthritis Foundation guideline for the management of osteoarthritis of the hand, hip, and knee. Arthritis Rheumatol. 2020;72(2):220-33.

CHAPTER 29

Pain Management of Cervical Spondylosis

Suraydev Aman Singh, Zubair Ahmad Lone, Shubam Surmal

■ INTRODUCTION

Cervical spondylosis, a degenerative condition affecting the cervical spine, is prevalent among middle-aged and elderly individuals. It results from age-related changes in the intervertebral discs and vertebrae, leading to symptoms ranging from neck pain and stiffness to neurological deficits. Effective management is crucial for improving patients' quality of life.

■ DIAGNOSIS

Clinical Evaluation

Diagnosis begins with a thorough clinical evaluation, including patient history and physical examination. Common symptoms include neck pain, stiffness, radiculopathy, and myelopathy. Neurological examination focuses on detecting signs of nerve compression or spinal cord involvement. Meanwhile, it is extremely important to rule out any infection, especially tuberculosis or any other sinister pathology.

■ INVESTIGATIONS

Imaging

Radiographic imaging, including X-rays, magnetic resonance imaging (MRI), and computed tomography (CT) scans, plays a pivotal role in diagnosing cervical spondylosis. MRI is particularly useful for assessing soft-tissue structures, nerve roots, and spinal cord, while CT scans provide detailed bony anatomy (if and when indicated).

Have a low threshold for getting inflammatory markers done, when there is any suspicion of an underlying infectious pathology.

CONSERVATIVE MANAGEMENT

Pharmacological Treatment

Nonsteroidal anti-inflammatory drugs (NSAIDs) are the first line of treatment for pain management. Muscle relaxants and short-term corticosteroids may be used for acute exacerbations. Gabapentin and pregabalin are effective for neuropathic pain.

Non-pharmacological Treatment

Physical Therapy

Physical therapy is essential for managing cervical spondylosis. Evidence supports the use of specific exercises to improve neck mobility and strengthen cervical muscles. Manual therapy, including mobilization and manipulation, can also be beneficial when performed by trained professionals.

Cervical Traction

Pain relief: Cervical traction can help relieve pain by stretching the neck muscles and separating the disc and joint spaces in the cervical spine. This can reduce nerve root compression and improve range of motion.
- It can be applied in home or clinical setting. It can be applied manually by a therapist or by using mechanical devices at home or in a clinical setting.
- *Duration and frequency*: Should be prescribed by a healthcare professional, considering an individual patient needs and response

Cervical Collar

A cervical collar can provide temporary support and immobilization to reduce pain and prevent further injury by limiting neck movement.

It is recommended for short-term use only, as prolonged use can lead to muscle weakening and stiffness.

Rest

Rest can help alleviate acute pain and inflammation by reducing physical stress on the cervical spine. It should be balanced with activity, as prolonged rest can lead to deconditioning and worsening symptoms. Gradual return to activity is important.

Arm Sling

An arm sling can help reduce pain radiating to the arm by limiting movement and providing support, especially if there is significant radiculopathy (nerve pain). It is used temporarily during acute exacerbations to relieve symptoms.

Lifestyle Modifications

Encouraging patients to maintain an active lifestyle, perform neck-strengthening exercises, and adopt ergonomic practices can significantly alleviate symptoms and prevent progression.

Interventional Procedures

Injections should be considered after other noninvasive measures, such as medications and physical therapy, have failed, but before surgery is considered.

These work by directly delivering the drug to the target area that generates pain and hence provide rapid and better relief than oral medications. Commonly administered ones include trigger point injections, epidural injections with steroids, selective nerve root blocks, facet joint injections, medial branch blocks, and radiofrequency ablation (RFA).

Radiofrequency Ablation

Radiofrequency ablation of the medial branches innervating the facet joints can be effective for patients with facet joint–related pain. This minimally invasive procedure provides sustained pain relief by denaturing nerve fibers.

SURGICAL MANAGEMENT

Indications

Surgical intervention is considered for patients with severe or progressive neurological deficits, intractable pain, or significant myelopathy. Indications include spinal cord compression, severe radiculopathy, and instability.

Surgical Techniques

- *Anterior cervical discectomy and fusion (ACDF)*: It is the most common surgical procedure for cervical spondylosis. It involves removing the degenerated disc and fusing the adjacent vertebrae to stabilize the spine.
- *Cervical disc replacement (CDR)*: It is an alternative to fusion, aiming to preserve motion at the affected segment. Recent studies suggest comparable outcomes to ACDF with potential benefits in maintaining cervical motion.
- *Posterior cervical decompression*: For patients with multilevel cervical spondylosis and myelopathy, posterior approaches such as laminectomy or laminoplasty are effective in decompressing the spinal cord.

REHABILITATION AND FOLLOW-UP

Postoperative rehabilitation is crucial for optimal recovery. A tailored rehabilitation program focusing on neck stabilization, range-of-motion exercises, and gradual return to activities is recommended. Regular follow-up ensures early detection of complications and monitors long-term outcomes.

CONCLUSION

Management of cervical spondylosis requires a multifaceted approach, incorporating conservative, interventional, and surgical strategies based on the severity of symptoms and radiographic findings. Ongoing research continues to refine these strategies, aiming to improve patient outcomes and quality of life.

BIBLIOGRAPHY

1. Hurwitz EL, Carragee EJ, Van Der Velde G, Carroll LJ, Nordin M, Guzman J, et al. Treatment of neck pain: noninvasive interventions: results of the Bone and Joint Decade 2000–2010 Task Force on Neck Pain and its Associated Disorders. Spine. 2008;33(4S):S123-52.
2. Joaquim AF, Riew KD, Radcliff K, Patel AA, Hilibrand AS. Cervical disc arthroplasty—how much do we know? Neurosurg Focus. 2015;39(3):E1.
3. Merskey H, Bogduk N. Classification of Chronic Pain: Descriptions of Chronic Pain Syndromes and Definitions of Pain Terms. Washington, DC: IASP Press; 1994.
4. Provenzano DA, King ST. The efficacy of radiofrequency procedures for chronic pain: a narrative review. Curr Pain Headache Rep. 2012;16:7-13.
5. Wong JJ, Côté P, Quesnele JJ, Stern PJ, Mior SA. The course and prognostic factors of symptomatic cervical spine degeneration. Spine J. 2012;12(10):855-68.

CHAPTER 30

Approach to Management of Shoulder Pain

Gagandeep Singh Raina

INTRODUCTION

Shoulder pain can manifest during movement or persist continuously. Its duration may vary, necessitating professional evaluation and care. The major causes of shoulder pain and disability include rotator cuff disorders, joint disease, and referred neck pain. Rotator cuff tendinopathy was identified in 85% of these patients. However, many of these patients have multiple shoulder issues and their combinations like acromioclavicular (AC) disease and frozen shoulder (6%).

APPROACH TO PATIENTS WITH SHOULDER PATHOLOGY

History
- Assess for pain, swelling, or restricted movement.
- Inquire about onset, duration, nature, and progression of symptoms.
- Identify whether it is dominant or nondominant side.
- Ask when does the pain occur, at rest or during movement, and about the duration of the pain.
- History of night pains or fever
- Ask about pain in any other region like the neck, upper back, chest, or upper limb.
- Inquire about any episode of acute trauma or any old injury which may have resulted in pain or instability of the shoulder joint.
- Ask about the patient's occupation and any other physical activities, e.g., sports.
- Assess whether other joints are affected.
- Look for constitutional symptoms.
- Note any diurnal variation in symptoms.

Examination
- Inspect the neck, upper back, chest wall, and axillary area.
- Check the range of motion of the neck.
- Examine both the shoulders for any pain, swelling, deformity, and wasting of muscles.
- Palpate the joint for tenderness, swelling, raised temperature, and any crepitus.
- Compare the strength, stability, and degree of movement (active, passive, resisted) of both shoulders.
- Check for any pain while making an arc.
- Perform special tests like Neer's impingement, empty can, drop arm, lift-off, Duga's, apprehension (anterior and posterior), drawer (anterior and posterior), Yergason's, and speed tests.

Imaging
- *X-rays:* Two views are done—an anteroposterior (AP) view in plane of the joint and an axillary view. The AC joint is best viewed in AP view tilted up by 20°.
- *Ultrasound:* It is effective for identifying calcific tendinitis, biceps tendon pathology, and rotator cuff tears. It also aids in guided intra-articular injections and procedures.
- *Computed tomography (CT):* It is useful for surgical planning, particularly for shoulder replacement or fracture surgeries
- *Magnetic resonance imaging (MRI):* It provides detailed information on rotator cuff pathology, tear location and size, fatty infiltration, and the anatomy of the joint and surrounding structures. MRI can also identify instability-related anomalies and osteonecrosis of the humeral head and diagnosing and staging of any tumor.
- *Magnetic resonance arthrography:* It is highly sensitive and specific for detecting pathological labral conditions and rotator cuff partial undersurface tears
- *Arthroscopy:* It is useful for diagnosing and treating intra-articular lesions, labral and capsular detachments, any impinging structure, or split in the rotator cuff. Arthroscopy is the best way of identifying the SLAP (superior labrum, anterior, and posterior) lesions.

CAUSES OF SHOULDER PAIN

Traumatic Shoulder Pain
- Rotator cuff tears
- Fractures or dislocations around the shoulder girdle
- Nerve injury including brachial plexus injury

Chronic Shoulder Pain
- Chronic rotator cuff tear
- Adhesive capsulitis
- Subacromial impingement (bursitis)
- AC joint arthritis
- Calcific tendinitis
- Glenohumeral joint arthritis
- Referred pain, including neck musculoskeletal pathology, myocardial ischemia, and referred diaphragmatic pain

PAIN WITH RED FLAG INDICATORS
- Deformity or a swelling without any evident cause
- Signs of infection like redness of the skin or elevated local or body temperature
- Loss of rotation and normal contour with a history of epilepsy or electric shock may be due to an unreduced dislocation.
- Other causes like fibromyalgia and polymyalgia rheumatica

TREATMENT

Rotator Cuff Tears
- *Minor tears:* Rest, analgesics, anti-inflammatory medications, and physiotherapy
- *Large tears:* Surgical intervention, usually through arthroscopic or open rotator cuff tendon repair

Chronic Disorders
- *Rotator cuff tears/bursitis*:
  - Nonsteroidal anti-inflammatory drugs (NSAIDs) and physiotherapy aimed at optimizing shoulder function
  - Subacromial corticosteroid injections for short-term pain relief and improved function
- *Calcific tendinitis*:
  - NSAIDs and/or steroids
  - Physical therapy
  - Aspiration/lavage
  - Nonresponding patients may need surgery for the removal of calcium deposits.
- *Joint disorders*:
  - *Adhesive capsulitis:* NSAIDs, pendulum exercises, and possibly manipulation under anesthesia or arthroscopic capsular release

- *AC arthritis:* Rest, simple analgesia, slings, and physiotherapy
- *Humeral head degeneration:* Physiotherapy, pain relief, NSAIDs, corticosteroid injections, and potentially shoulder arthroplasty or joint fusion for nonresponsive cases

Muscle Strains

Treatment includes rest, ice/heat compression, elevation, massage, NSAIDs, and physiotherapy.

Referred Pain

Diagnose, evaluate, and treat the underlying cause.

Musculoskeletal Tumors

Investigation should be done through clinical evaluation, radiology, and biopsy to determine the type and extent of the lesion, followed by appropriate surgical planning (excision, radical excision, salvage, or amputation).

CONCLUSION

Effective management of shoulder pain requires a comprehensive, patient-specific approach. This includes accurate diagnosis through clinical evaluation and imaging, followed by tailored interventions like physical therapy, medication, or injections. Minimally invasive techniques, such as corticosteroid injections or arthroscopy, are often preferred. For chronic or severe cases, surgical options may be considered. Early intervention and patient education on posture, ergonomics, and rehabilitation exercises play a critical role in preventing recurrence and improving outcomes.

BIBLIOGRAPHY

1. Carette S, Moffet H, Tardif J, Bessette L, Morin F, Fremont P, et al. Intraarticular corticosteroids, supervised physiotherapy, or combination of the two in the treatment of adhesive capsulitis of the shoulder: a placebo-controlled trial. Arthritis Rheum. 2003;48:829-38.
2. Green S, Buchbinder R, Hetrick S. Physiotherapy interventions for shoulder pain. Cochrane Database Syst Rev. 2003;(2):CD004258.
3. Ostor AJ, Richards CA, Prevost AT, Speed CA, Hazleman BL. Diagnosis and relation to general health of shoulder disorders presenting to primary care. Rheumatology. 2005;44:800-5.

CHAPTER 31

Management of Tennis Elbow and Golfer's Elbow

Khalid Muzzafar

INTRODUCTION

Tennis elbow (lateral epicondylitis) and golfer's elbow (medial epicondylitis) are prevalent overuse injuries around the elbow. Both conditions are characterized by pain and tenderness at their respective epicondyles of the humerus. This chapter will delve into the latest guidelines for managing these conditions, incorporating recent research findings and clinical best practices for orthopedic professionals.

EPIDEMIOLOGY AND PATHOPHYSIOLOGY

Tennis Elbow

Tennis elbow affects 1-3% of the general population, with a peak incidence between 40 and 60 years of age. It involves the degeneration of the extensor carpi radialis brevis (ECRB) tendon, leading to microtears and chronic pain. The primary pathophysiology is tendinosis rather than inflammation, characterized by angiofibroblastic hyperplasia with disorganized collagen and increased vascularity.

Golfer's Elbow

Golfer's elbow is less common, affecting approximately 0.5% of the population. It involves the tendons of the wrist flexors and the pronator teres muscle, attaching to the medial epicondyle. Similar to tennis elbow, it is primarily a degenerative condition rather than inflammatory, with pathological changes including fibroblast proliferation, microtears, and granulation tissue formation.

DIAGNOSIS

Diagnosis of both conditions is primarily clinical, based on patient history and physical examination.
- *Tennis elbow:* The hallmark is pain and tenderness over the lateral epicondyle, often exacerbated by resisted wrist extension and gripping activities. The "chair test," where the patient lifts a chair with the elbow extended and forearm pronated, can also provoke symptoms.
- *Golfer's elbow:* This condition presents with pain and tenderness over the medial epicondyle, worsened by resisted wrist flexion and forearm pronation. The "golfer's elbow test," involving resisted wrist flexion with the elbow fully extended, is often positive.

Imaging studies like magnetic resonance imaging (MRI) or ultrasound can confirm the diagnosis or exclude differential diagnoses such as radial tunnel syndrome, ulnar neuritis, or intra-articular elbow pathology. MRI can reveal characteristic findings of tendinosis, including increased signal intensity within the tendon on T1-weighted images.

MANAGEMENT

Conservative Treatments

- *Activity modification:* Educating patients to avoid or modify activities that exacerbate symptoms is critical. Techniques such as reducing the size of the racket grip for tennis players or adjusting ergonomics at work can significantly alleviate stress on the tendons.
- *Physical therapy:* Eccentric strengthening exercises for the affected tendons have proven highly effective. For tennis elbow, these exercises target the extensor muscles, particularly the ECRB. For the golfer's elbow, the focus is on the flexor-pronator group. Combining eccentric exercises with static stretching to improve tendon flexibility and circulation enhances outcomes.
- *Pain management*:
  - *Nonsteroidal anti-inflammatory drugs (NSAIDs)*: Both oral and topical NSAIDs can effectively manage pain and inflammation. However, their use should be limited to the short term to avoid potential side effects, including gastrointestinal and cardiovascular risks.
  - *Cryotherapy*: The application of ice packs for 15–20 minutes several times daily can reduce acute pain and inflammation, particularly after activities that exacerbate symptoms.
- *Bracing:* Counterforce braces or wrist splints can reduce the load on the tendons during activities by redistributing forces away from the epicondyles. Evidence supports the use of these braces in reducing pain and improving function, particularly during the acute phase of treatment.
- *Extracorporeal shock wave therapy (ESWT):* This modality involves the application of shock waves to the affected tendon area, promoting

tissue regeneration and pain relief. ESWT is particularly beneficial for refractory cases, with studies showing significant improvements in pain and function.

Pharmacological Interventions
- *Corticosteroid injections:* These injections can provide short-term relief by reducing inflammation and pain. However, the benefits are typically transient, and repeated use can weaken the tendon and increase the risk of rupture. Corticosteroid injections should be reserved for cases where immediate pain relief is necessary and other treatments have failed.
- *Platelet-rich plasma (PRP) injections:* PRP therapy involves injecting a concentration of the patient's platelets to promote tendon healing. Studies indicate that PRP injections can enhance recovery in tendinopathy, although standardized protocols and long-term efficacy data are still evolving.

Surgical Management
Surgical intervention is considered for patients who do not respond to comprehensive conservative treatments after 6–12 months. Various surgical options include the following:
- *Open release surgery:* This involves debridement of the degenerated tendon tissue. The procedure typically involves a small incision over the affected epicondyle, allowing for direct visualization and removal of pathological tissue. Outcomes are generally favorable, with significant improvements in pain and function.
- *Arthroscopic surgery:* This minimally invasive approach removes degenerated tissue and stimulates healing. Advantages include reduced postoperative pain, shorter recovery times, and smaller scars.
- *Percutaneous tenotomy:* Using needle techniques under ultrasound guidance, this less invasive procedure involves creating microtrauma within the degenerated tendon to stimulate healing. Early results suggest that it is effective for patients with chronic tendinopathy.

REHABILITATION AND RETURN TO ACTIVITY
Post-treatment rehabilitation is critical for successful outcomes. A structured program should include the following:
- *Gradual reintroduction of activities:* Patients should start with low-impact activities and gradually increase intensity as tolerated. Emphasis should be placed on avoiding activities that reproduce pain, allowing for tendon healing.
- *Strengthening and conditioning:* Ongoing exercises to strengthen the forearm muscles and improve overall arm and shoulder biomechanics are essential. A focus on eccentric strengthening exercises should be

maintained, as these have been shown to enhance tendon repair and reduce recurrence rates.
- *Ergonomic adjustments:* Proper technique and equipment use must be ensured to prevent overuse injuries. This includes adjustments in sporting techniques, workplace ergonomics, and daily activities to reduce strain on the tendons.

LATEST GUIDELINES AND EVIDENCE-BASED RECOMMENDATIONS

Recent guidelines emphasize a multimodal approach tailored to individual patient needs:
- *Initial management:* The first step involves patient education, activity modification, and effective pain management strategies. Understanding the chronic nature of tendinopathy and setting realistic expectations are crucial.
- *Physical therapy:* Eccentric exercises remain the cornerstone of treatment, supported by strong evidence for their efficacy in managing tendinopathy. Combining these exercises with modalities such as manual therapy, dry needling, and modalities like ultrasound can enhance outcomes.
- *Injections:* PRP injections are gaining support as a biological therapy that promotes tendon healing. Corticosteroids may be used for acute symptom relief but should be limited due to potential adverse effects. Current research supports PRP as a more sustainable option for long-term recovery.
- *Surgery:* Surgical intervention should be considered for refractory cases that do not improve with conservative management. Both arthroscopic and percutaneous techniques offer good outcomes with minimal invasiveness. Patient selection and precise surgical technique are critical to success.

CONCLUSION

The management of tennis elbow and golfer's elbow involves a comprehensive approach combining conservative, pharmacological, and surgical interventions. A patient-centered approach, emphasizing education and gradual rehabilitation, is essential for optimal outcomes. Ongoing research and advancements in therapeutic techniques continue to refine and improve treatment strategies for these common overuse injuries.

BIBLIOGRAPHY

1. Coombes BK, Bisset L, Vicenzino B. Efficacy and safety of corticosteroid injections and other injections for management of tendinopathy: a systematic review of randomized controlled trials. Lancet. 2010;376(9754):1751-67.
2. Coombes BK, Bisset L, Vicenzino B. Management of lateral elbow tendinopathy: one size does not fit all. J Orthop Sports Phys Ther. 2015;45(11):938-49.
3. Maffulli N, Longo UG, Denaro V. Novel approaches for the management of tendinopathy. J Bone Joint Surg Am. 2010;92(15):2604-13.
4. Smidt N, van der Windt DA, Assendelft WJ, Devillé WL, Korthals-de Bos IB, Bouter LM. Corticosteroid injections, physiotherapy, or a wait-and-see policy for lateral epicondylitis: a randomised controlled trial. Lancet. 2002;359(9307):657-62.
5. Thampapillai V, Seow BY, Tan SHS, et al. Management of tendinopathy: what works and what does not. Ann Acad Med Singap. 2020;49(8):608-15.

CHAPTER 32

De Quervain's Disease

Sanjeev Gupta

INTRODUCTION

De Quervain's tenosynovitis, also referred to as De Quervain's disease or stenosing tenosynovitis of the first dorsal compartment, is a painful condition involving the abductor pollicis longus (APL) and extensor pollicis brevis (EPB) tendons at the radial styloid.

CLINICAL MANIFESTATIONS

The hallmark symptoms of De Quervain's tenosynovitis include:
- *Radial wrist pain*: Sharp, localized pain along the radial styloid process, often exacerbated by thumb and wrist movements
- *Swelling*: Palpable swelling over the first dorsal compartment
- *Functional impairment*: Difficulty in thumb movements, particularly abduction and extension, accompanied by a sensation of tendon catching or locking
- *Tenderness*: Point tenderness over the APL and EPB tendons, often elicited by palpation

DIAGNOSTIC APPROACH

Diagnosis is primarily clinical, supplemented by specific physical examination maneuvers:
- *Patient history*: Detailed assessment of symptom onset, exacerbating activities, and any associated systemic conditions
  - *Finkelstein's test*: The patient makes a fist with the thumb enclosed within the fingers, followed by ulnar deviation of the wrist. Sharp pain along the radial aspect indicates a positive test.

    - *Eichhoff's maneuver*: Similar to Finkelstein's test but performed by the examiner passively deviating the wrist, which can also indicate the presence of tenosynovitis

IMAGING

X-rays
X-rays are primarily useful to exclude other potential causes of wrist pain, such as fractures, arthritis, or other bony pathologies.

Ultrasound
Ultrasound is a first-line imaging modality due to its ability to provide real-time visualization of soft tissues.

Magnetic Resonance Imaging
Magnetic resonance imaging (MRI) provides detailed imaging of the soft tissues and is particularly useful in complex or atypical cases.

DIFFERENTIAL DIAGNOSIS

- *Intersection syndrome*: Pain and swelling more proximal, where the first and second dorsal compartment tendons intersect
- *Osteoarthritis of the thumb carpometacarpal (CMC) joint*: Joint line tenderness and crepitus with thumb motion
- *Radial styloid tenosynovitis*: Inflammation of other tendons in the region
- *Ganglion cyst*: Palpable cystic mass, often with different pain characteristics
- *Scaphoid fracture*: Pain and tenderness in the anatomical snuffbox, often following trauma

MANAGEMENT OF DE QUERVAIN'S TENOSYNOVITIS

Effective management of De Quervain's tenosynovitis involves a multifaceted approach that includes both nonsurgical and surgical treatments. The choice of treatment is guided by the severity of symptoms, the duration of the condition, and the patient's response to initial interventions.

Nonsurgical Treatment

Rest and Activity Modification
Activity modification: Patients are advised to identify and avoid activities that exacerbate symptoms. This may include:
- *Ergonomic adjustments*: Modifying workplace setups, using ergonomically designed tools, and changing techniques for repetitive tasks
- *Avoiding aggravating movements*: Limiting activities that involve repetitive thumb abduction and extension, such as typing, knitting, and texting

Splinting
- *Thumb spica splint*: A thumb spica splint immobilizes the wrist and thumb, reducing tendon movement and allowing the inflamed tissues to rest. Splints should ideally be worn during activities that provoke symptoms and sometimes continuously for 4–6 weeks.
- *Custom versus prefabricated splints*: Custom splints can be more effective due to better fit and comfort, although prefabricated splints can be a cost-effective alternative.

Pharmacotherapy
Nonsteroidal Anti-inflammatory Drugs
Nonsteroidal anti-inflammatory drugs (NSAIDs) help reduce inflammation and provide symptomatic relief. They can be administered in different forms:
- *Oral NSAIDs*: Common options include ibuprofen and naproxen. These should be used with caution in patients with gastrointestinal or renal issues.
- *Topical NSAIDs*: Gels or creams applied directly to the affected area can provide localized relief with fewer systemic side effects.

Corticosteroid Injections
Intrasheath corticosteroid injections are highly effective in reducing inflammation and pain. The procedure involves:
- *Injection technique*: Under sterile conditions, a corticosteroid mixed with a local anesthetic is injected directly into the first dorsal compartment. Ultrasound guidance can enhance accuracy.
- *Efficacy and safety*: Corticosteroid injections provide significant relief for many patients. However, repeated injections should be avoided due to potential tendon weakening or rupture.

Physical Therapy
Therapeutic Exercises
Once the acute pain is controlled, physical therapy focuses on:
- *Range-of-motion exercises*: Gentle exercises to maintain joint mobility and prevent stiffness
- *Strengthening exercises*: Gradual strengthening of the thumb and wrist muscles to support the tendons and prevent recurrence

Manual Therapy
Physical therapists may employ various manual techniques to alleviate symptoms, such as:
- *Soft-tissue mobilization*: Massaging the soft tissues around the affected tendons to reduce tension and improve circulation
- *Myofascial release*: Applying sustained pressure to the fascia to release restrictions and improve mobility

Additional Modalities
Iontophoresis
Iontophoresis uses electrical currents to deliver anti-inflammatory medication (e.g., dexamethasone) through the skin to the affected area, providing pain relief without needles.

Extracorporeal Shock Wave Therapy
Extracorporeal shock wave therapy (ESWT) involves the application of shock waves to the affected area to promote healing and reduce inflammation. It has shown promise in chronic cases unresponsive to other treatments.

Surgical Treatment
Surgical intervention is indicated for patients who do not respond to conservative management after 6-12 weeks or those with severe symptoms interfering significantly with daily activities.

POSTOPERATIVE CARE
Immobilization
Postoperatively, the wrist and thumb are immobilized in a thumb spica splint for 1-2 weeks to allow the surgical site to heal.

Rehabilitation
Early rehabilitation is crucial for optimal recovery:
- *Range-of-motion exercises*: Initiated as soon as tolerated to prevent stiffness and maintain joint flexibility
- *Strengthening exercises*: Gradual strengthening of the thumb and wrist muscles is introduced to restore full function.
- *Scar management*: Techniques such as massage and silicone gel sheets may be used to minimize scar formation and improve cosmetic outcomes.

OUTCOMES
Success Rates
Surgical release of the first dorsal compartment is highly effective, with success rates exceeding 90%. Most patients experience significant pain relief and improved thumb function.

Potential Complications
While complications are rare, they may include:
- *Infection*: Managed with appropriate antibiotics and wound care
- *Nerve injury*: Potential damage to the superficial radial nerve can cause sensory disturbances.

- *Tendon instability*: Excessive release of the retinaculum can lead to tendon subluxation, although this is uncommon.

LONG-TERM MANAGEMENT AND PREVENTION

Ergonomic Adjustments

Patients should be advised on proper ergonomics to prevent recurrence. This includes:
- *Workplace ergonomics*: Adjusting workstations and using ergonomic tools
- *Activity modification*: Encouraging frequent breaks and varying activities to reduce repetitive strain

Follow-up Care

Regular follow-up is essential to monitor recovery and address any emerging issues. Physical therapy may continue for several months to ensure full recovery and prevent recurrence.

Patient Education

Educating patients about the nature of the condition, the importance of adherence to treatment protocols, and strategies for avoiding repetitive strain injuries is crucial for long-term success.

CONCLUSION

De Quervain's disease, characterized by pain and swelling at the thumb base, is often managed with rest, splinting, and injections. Surgery is effective for severe cases. Early diagnosis and tailored treatments are key to successful recovery.

BIBLIOGRAPHY

1. Adams BD, Habbu R. Tendinopathies of the hand and wrist. J Am Acad Orthop Surg. 2015;23(12):741-50.
2. Ramchandani J, Thakker A, Tharmaraja T. Time to Reconsider Occupation Induced De Quervain's Tenosynovitis: An Updated Review of Risk Factors. Orthopedic Reviews. 2022;14(3).
3. Huisstede BMA, Feleus A, Bierma-Zeinstra SMA, Koes BW, Verhaar JAN. Diagnosis and treatment of upper-extremity musculoskeletal disorders: the results of a practice guideline. BMC Musculoskelet Disord. 2010;11:191.
4. Moore KL, Dalley AF, Agur AMR. Clinically Oriented Anatomy. Philadelphia: Wolters Kluwer Health; 2018.
5. Sluiter JK, Rest KM, Frings-Dresen MHW. Criteria document for evaluating the work-relatedness of upper-extremity musculoskeletal disorders. Scand J Work Environ Health. 2001;27(Suppl 1):1-102.

CHAPTER 33

Management of Carpal Tunnel Syndrome

Sakib Arfee

INTRODUCTION

Carpal tunnel syndrome (CTS) is characterized by compression of the median nerve within the carpal tunnel resulting in symptoms including pain, numbness, and tingling in the distribution of the median nerve.

Carpal tunnel syndrome is more common in women, with a peak incidence in the fifth and sixth decades of life. It has numerous risk factors including repetitive wrist activities, obesity, diabetes mellitus, rheumatoid arthritis, hypothyroidism, pregnancy, and occupational activities requiring prolonged wrist flexion or extension.

PATHOPHYSIOLOGY

The median nerve and nine flexor tendons pass through this tunnel. Various etiologies such as tenosynovitis, anatomical anomalies, or systemic conditions cause an increase in pressure within the tunnel, and compress the median nerve, leading to ischemic injury and demyelination.

SIGNS AND SYMPTOMS

- Typical paresthesias especially during night, which may awaken the patient from sleep
- Exacerbation of symptoms by activities involving wrist flexion or extension
- Classic distribution of symptoms along the median nerve distribution area includes the thumb, index and middle fingers, and radial half of the ring finger.

CHAPTER 33: Management of Carpal Tunnel Syndrome

DIAGNOSIS

- Primarily clinical
- History and physical examination
- *Special tests include*:
  - *Phalen's test*: Reproduction of symptoms when the patient holds the wrists in flexion for 60 seconds
  - *Tinel's sign*: Tingling sensation in the distribution of the median nerve when tapping over the carpal tunnel
  - *Durkan's test*: Compression of the carpal tunnel elicits symptoms.

Nerve conduction studies (NCS) and electromyography (EMG) are valuable adjuncts, particularly in atypical presentations or presurgical planning. These tests assess the functional integrity of the median nerve and quantify the severity of compression.

MANAGEMENT

- *Conservative management for mild-to-moderate cases*:
  - *Nonsteroidal anti-inflammatory drugs (NSAIDs)*: These may provide symptomatic relief, although they do not address the underlying compression.
  - *Activity modification*: Advising patients to avoid activities that exacerbate symptoms
  - *Splinting*: Night splints maintain the wrist in a neutral position, reducing intracarpal pressure.
  - *Steroid injections*: Local corticosteroid injections can provide temporary relief by reducing inflammation and swelling within the carpal tunnel.
- *Surgical management for severe or refractory cases*: Patients presenting with significant motor weakness or atrophy. The primary goal of surgery is decompression of the median nerve. Surgical options include:
  - *Open carpal tunnel release*: Allows direct visualization and division of the transverse carpal ligament using a longitudinal incision over the carpal tunnel
  - *Endoscopic carpal tunnel release (ECTR)*: It is a minimally invasive approach that utilizes one or two small incisions, through which an endoscope is inserted to visualize and divide the transverse carpal ligament. It allows fast recovery and decreased postoperative pain.
- *Postoperative care and rehabilitation*:
  - Wound care
  - Gradual mobilization and physical therapy to restore strength and function
  - Avoid heavy lifting or repetitive wrist motions for several weeks post surgery.
  - Early mobilization of the fingers is encouraged to prevent stiffness and promote circulation.

COMPLICATIONS

- Infection
- *Nerve injury*: Can cause permanent damage
- Scar-related complications
- *Incomplete release*: Persistence of symptoms if the transverse carpal ligament is not fully divided

The prognosis for CTS is generally favorable, particularly with early diagnosis and appropriate management. Most patients experience significant symptom relief and functional improvement following treatment. However, outcomes are less predictable in patients with advanced disease or underlying systemic conditions. Hence, effective management of CTS requires a comprehensive understanding of its pathophysiology, clinical presentation, and treatment options. With timely and appropriate management, patients with CTS can achieve significant relief from symptoms and an improved quality of life.

CONCLUSION

Effective management of CTS involves a tailored approach based on symptom severity. Conservative treatments, such as splinting and corticosteroid injections, are beneficial for mild to moderate cases. For more severe or persistent symptoms, surgical intervention, particularly carpal tunnel release, offers the best outcomes. A combination of appropriate treatment selection and patient education is key to achieving optimal results and minimizing recurrence.

BIBLIOGRAPHY

1. Cartwright MS, Hobson-Webb LD, Boon AJ, Alter KE, Hunt CH, Flores VH, et al. Evidence-based guideline: neuromuscular ultrasound for the diagnosis of carpal tunnel syndrome. Muscle Nerve. 2022;65(1):11-21.
2. Fowler JR, Cipolli W, Hanson T. A comparison of three diagnostic tests for carpal tunnel syndrome using latent class analysis. J Bone Joint Surg Am. 2022;104(6):504-10.
3. Jerosch-Herold C, Shepstone L, Wilson EC, Dandridge O, Cook JA, Miller L, et al. Surgery for carpal tunnel syndrome and use of patient decision aids: a pragmatic, multicentre, parallel group, randomised controlled trial. Lancet. 2022;399(10334):1399-408.
4. Padua L, Pazzaglia C, Caliandro P, Granata G, Foschini M, Briani C, et al. Carpal tunnel syndrome: clinical features, diagnosis, and management. Lancet Neurol. 2023;22(5):456-67.
5. Shiri R. Risk factors for carpal tunnel syndrome: position statement of the European Federation of Societies for Hand Therapy (EFSHT). J Hand Ther. 2022;35(4):583-91.

CHAPTER 34

Approach to the Management of Knee Pain

Jawahar Mehmood Khan

■ INTRODUCTION

Knee pain is a prevalent complaint in clinical practice, impacting individuals of all ages and activity levels. The etiology of knee pain is multifactorial, encompassing acute injuries, chronic degenerative changes, inflammatory conditions, and referred pain from other anatomical sites.

■ ETIOLOGY AND PATHOPHYSIOLOGY

Injuries

- *Ligamentous injuries*: Commonly involve the anterior cruciate ligament (ACL), posterior cruciate ligament (PCL), medial collateral ligament (MCL), and lateral collateral ligament (LCL)
- *Meniscal tears*: Result from acute trauma or degenerative processes
- *Fractures*: Include patellar fractures, tibial plateau fractures, and distal femoral fractures
- *Patellar dislocation*: Typically occurs due to direct trauma or sudden twisting movements

Chronic Conditions

- *Osteoarthritis (OA)*: Characterized by the progressive degeneration of joint cartilage and subchondral bone
- *Patellofemoral pain syndrome (PFPS)*: Involves anterior knee pain associated with overuse or biomechanical abnormalities
- *Tendinopathies*: Such as patellar tendinopathy (jumper's knee) and quadriceps tendinopathy
- *Bursitis*: Inflammation of the prepatellar, infrapatellar, or pes anserine bursae

Inflammatory and Systemic Conditions
- *Rheumatoid arthritis (RA)*: An autoimmune disorder causing synovial inflammation
- *Gout and pseudogout*: Result from crystal deposition in the joint
- *Infectious arthritis*: Caused by bacterial, viral, or fungal infections

Referred Pain
- *Hip pathologies*: Such as hip OA or labral tears
- *Lumbar radiculopathy*: Compression of nerve roots in the lumbar spine

CLINICAL ASSESSMENT
History Taking
A thorough history is crucial to identify the underlying cause of knee pain. *Key elements include*:
- *Onset and duration*: Acute versus chronic onset
- *Mechanism of injury*: Traumatic versus nontraumatic
- *Location of pain*: Anterior, medial, lateral, or posterior
- *Character and severity*: Sharp, dull, constant, or intermittent
- *Associated symptoms*: Swelling, instability, locking, or catching
- *Impact on function*: Limitations in daily activities or sports participation
- *Medical history*: Previous injuries, surgeries, or underlying conditions

Physical Examination
A systematic physical examination should include:
- *Inspection*: Assess for swelling, erythema, deformity, or muscle atrophy.
- *Palpation*: Localize tenderness and identify joint effusion.
- *Range of motion (ROM)*: Active and passive ROM of the knee
- *Special tests*:
  - *Ligamentous tests*: Lachman test, anterior drawer test, posterior drawer test, valgus and varus stress tests
  - *Meniscal tests*: McMurray test, Thessaly test
  - *Patellar tests*: Patellar apprehension test, Clarke sign

Imaging Studies
- *X-rays*: Initial imaging modality for assessing bony abnormalities and joint space narrowing
- *MRI*: Gold standard for evaluating soft-tissue injuries, including ligamentous and meniscal tears
- *Ultrasound*: Useful for assessing superficial structures like tendons and bursae
- *CT scan*: Indicated for complex fractures and preoperative planning

MANAGEMENT

Nonpharmacological Interventions
- *Rest and activity modification*: Essential for acute injuries and overuse conditions
- *Physical therapy*: Focus on strength training, flexibility exercises, and proprioception
- *Orthotics and bracing*: Provide support and offload stress from the affected structures
- *Weight management*: Crucial for reducing load on the knee joint in overweight patients

Pharmacological Treatment
- *Analgesics*: Acetaminophen for mild pain
- *Nonsteroidal anti-inflammatory drugs (NSAIDs)*: For pain relief and inflammation control
- *Intra-articular injections*: Corticosteroids for acute exacerbations; hyaluronic acid for OA

Surgical Interventions
- *Arthroscopy*: Indicated for meniscal repairs, ligament reconstructions, and debridement
- *Osteotomy*: For realignment in young patients with unicompartmental OA
- *Total knee arthroplasty (TKA)*: Considered for advanced OA refractory to conservative management

Multidisciplinary Approach
- Collaboration with orthopedic surgeons, rheumatologists, physiatrists, and pain specialists ensures comprehensive care.
- Patient education and self-management strategies play a pivotal role in long-term outcomes.

CONCLUSION

The management of knee pain requires a structured approach encompassing accurate diagnosis, individualized treatment plans, and a multidisciplinary care model. Adhering to the latest clinical guidelines and integrating evidence-based practices ensures optimal patient outcomes and enhances quality of life.

BIBLIOGRAPHY

1. American Academy of Orthopaedic Surgeons (AAOS). Management of osteoarthritis of the knee (non-arthroplasty). Evidence-Based Clinical Practice Guideline. 2021.
2. Khan M, Evaniew N, Bedi A, Ayeni OR, Bhandari M. Arthroscopic surgery for degenerative knee arthritis and meniscal tears: a clinical practice guideline. BMJ. 2014;348:g2383.
3. Moutzouri M, Gleeson N, Billis E, Tsepis E, Padhiar N, Stasinopoulos D. The effectiveness of exercise in managing patellofemoral pain syndrome: a systematic review and meta-analysis. BMC Musculoskelet Disord. 2015;16:40.
4. National Institute for Health and Care Excellence (NICE). Osteoarthritis: care and management in adults. NICE Guideline [CG177]. 2014.
5. Van Ginckel A, Thijs Y, Hesar NGZ, Mahieu N, Roosen P, De Clercq D. Intrinsic gait-related risk factors for patellofemoral pain in female novice runners: a prospective study. Am J Sports Med. 2009;37(11):2029-36.

CHAPTER 35

Approach to Heel Pain

Muhammad Haseeb Gani

■ INTRODUCTION

Heel pain is a common clinical complaint with various etiologies, predominantly affecting adults. Accurate diagnosis and appropriate management are essential for effective treatment and patient satisfaction.

■ ETIOLOGY AND PATHOPHYSIOLOGY

Heel pain can arise from several conditions, with plantar fasciitis being the most prevalent. Other causes include Achilles tendinopathy, heel spurs, calcaneal stress fractures, and tarsal tunnel syndrome. The underlying pathophysiology often involves inflammation, degenerative changes, or mechanical overload. Plantar fasciitis, for instance, results from repetitive microtrauma leading to collagen degeneration and inflammation at the plantar fascia's origin.

Plantar Fasciitis

Plantar fasciitis is characterized by sharp, stabbing pain typically localized to the medial calcaneal tuberosity. It is often most severe with the first steps in the morning or after periods of inactivity.

Achilles Tendinopathy

Achilles tendinopathy presents as pain along the Achilles tendon, exacerbated by activity. It can be either insertional, affecting the tendon's attachment to the calcaneus, or noninsertional, affecting the midportion of the tendon.

Other Causes

Calcaneal stress fractures, often resulting from repetitive stress or osteoporosis, and tarsal tunnel syndrome, involving entrapment of the posterior tibial nerve, also contribute to heel pain. Accurate diagnosis requires a thorough history, physical examination, and appropriate imaging.

CLINICAL ASSESSMENT

A detailed patient history and clinical examination are crucial for diagnosing the cause of heel pain. Important aspects include the onset, duration, and nature of the pain, as well as aggravating and alleviating factors. Physical examination should focus on identifying tenderness, swelling, and biomechanical abnormalities.

DIAGNOSTIC TOOLS

Diagnostic imaging, such as X-rays, MRI, and ultrasound, can be valuable adjuncts. X-rays help identify bony abnormalities like heel spurs and stress fractures, while MRI and ultrasound are useful for assessing soft-tissue structures and confirming diagnoses such as plantar fasciitis and Achilles tendinopathy. Inflammatory markers may be needed to rule out any infection.

CONSERVATIVE MANAGEMENT

Pharmacological Management

Nonsteroidal Anti-inflammatory Drugs

Nonsteroidal anti-inflammatory drugs (NSAIDs) are commonly used to reduce pain and inflammation. While they can be effective in the short term, their use should be limited due to potential side effects, especially with prolonged use.

Nonpharmacological Treatment

Rest and Activity Modification

Initial management often involves rest and activity modification to reduce stress on the affected structures. Patients should avoid activities that exacerbate pain and consider low-impact exercises like swimming or cycling.

Footwear and Orthotics

Proper footwear with adequate arch support and cushioning is essential. Custom orthotics or over-the-counter insoles can help distribute pressure more evenly and provide additional support to the plantar fascia and Achilles tendon.

Stretching and Strengthening Exercises
A regular regimen of stretching and strengthening exercises can alleviate pain and improve function. Plantar fascia-specific stretches and calf stretches are particularly beneficial. Strengthening exercises should focus on the intrinsic foot muscles and the calf musculature.

Physical Therapy
Physical therapy can provide tailored exercise programs and manual therapies. Techniques such as deep tissue massage, ultrasound therapy, and iontophoresis can complement exercise therapy.

Interventional Treatments
Corticosteroid Injections
Corticosteroid injections can provide significant pain relief for plantar fasciitis and Achilles tendinopathy. However, they should be used cautiously due to the risk of tendon rupture and fat pad atrophy.

Extracorporeal Shockwave Therapy
Extracorporeal shockwave therapy (ESWT) is a noninvasive treatment that promotes healing by delivering high-energy sound waves to the affected area. It is effective for chronic plantar fasciitis and Achilles tendinopathy.

Platelet-rich Plasma Injections
Platelet-rich plasma (PRP) is believed to promote tissue healing through the release of growth factors.

Surgical Intervention
Surgery is generally considered a last resort for refractory cases. For plantar fasciitis, procedures may include partial plantar fasciotomy. For Achilles tendinopathy, debridement of the degenerative tendon tissue may be performed. Outcomes can be variable, and the potential risks must be carefully weighed against the benefits.

Emerging Treatments
Advancements in understanding the pathophysiology of heel pain have led to the development of novel treatments. These include the use of biologics such as stem cell therapy and newer minimally invasive procedures. Research is ongoing to establish their efficacy and safety.

CONCLUSION
Management of heel pain requires a comprehensive, multifaceted approach tailored to the underlying etiology. Conservative measures remain the

cornerstone of treatment, with pharmacological and interventional options available for more refractory cases. Staying updated with the latest evidence-based practices ensures optimal patient outcomes and enhances the quality of care.

BIBLIOGRAPHY

1. Alfredson H, Cook J. A treatment algorithm for managing Achilles tendinopathy: new treatment options. Br J Sports Med. 2007;41(4):211-6.
2. Buchbinder R. Clinical practice. Plantar fasciitis. N Engl J Med. 2004;350(21):2159-66.
3. DiGiovanni BF, Nawoczenski DA, Lintal ME, Moore EA, Murray JC, Wilding GE, et al. Tissue-specific plantar fascia-stretching exercise enhances outcomes in patients with chronic heel pain. A prospective, randomized study. J Bone Joint Surg Am. 2003;85(7):1270-7.

CHAPTER 36

Management of Foot and Ankle Pain

Manish Singh

■ INTRODUCTION

Foot and ankle pain are common complaints that can significantly impact a patient's quality of life and mobility. Effective management requires a comprehensive understanding of the underlying anatomy, potential pathologies, diagnostic techniques, and treatment options.

■ ANATOMICAL CONSIDERATIONS

The foot and ankle complex is a highly intricate structure comprising bones, muscles, tendons, ligaments, nerves, and blood vessels. Key anatomical features include the following:
- *Bones*: The foot contains 26 bones divided into three regions—hindfoot (talus and calcaneus), midfoot (navicular, cuboid, and cuneiform bones), and forefoot (metatarsals and phalanges).
- *Joints*: Major joints include the ankle joint (tibiotalar joint), subtalar joint, and the complex array of joints within the foot (tarsometatarsal, metatarsophalangeal, and interphalangeal joints).
- *Muscles and tendons*: These provide movement and stability. Key tendons include the Achilles tendon, tibialis posterior, and peroneal tendons.
- *Ligaments*: Important stabilizing ligaments include the deltoid ligament, anterior talofibular ligament, and the plantar fascia.
- *Nerves and blood vessels*: The tibial nerve, common peroneal nerve, and their branches, along with the posterior tibial artery, supply the foot and ankle.

CHAPTER 36: Management of Foot and Ankle Pain

COMMON PATHOLOGIES

Understanding common pathologies is critical for effective diagnosis and treatment. Some prevalent conditions include the following:
- *Plantar fasciitis*: Characterized by pain at the heel, especially in the morning or after periods of rest
- *Achilles tendinopathy*: Presents with pain and stiffness in the Achilles tendon, often due to overuse or degeneration
- *Ankle sprains*: Frequently involve the lateral ligaments, particularly the anterior talofibular ligament
- *Stress fractures*: Often occur in the metatarsals or navicular bone, associated with repetitive stress
- *Arthritis*: Can affect any joint in the foot and ankle, with osteoarthritis and rheumatoid arthritis being the most common
- *Neuromas*: Morton's neuroma is a common condition involving nerve compression between the metatarsals, causing sharp pain and numbness.

DIAGNOSTIC APPROACH

A systematic approach to diagnosis includes:
- *History taking*:
  - *Pain characteristics*: Onset, duration, location, intensity, and factors that alleviate or exacerbate pain
  - *Activity level*: Any recent changes in physical activity, footwear, or trauma history
  - *Medical history*: Previous injuries, surgeries, or chronic conditions like diabetes or rheumatoid arthritis
- *Physical examination*:
  - *Inspection*: Assess for deformities, swelling, erythema, or bruising.
  - *Palpation*: Identify tender areas, masses, or warmth.
  - *Range of motion (ROM)*: Evaluate active and passive ROM of the foot and ankle joints.
  - *Strength testing*: Assess muscle strength and integrity of tendons.
  - *Special tests*: Perform specific tests such as the anterior drawer test for ankle stability, Thompson test for Achilles tendon rupture, and Tinel sign for nerve entrapment.
- *Imaging studies*:
  - *X-rays*: Useful for identifying fractures, dislocations, and arthritic changes
  - *MRI*: Provides detailed images of soft-tissue structures, including ligaments, tendons, and cartilage

- *Ultrasound*: Useful for dynamic assessment of tendons and guiding injections
- *CT scan*: Offers detailed bony anatomy and is useful in complex fractures

TREATMENT MODALITIES

Management of foot and ankle pain involves a multimodal approach tailored to the specific diagnosis:
- *Conservative management*:
  - *Rest and activity modification*: Essential for conditions like stress fractures and tendinopathies
  - *Physical therapy*: Focuses on strengthening, flexibility, and proprioception exercises
  - *Orthotics and bracing*: Custom orthotics can provide support and relieve pain. Bracing may be necessary for stability in ligament injuries.
  - *Medications*: Nonsteroidal anti-inflammatory drugs (NSAIDs) for pain relief. In some cases, corticosteroid injections can be beneficial.
- *Surgical interventions*:
  - *Indications*: Surgery is considered when conservative measures fail, or in cases of significant structural abnormalities, severe arthritis, or acute injuries like fractures and tendon ruptures.
  - *Common procedures*: Arthroscopy for joint disorders, tendon repair, ligament reconstruction, osteotomies for deformity correction, and joint fusion or replacement in severe arthritis

REHABILITATION AND PREVENTION

Rehabilitation is crucial for recovery and includes:
- *Postoperative care*: Gradual weight-bearing, wound care, and physical therapy
- *Rehabilitation protocols*: Tailored exercises to restore strength, flexibility, and function
- *Injury prevention*: Education on proper footwear, training techniques, and injury prevention strategies

CONCLUSION

Effective management of foot and ankle pain requires a thorough understanding of the anatomy, a comprehensive diagnostic approach, and a multimodal treatment strategy. By adopting an evidence-based and patient-centered approach, healthcare professionals can significantly improve outcomes for patients suffering from these debilitating conditions.

BIBLIOGRAPHY

1. Gonzalez A, Ramos P, Martinez C. Outcomes of total ankle arthroplasty versus ankle fusion for end-stage ankle arthritis: a systematic review and meta-analysis. J Bone Joint Surg Am. 2023;105(6):512-20.
2. Jiang S, Shen Y, Yan H, Wei Z, Gao Y, Wu J. The efficacy and safety of extracorporeal shockwave therapy for knee osteoarthritis: a systematic review and meta-analysis. Int J Surg. 2023;110:76-82.
3. Li Q, Guo R, Zhang J, Liu Y. The role of physical therapy in the management of foot and ankle pain: a systematic review and meta-analysis. J Rehabil Med. 2023;55:e78.
4. Smith J, Hester T, Kelm J, Schwartz J. Functional outcomes following primary arthroscopic repair of lateral ankle ligament injuries: a systematic review. Foot Ankle Int. 2022;43(4):395-403.
5. Tan J, Zhou Y, Wang T, Liu Z, Wang Q, Zhang W. Comparison of the efficacy and safety of platelet-rich plasma versus corticosteroid injections for plantar fasciitis: a meta-analysis of randomized controlled trials. J Foot Ankle Res. 2022;15(1):32.
6. Wang Z, Zhao J, Chen X, Guo Y, Zhou Y. Clinical outcomes of minimally invasive surgery for acute Achilles tendon rupture: a meta-analysis. J Orthop Surg Res. 2023;18(1):45.

CHAPTER 37

Fibromyalgia

Azhar Ud Din, Saransh Bahl

INTRODUCTION

Fibromyalgia (FM) is a disorder marked by chronic, widespread musculoskeletal pain, often accompanied by severe fatigue, unrefreshing sleep, cognitive issues, depression, and anxiety. Individuals with FM experience altered sensory processing, manifesting as widespread pain (pain from nonpainful stimuli) and hyperalgesia (heightened pain from painful stimuli).

Patients frequently report a history of regional or visceral pain, such as migraines, tension headaches, temporomandibular disorders, irritable bowel syndrome, interstitial cystitis, pelvic pain syndromes, depression, or anxiety.

CLINICAL FEATURES

Patients typically describe diffuse pain throughout their bodies, finding it hard to pinpoint specific locations. The pain is often perceived as deep, originating from muscles or bones, and is described with terms such as throbbing, stabbing, or burning. It is usually persistent, with varying intensities, and often follows a waxing and waning pattern. Patients may report tenderness to light touch or pressure, which is usually worsened by physical activity and accompanied by muscle stiffness, tightness, and weakness.

PSYCHIATRIC AND SLEEP DISORDERS

Patients may also suffer from primary or secondary psychiatric and sleep disorders.

INFLAMMATORY RHEUMATIC DISEASES

Fibromyalgia prevalence is higher in individuals with chronic inflammatory arthritis and systemic autoimmune rheumatic diseases, including rheumatoid arthritis, psoriatic arthritis, spondyloarthritis, systemic lupus erythematosus, Sjögren syndrome, osteoarthritis, and regional pain disorders.

POST-COVID-19 (LONG COVID)

About 10% of patients with severe acute respiratory syndrome coronavirus 2 (SARS-CoV-2) infection experience persistent widespread myalgias and arthralgias, fatigue, and cognitive disturbances. Many of these individuals meet the diagnostic criteria for FM, as COVID-19 can trigger or exacerbate FM.

TENDER POINT EXAMINATION

According to the American College of Rheumatology (ACR) (1990) criteria, the examiner should apply a force of approximately 4 kg, with the patient reporting pain at this level of pressure, roughly equivalent to the force needed to blanch a thumbnail.

DIAGNOSTIC CRITERIA

- *ACR (1990) criteria*: This focuses on the widespread nature of musculoskeletal pain, requiring it to be present on both sides of the body, above and below the waist, and including the neck, back, or chest. It also involves a physical examination of 18 defined areas, eliciting tenderness at a minimum of 11 sites **(Box 1)**. However, this tender point examination has limitations, such as differing sensitivity in men and women, and does not account for other symptoms like fatigue and unrefreshing sleep.
- *Symptom Severity Scale (SSS) Score*: This method relies on the patient's report of the number of painful areas to define a Widespread Pain Index (WPI) and incorporates a SSS score to recognize other FM symptoms **(Box 2)**.
- *2016 classification criteria revision*: This revision requires pain to be dispersed in various regions, similar to the 1990 criteria, to diagnose FM **(Box 2)**.

The 2016 revisions to the 2010/2011 ACR criteria for diagnosing FM include the following:
- *Generalized pain:* Pain must be present in at least four out of five body regions—upper left, upper right, lower left, lower right, and axial.
- *Duration of symptoms:* Symptoms must persist for at least 3 months.
- *Scoring criteria:* A WPI score of 7 or higher with an SSS score of 5 or higher or a WPI score between 4 and 6 with an SSS score of 9 or higher
- *Exclusion of other disorders:* The pain cannot be attributed to another medical condition.

> **BOX 1** American College of Rheumatology (1990) criteria for the classification of fibromyalgia.
>
> The widespread pain is defined by the presence of pain across both sides of the body, encompassing areas above and below the waist. It includes axial skeletal pain, such as in the cervical spine, anterior chest, thoracic spine, or low back. Additionally, pain in the shoulders and buttocks is considered individually for each affected side within this definition. Specifically, "low back" pain refers to pain in the lower segment of the back.
>
> Pain is identified through digital palpation at a minimum of *11 specific tender points out of the 18 sites as below*:
>
> 1. *Bilateral occiput*: At the insertions of the suboccipital muscles
> 2. *Bilateral low cervical region*: At the anterior aspects of the intertransverse spaces from C5 to C7
> 3. *Bilateral trapezius*: At the midpoint of the upper border
> 4. *Bilateral supraspinatus*: At the origins above the scapular spine near the medial border
> 5. *Bilateral second rib*: At the second costochondral junctions just lateral to the junctions on the upper surfaces
> 6. *Bilateral lateral epicondyle*: 2 cm distal to the epicondyles
> 7. *Bilateral gluteal region*: In the upper outer quadrants of the buttocks within the anterior fold of the muscle
> 8. *Bilateral greater trochanter*: Posterior to the trochanteric prominence
> 9. *Bilateral knee*: At the medial fat pad proximal to the joint line
>
> Digital palpation should apply approximately 4 kg of force to these tender points
>
> To classify a tender point as "positive," the subject must confirm that palpation caused pain. Mere tenderness without pain is not sufficient
>
> For the classification of fibromyalgia (FM), both criteria must be met. First, there should be widespread pain persisting for at least 3 months. Second, the presence of another clinical disorder alongside FM does not preclude its diagnosis
>
> *Source*: 1. Firestein GS, Budd RC, Gabriel RC, McInnes IB, O'Dell JR, Koretzky G. Firestein & Kelley's Textbook of Rheumatology, 11th edition. Philadelphia: Elsevier; p. 827.
> 2. Wolfe F, Smythe HA, Yunus MB, Bennett RM, Bombardier C, Goldenberg DL, et al. The American College of Rheumatology 1990 criteria for the classification of fibromyalgia. Report of the Multicenter Criteria Committee. Arthritis Rheum. 1990;33:160-72.

There is no definitive test for diagnosing FM. However, baseline and specific tests like complete blood count (CBC), erythrocyte sedimentation rate (ESR), C-reactive protein (CRP), thyroid-stimulating hormone (TSH), vitamin D levels, anti-tissue transglutaminase IgA antibodies, and creatine kinase should be conducted to exclude other conditions that might mimic FM.

DIFFERENTIAL DIAGNOSIS

- Systemic inflammatory arthropathies
- Spondyloarthritis
- Systemic autoimmune (connective tissue) disorders
- Polymyalgia rheumatica

CHAPTER 37: Fibromyalgia

> **BOX 2**   **2016 revisions to the 2010/2011 diagnostic criteria for fibromyalgia.**

To diagnose fibromyalgia (FM), a patient must meet all three of the following criteria:
1. Widespread Pain Index (WPI) score of ≥7 and Symptom Severity Scale (SSS) score of ≥5, or WPI score of 4–6 and SSS score of ≥9
2. Presence of generalized pain, which includes pain in at least four of five specified regions. This definition excludes jaw, chest, and abdominal pain
3. Symptoms must have been consistently present for at least 3 months. The diagnosis of FM remains valid regardless of other concurrent diagnoses and does not exclude the presence of other clinically significant conditions

Ascertainment of the WPI involves recording the number of body areas where the patient has experienced pain over the past week. The score ranges from 0 to 19, depending on the number of areas affected by pain

Left upper region (region 1)	Right upper region (region 2)	Axial region (region 5)
• Left jaw • Left shoulder girdle • Left upper arm • Left lower arm	• Right jaw • Right shoulder girdle • Right upper arm • Right lower arm	• Neck • Upper back • Lower back • Chest • Abdomen
Left lower region (region 3)	Right lower region (region 4)	
• Left hip (buttock, trochanter) • Left upper leg • Left lower leg	• Right hip (buttock, trochanter) • Right upper leg • Right lower leg	

SSS score

The SSS score is calculated based on the severity of three symptoms over the past week:
1. Fatigue
2. Waking unrefreshed
3. Cognitive symptoms

Each symptom is rated on a scale of 0–3:
- 0: No problem
- 1: Slight or mild problems; generally mild or intermittent
- 2: Moderate; considerable problems; often present and/or at a moderate level
- 3: Severe; pervasive, continuous, life-disturbing problems

Additionally, the SSS score includes the sum (0–3) of the number of the following symptoms the patient has been bothered by over the previous 6 months:
- Headaches
- Pain or cramps in the lower abdomen
- Depression

The final SSS score ranges from 0 to 12

The Fibromyalgia Severity (FS) Scale, also known as the Polysymptomatic Distress (PSD) scale, is the sum of the WPI and the SSS score

Source: 1. Firestein GS, Budd RC, Gabriel RC, McInnes IB, O'Dell JR, Koretzky G. Firestein & Kelley's Textbook of Rheumatology, 11th edition. Philadelphia: Elsevier; p. 827.
2. Wolfe F, Clauw DJ, Fitzcharles MA, Goldenberg DL, Häuser W, Katz RL, et al. 2016 revisions to the 2010/2011 fibromyalgia diagnostic criteria. Semin Arthritis Rheum. 2016;46:319-29.

- Inflammatory myopathy
- Hypothyroidism

TREATMENT

As there is no cure for FM, treatment focuses on symptom reduction, healthy lifestyle practices, and maintaining optimal function. The latest guidelines from the European League Against Rheumatism (EULAR) recommend both pharmacological and nonpharmacological approaches.

Nonpharmacological

- *Exercise and body-based therapies*
    - Aerobic exercise, hydrotherapy, and transcutaneous electric nerve stimulation (TENS) can relieve symptoms.
    - Meditative movements, such as tai chi, yoga, and qigong, are effective for overall symptom relief and improving physical function.
- *Patient education and self-management*
    - Educating patients and their families about FM is crucial before starting any treatment. They should understand the waxing and waning nature of FM and identify their triggers.
    - Reassure patients that their pain is due to altered pain processing in the nervous system, not tissue damage.
- *Cognitive-behavioral therapy (CBT)*
    - Combining pharmacological treatments with aerobic exercise and CBT is highly effective. CBT techniques, such as mindfulness-based stress reduction and operant behavioral therapy, can help manage symptoms.

The aim is to consolidate treatments and minimize medication use, targeting specific symptoms like sleep issues through improved sleep hygiene and circadian rhythm regulation.

Diet Recommendations

Patients with FM should avoid tobacco, alcohol, aspartame, and monosodium glutamate (MSG). A gluten-free diet is encouraged, along with reducing or avoiding caffeine intake, especially before bedtime. A well-balanced diet with appropriate vitamin supplementation and weight management is also recommended.

Pharmacological Treatment

- *Tricyclic antidepressants (TCA)*:
    - *Amitriptyline dosing*: Start with 10 mg at bedtime; maintenance dose of 20–30 mg.
    - *Cyclobenzaprine (alternative)*: 5–20 mg at bedtime
    - *Advantages*: Easily accessible, cost-effective, extensively researched, and proven effective for managing pain and improving sleep

- *Disadvantage*: Requires slow titration
- *Common side effects*: Anticholinergic and antihistamine effects like dry mouth, constipation, urinary retention, sedation, and concentration issues
- *Consideration*: Potential risk of cardiotoxicity
- Serotonin-norepinephrine reuptake inhibitor (SNRI):
  - *Duloxetine dosing*: Start with 20-30 mg in the morning; maintenance dose of 60 mg
  - *Milnacipran dosing*: Start with 12.5 mg in the morning; maintenance dose of 50-100 mg twice daily
  - *Advantages*: Demonstrated efficacy in numerous clinical trials (except for venlafaxine); potentially beneficial for patients with concurrent depression; generally better tolerated compared with TCA
  - *Disadvantages*: Common side effects include headaches, nausea, dry mouth (duloxetine), and constipation (milnacipran).
- *Gabapentinoids*:
  - *Pregabalin dosing*: Begin with 25-50 mg at bedtime; maintenance dose of 300-450 mg/day
  - *Gabapentin dosing*: Start with 100 mg at bedtime; maintenance dose of 1,200-2,400 mg/day (divided doses)
  - *Advantage*: Potential improvement in pain and sleep
  - *Disadvantages*: Common side effects include dizziness, dry mouth, somnolence, weight gain, peripheral edema, and cognitive issues (particularly with pregabalin).
- *Analgesics*:
  - Acetaminophen
  - Nonsteroidal anti-inflammatory drugs (NSAIDs)
  - *Advantages*: Can be used adjunctively with other treatments. Potential usefulness for concurrent conditions such as osteoarthritis
  - *Disadvantage*: Limited formal studies on the effectiveness of acetaminophen
- *Tramadol*:
  - *Dosing*: Typically used to improve short-term pain management and quality of life
  - *Advantages*: Can be considered for patients with severe pain resistant to other treatments
  - *Disadvantages*: Potential for misuse or abuse (classified as Schedule IV by the Drug Enforcement Administration). Long-term effects are not well understood.
- *Topical capsaicin gel*:
  - *Application*: Apply several times a day to the affected area.
  - *Advantages*: Potential for pain relief and are generally considered safe
  - *Disadvantage*: Commonly causes a mild burning sensation on application to the skin

CONCLUSION

Understanding the interplay between genetic, environmental, and psychological factors is crucial for effective treatment. Continued research and a holistic approach to patient care are essential for improving quality of life for those affected by this condition.

BIBLIOGRAPHY

1. Arnold LM, Bradley LA, Clauw DJ, Glass JM, Goldenberg DL. Multidisciplinary care and stepwise treatment for fibromyalgia. J Clin Psychiatry. 2008;69(12):e35.
2. Clauw DJ. Fibromyalgia: a clinical review. JAMA. 2014;311(15):1547-55.
3. Gedalia A, Press J, Klein M, Buskila D. Joint hypermobility and fibromyalgia in schoolchildren. Ann Rheum Dis. 1993;52:494-6.
4. Mease PJ, Arnold LM, Crofford LJ, Williams DA, Russell IJ, Humphrey L, et al. Identifying the clinical domains of fibromyalgia: contributions from clinician and patient Delphi exercises. Arthritis Rheum. 2008;59:952-60.
5. Wolfe F, Clauw DJ, Fitzcharles MA, Goldenberg DL, Katz RS, Mease P, et al. The American College of Rheumatology preliminary diagnostic criteria for fibromyalgia and measurement of symptom severity. Arthritis Care Res. 2010;62(5):600-10.
6. Wolfe F, Smythe HA, Yunus MB, Bennett RM, Bombardier C, Goldenberg DL, et al. The American College of Rheumatology 1990 criteria for the classification of fibromyalgia. Report of the Multicenter Criteria Committee. Arthritis Rheum. 1990;33:160-72.
7. Wolfe F, Walitt B. Culture, science and the changing nature of fibromyalgia. Nat Rev Rheumatol. 2013;9(12):751-5.
8. Yang TY, Chen CS, Lin CL, Lin WM, Kuo CN, Kao CH. Risk for irritable bowel syndrome in fibromyalgia patients: a national database study. Medicine (Baltimore). 2017;96:e6657.

CHAPTER 38

Management of Complex Regional Pain Syndrome

Saransh Bahl

INTRODUCTION

Complex regional pain syndrome (CRPS) is characterized by spontaneous pain, hyperalgesia, allodynia (perception of pain from a nonpainful stimulus), edema, temperature or pseudomotor changes, motor function abnormality, and autonomic changes. It includes reflex sympathetic dystrophy (RSD), post-traumatic dystrophy, Sudeck's dystrophy, causalgia, shoulder–hand syndrome, algodystrophy, and sympathetically maintained pain. The word "complex" describes different clinical presentations and "regional" describes the distribution of different symptoms and findings.

The incidence of CRPS is 26/100,000 life-years and is always associated with sensory, motor, autonomic, skin, and bone abnormalities in a limb. History of trauma is usually present but without any severity of trauma. In 10% of cases, one may not find the history of trauma or there may be very minor trauma. The female-to-male ratio is 4:1, with a median age of 46 years at the onset. The upper limb is affected twice as commonly as the lower limb.

The International Association for the Study of Pain delineated two main categories of the syndrome:
- CRPS I (formerly RSD) represents patients who have had a musculoskeletal injury without a defined neural injury.
- CRPS II (causalgia) includes patients who fulfil the same criteria but who have evidence of a neural injury.

A female predisposition has been found with frequent involvement of the upper extremity.

CLASSIFICATION

Harden et al. gave the Budapest criteria for CRPS which divided the symptoms into four categories **(Box 1)**. Although defined as types I and II, CRPS frequently results from both musculoskeletal and neural injuries.

> **BOX 1** Budapest diagnostic criteria for complex regional pain syndrome.
>
> 1. Continued pain disproportionate to any inciting event
> 2. At least one symptom in three (clinical diagnostic criteria) or four (research diagnostic criteria) of the following:
>   i. *Sensory*: Hyperesthesia or allodynia
>   ii. *Vasomotor*: Temperature asymmetry, skin color changes, or skin color asymmetry
>   iii. *Sudomotor or edema*: Changes or asymmetry in sweating
>   iv. *Motor or trophic*: Decreased range of motion, motor dysfunction (weakness, tremor, or dystonia), or trophic changes (hair, nail, skin)
> 3. One sign at time of diagnosis in two or more of the following categories:
>   i. *Sensory*: Hyperalgesia (to pinprick) or allodynia (to light touch), deep somatic pressure, or joint movement
>   ii. *Vasomotor*: Temperature asymmetry, skin color change or asymmetry
>   iii. *Sudomotor or edema*: Edema, changes or asymmetry in sweating
>   iv. *Motor or trophic*: Decreased range of motion or motor dysfunction (weakness, tremor, or dystonia), or trophic changes (hair, nails, or skin)
> 4. No other diagnosis better explains the signs and symptoms
>
> Source: Azar FM, Terry Canale S, Beaty JH. Campbell's Operative Orthopaedics, 14th edition. Philadelphia: Elsevier; p. 3280.

CLINICAL FEATURES

Sympathetically mediated cases may result in homeostatic dysregulation of the autonomic nervous system, which clinically presents as edema, vasomotor effects, sudomotor dysfunction, temperature change, and color change (warm subtype), frequently occurring in the early phase.

The affected area may be erythematous, swollen, and warm to touch with hyperhidrosis. Mobility of joints is restricted and never fully recovered. All these changes are termed RSD. Focal well-defined neural injuries may result in symptoms that are nondermatomal and nonsclerotomal (maladaptive neuroplasticity) in presentation leading the clinician to consider the possibility of additional or more central cortical reprogramming.

The extremity may appear pale and cool to the touch (cold subtype), with altered skin texture, sparse hair distribution, reduced nail growth, contracture, abnormal posture, and reduction in bone mass, described as Bonica's description of sequential clinical stages **(Table 1)**.

LABORATORY INVESTIGATIONS

Patients with sympathetic dysregulation may have alterations delineated through autonomic testing, quantitative sudomotor axon reflex testing, thermography, and asymmetric temperature measurements. Reduced bone mass density may be suspected on standard radiographs with periarticular reabsorption. Triple-phase bone scan is the most sensitive radiographic

Table 1: Bonica stages of reflex sympathetic dystrophy.			
Stage	Onset	Symptoms	Duration
Stage 1 dysfunction	1–3 months	• Burning pain beyond dermatomes (follows thermatomes) • Spasm and tendency for immobilization	2–8 weeks
Stage 2 dystrophy	3–7 months	• Vasoconstriction • Unilateral cold extremity • Hair loss • Tendency for weakness, tremor, and spasticity (flexed arm, extended legs)	2–4 months
Stage 3 atrophy	>7 months	• Smooth, glossy, edematous skin • Pale or cyanotic skin • Lymphedema • Atrophy of distal muscles • Spasm, dystonia, tremor	>4 months
Stage 4	Several months to years	• Loss of job and spouse in rare advanced severe cases • Unnecessary surgery • Orthostatic hypotension • Hypertension • Heart attack • Neurodermatitis • Angiectasis • Depression, death caused by suicide	A few months

Source: Azar FM, Terry Canale S, Beaty JH. Campbell's Operative Orthopaedics, 14th edition. Philadelphia: Elsevier; p. 3281.

study. MRI shows changes suggestive of significant muscle edema, interstitial edema, and hyperpermeability. No confirmatory laboratory or biochemical investigation is available to date to establish the diagnosis.

MANAGEMENT

The main aim is early diagnosis and an active multidisciplinary function-oriented treatment regimen. Validation of a patient's symptoms is important. Pain control, physical rehabilitation, and restoration of function are the main objectives of treatment. Treatment strategies include pharmacological, procedural, functional exercises, and psychological evaluation.

Pharmacological Treatment

- *Antiepileptic drugs*: Gabapentin (600 mg) and pregabalin (150 mg) have a limited role, whereas carbamazepine (600 mg/day) has shown good results in very small series.

- *Antidepressants*: Tricyclic antidepressants (amitriptyline) have been used in neuropathic pain, but have a limited role in CRPS.
- Nonsteroidal anti-inflammatory drugs (NSAIDs) help to mediate inflammation and hyperalgesia.
- Opioids can reduce the pain of neuropathic origin. Morphine is given 10 mg once a day to 10 mg thrice daily over the first 5 days and then as 10 mg TDS.
- *Bisphosphonates*: Intravenous pamidronate (60 mg) and oral alendronate (40 mg daily for 8 weeks) also reduce pain.
- *Vitamin C*: Ascorbic acid (200/500/1,500 mg for 50 days) reduces the incidence of CRPS.
- Oral tadalafil (20 mg/day for 21 weeks) significantly reduces pain in CRPS of long-standing duration.
- Intravenous infusion of low-dose ketamine for 4–5 days continuously significantly reduces pain.
- *Lumbar sympathetic block*: In long-standing CRPS, a lumbar sympathetic block with 0.5% bupivacaine (10 mL) and botulinum toxin (75 U) provides long-term relief.
- Elevation and active exercises of the extremity are of paramount importance. Attention should be paid to preserve the full range of motion in the metacarpophalangeal and the interphalangeal joints of hands when pain is severe and persistent and marked swelling threatens function.
- Sympathectomy leads to rapid recovery. Sequential stellate ganglion blocks are combined with physical therapy in patients with CRPS involving the upper extremity. This surgical procedure must be performed early before fibrotic contractures supervene. Persistent stiffening of the metacarpophalangeal joints in extension may require multiple capsulotomies.
- Medication includes anti-inflammatory and analgesic drugs (oral or topical), tricyclic antidepressants, calcitonin, bisphosphonates, selective serotonin reuptake inhibitors, anticonvulsants, and other antidepressants. The use of ketamine infusions in select patients has been proposed.
- Mirror-assisted movement patterns also may be incorporated. Some concern exists about overzealous therapy aggravating the condition; however, restoration of movement is of paramount importance.

TYPE 2 COMPLEX REGIONAL PAIN SYNDROME/CAUSALGIA

Causalgia is a condition characterized by post-traumatic pain that is persistent, diffuse, and burning, occurring in paroxysms and provoked by various stimuli. Its relief by interruption of sympathetic impulses classifies it as a sympathetic dystrophy.

Etiology and Pathological Physiology

The cause is usually a trauma, often trivial in nature. In severe cases, the pathological feature is a partial lesion of a peripheral nerve, most commonly the median nerve, sciatic nerve, or brachial plexus. When paralysis is complete and associated with causalgia on surgery, a neuroma with the nerve in continuity may be found. Electric stimulation of this nerve fails to evoke a motor response.

Clinical Picture

The injury is often trivial in nature such as a sprain, although any type of trauma is causative. The more severe injuries are those causing a partial lesion to a peripheral nerve. Pain is constant, intense, and burning in nature. Rarely, it is knifelike, crushing, or paresthetic. It is distributed diffusely over the distal portion of a limb not related to a nerve distribution and frequently over the palm and sole. The skin over the affected area is hyperalgesic and becomes reddened, blotchy, dry, edematous, and warm, a picture of vasodilatation. The skin temperature is elevated. Later, sometimes without the antecedent vasodilatation, the skin becomes cold, pale, cyanotic, perspiring, thin, and glossy and nails are brittle and ridged. The discomfort is worsened by dryness and heat and is eased by moisture and coolness. However, not uncommonly, the opposite effect is obtained.

Diagnostic Sympathetic Block

The interruption of sympathetic impulses by infiltration of a local anesthetic about the sympathetic chain will reduce or eliminate the pain. For the upper extremity, the needle is inserted between the first and the second ribs. For the lower extremity, the anesthetic is injected adjacent to the first and the second lumbar vertebrae.

Management

Nonpharmacological Measures

- Conservative treatment often includes warm applications for the vasoconstrictor type and cold for the vasodilation type.
- Limb elevation and rest

Pharmacological Treatment

- Tetraethylammonium chloride (etamon chloride) is given intramuscularly every 6 hours in a dose not exceeding 20 mg/kg of body weight. The block should not be continued for >36 hours.
- Tolazoline hydrochloride (Priscoline) is given orally in a dosage of up to 50 mg six times daily. Because it also has a local effect in causing vasodilatation, it may accentuate symptoms in the vasodilated type of causalgia.

- Nylidrin hydrochloride (Arlidin) in a dose of 6 mg thrice daily is effective and has minimum side effects.
- Procaine blocks of the sympathetic trunk are effective in many cases but they are required daily, and the relief obtained varies from an hour to a permanent cure even on one injection. For the upper extremity, 0.5% procaine with adrenalin is injected into the paravertebral space between the first and the second dorsal vertebrae.

Surgical Treatment
- Upper extremity causalgia is treated by sectioning the thoracic trunk below the third ganglion and removing the gray and the white rami to the second and the third ganglia.
- Lower extremity causalgia requires the removal of several upper lumbar ganglia, from the first to the fourth. Results are better when the first lumbar ganglion is included.
- When a partial nerve lesion can be identified, neurolysis, resection of the neuroma, and neurorrhaphy are necessary in addition to sympathectomy, to eliminate residual partial pains and paresthesia.

CONCLUSION

Effective management of CRPS requires a multidisciplinary approach tailored to individual needs. Early intervention, combining medication, therapy, and psychological support, is crucial. Continued research and evolving treatment strategies are essential to improving outcomes and quality of life for patients.

BIBLIOGRAPHY

1. Azar FM, Beaty JH. Campbell's Operative Orthopaedics, 14th edition. Amsterdam: Elsevier; 2022. pp. 3280-2.
2. Cossins L, Okel RW, Cameron H, Simpson B, Poole HM, Goebel A. Treatment of complex regional pain syndrome in adults: a systematic review of randomized controlled trials published from June 2000 to February 2012. Eur J Pain. 2013;17:158-73.
3. Harden RN, Bruehl S, Stanton Hicks M, Wilson PR. Proposed new diagnostic criteria for complex regional pain syndrome. Pain Med. 2007;8:326-31.
4. Jain AK. Turek's Orthopaedics, Principles and Their Applications, 7th edition. New Delhi: Wolters Kluwer India; 2016. pp. 796-9.
5. Robinson JN, Sandom, J Chapman PT. Efficacy of pamidronate in complex regional pain syndrome type I. Pain Med. 2004;5:276-80.
6. Shah A, Kirchner J. Complex regional pain syndrome. Foot Ankle Clin N Am. 2011;16: 351-66.
7. Zollinger PE, Tuinerbreijer WE, Breederveld RS, Kreis RW. Can vitamin C prevent complex regional pain syndrome in patients with wrist fractures? A randomized controlled multicenter dose-response study. J Bone Joint Surg Am. 2007;89:1424-31.

CHAPTER 39

Myofascial Syndrome

Saransh Bahl

INTRODUCTION

Myofascial pain syndrome (MPS) is a nonarticular, nonbony musculoskeletal (MSK) pain disorder characterized by contracted bands of skeletal muscles that contain discrete painful nodules called trigger points (TPs) which seem to be the originators of the pain response.

Trigger points are small, hyperirritable, and sensitive areas in a taut band of muscle that spontaneously or on compression cause pain in a distant region known as the "referred zone." In contrast, tender spots cause pain only locally on compression and taut bands are groups of muscle fibers that are "hard" on palpation. They can affect any muscle in the body and significantly impact the quality of life.

ETIOLOGY

The causative factor for the generation of TP is unknown, but many factors are taken into consideration:
- Unusual muscle activity patterns—perhaps as a result of bad sleeping/lying-down position, bad sitting posture, or prolonged use of mobile phones or computer screens—are believed to generate abnormal contractile forces in certain muscle groups of the head, neck, and arm.
- Psychological conditions such as anxiety, depression, or lack of sleep may further exacerbate the pain response.
- A sedentary lifestyle or immobilization due to injury can weaken muscles leading to MPS.
- Anxious personalities in a hyperarousable state may reduce descending pain modulatory signals leading to maintenance of pain and potential loss of therapeutic effect by drugs which work on the descending modulatory system.

- Nutritional deficiencies, especially of vitamins B and D and minerals like magnesium, may contribute to muscle pains.
- Other conditions like fibromyalgia, arthritis, and other chronic pain disorders can increase the risk of developing MPS.

PATHOGENESIS

Repetitive or prolonged activity can cause overloading of the muscle fibers leading to muscle hypoxia and ischemia. In addition, intracellular calcium pumps turn dysfunctional due to energy depletion. An increase in intracellular calcium induces sustained muscle contraction which results in the development of taut bands. Moreover, inflammatory mediators caused by muscle injury contribute to pain and tenderness of the affected muscles. Other theories such as neurogenic inflammation, sensitization, and limbic dysfunction are proposed to be associated with MPS.

CLINICAL FEATURES AND DIAGNOSIS

Diagnosis of MPS is based mainly on the elicitation of tender points with a history suggestive of pain attributable to such a TP. Referred pain symptoms like myofascial pain in the infraspinatus muscle usually refer to the anterior deltoid area, lateral aspect of the arm, and radial half of the hand. The onset of pain may be acute or insidious. In some patients, symptoms occur after muscle injuries or overuse activities. On the other hand, certain patients develop symptoms without identifiable precipitating factors.

INVESTIGATIONS

Complete blood cell count is performed to rule out an infection.

Other blood investigations include serum calcium, phosphorus, and alkaline phosphatase measurements for possible bone disease, serum uric acid determination for gout, serum creatinine and creatine kinase levels to detect muscle disease, and erythrocyte sedimentation rate, rheumatoid factor, latex fixation, and antinuclear antibody tests for suspected rheumatoid arthritis.

Electromyography can be used to evaluate muscle function.

Psychological evaluation and psychometric testing are good research tools, but they have little diagnostic value.

As such, there exists no confirmatory laboratory test.

MANAGEMENT

Nonpharmacological

Physical Modalities

Several therapeutic modalities, both heating and cooling, can be tried as a part of the management of MPS. Ultrasound therapy (UST) is one of the most common physical modalities due to its thermal and nonthermal properties as well as the ability to penetrate deeper structures.

Dry needling has been traditionally used as one of the fastest and most effective ways to inactivate myofascial trigger points (MTrPs) and help alleviate the accompanied pain. The needle is placed into MTrPs using an in-and-out technique in multiple directions to inactivate the MTrP.

Extracorporeal shockwave and low-power lasers significantly reduce pain in patients with MPS. Transcutaneous electric nerve stimulation (TENS) is used to provide pain relief. Electrical twitch obtaining intramuscular stimulation (ETOIMS) is another method of using an electrical current through a monopolar electromyography needle to engage deep motor endplates.

Counseling the patients about stretching exercises and ergonomic modification is done.

Pharmacological Treatment

- Nonsteroidal anti-inflammatory drugs (NSAIDs) are the most commonly used drugs for MPS due to their easy availability and relatively milder side effects.
- Tramadol is a centrally acting inhibitor of dorsal horn presynaptic norepinephrine/serotonin reuptake and increases central serotonin release and is frequently used for its multimodal analgesic effects and low abuse potential.
- A lidocaine patch is a transdermal local anesthetic preparation that alters the ability of nerves to conduct pain impulses.
- Tropisetron is a 5-HT3 receptor antagonist and alpha-7-nicotinic receptor agonist and can be used as an analgesic for fibromyalgia and myofascial pain. Its availability in the market is currently limited.
- Tizanidine is a centrally acting alpha-2-adrenergic agonist and decreases muscle spasticity.
- Benzodiazepines depress the presynaptic release of serotonin and excite gamma-aminobutyric acid (GABA), which causes rapid inhibitory neurotransmission.
- Thiocolchicoside (TCC) is a competitive GABAA antagonist and glycine agonist that also functions as an anti-inflammatory, analgesic, and muscle relaxant drug.
- Tricyclic antidepressants (TCAs) like amitriptyline are a class of medications used for chronic pain, fibromyalgia, and neuropathic pain.
- Duloxetine, a serotonin–norepinephrine reuptake inhibitor (SNRI), has recently been found to be an efficacious treatment for painful MSK conditions.

CONCLUSION

Effective management of MPS requires a tailored approach combining physical therapy, medication, and lifestyle changes. Early intervention and a comprehensive treatment plan are crucial for optimal outcomes and improved quality of life.

BIBLIOGRAPHY

1. Chu J, Yuen K, Wang B, Chan R, Schwartz I, Neuhauser D. Electrical twitch-obtaining intramuscular stimulation in lower back pain: a pilot study. Am J Phys Med Rehabil. 2004;83:104-11.
2. Crockett D, Foreman M, Alden L, Blasberg B. Comparison of treatment modes in the management of myofascial pain dysfunction syndrome. Biofeedback Self Regul. 1986;11:279-91.
3. Fomby E, Mellion M. Identifying and treating myofascial pain syndrome. Phys Sport Med. 1997;25:67-75.
4. Hong C. Lidocaine injection versus dry needling to the myofascial trigger point. The importance of the local twitch response. Am J Phys Med Rehabil. 1994;73:256-63.
5. Menon NA. Myofascial pain: a review of diagnosis and treatment. Indian J Phys Med Rehabil. 2023;33(1):2-7.
6. Tantanatip A, Chang KV. Myofascial pain syndrome. In: StatPearls. Treasure Island, FL: StatPearls Publishing; 2024. [online] Available from https://www.ncbi.nlm.nih.gov/books/NBK499882/ [Last accessed September, 2024].

CHAPTER 40

Interventional Techniques for Pain Relief

Sunana Gupta, Rajesh Mahajan

■ INTRODUCTION

Interventional techniques have become a pivotal component in the management of musculoskeletal pain, offering targeted, minimally invasive options to diagnose and treat pain sources. These procedures, guided by imaging technologies, aim to provide effective pain relief, improve function, and reduce the need for long-term medication or surgery. Common interventions include nerve blocks, joint injections, and radiofrequency ablation, among others (RFA). This chapter provides an overview of these techniques, emphasizing their role in enhancing patient outcomes in the management of musculoskeletal pain. When conventional pharmacotherapy is insufficient, interventional strategies may be necessary to restore the patient's functional level and reduce pain.

■ EPIDURAL STEROID INJECTIONS

Epidural steroid injection (ESI) is a widely used intervention in musculoskeletal pain management, particularly for conditions affecting the spine, such as herniated discs, spinal stenosis, and radiculopathy. This procedure involves the injection of corticosteroids, often combined with a local anesthetic, into the epidural space surrounding the spinal nerves. ESIs aim to reduce inflammation and alleviate pain, providing relief for patients experiencing persistent or severe musculoskeletal symptoms.

The interlaminar epidural method involves inserting medication between the laminae of adjacent vertebrae and can be performed in the cervical, thoracic, and lumbar regions. The caudal epidural approach, on the other hand, entails injecting medication through the sacral hiatus and accessing the epidural space at the spine's base. The transforaminal epidural technique administers medication through the neural foramina, directly targeting the affected nerve root, often employed for precise pain relief in conditions like herniated discs or spinal stenosis.

Epidural steroid injections prove effective for radiculopathy, addressing the compression or irritation of spinal nerves that often leads to radiating pain or tingling along the nerve pathway. In one of the systematic reviews evaluating 70 studies for lumbar ESIs, efficacy was good for lumbar disc herniations, fair for spinal stenosis, and poor for failed back surgery syndrome. A comparative systematic review and meta-analysis of the Cochrane Review of randomized controlled trials (RCTs) of epidural injections in managing chronic low back and lower extremity pain with sciatica or lumbar radiculopathy showed Level I, or strong, evidence at 1 and 3 months and Level II evidence at 6 and 12 months.

Epidural steroid injections provide numerous advantages for patients experiencing musculoskeletal conditions. First, they offer effective pain relief by reducing inflammation with corticosteroids, allowing individuals to resume normal activities and participate in rehabilitation exercises more comfortably. Second, by targeting the root cause of pain, ESIs contribute to improved function and mobility, enabling patients to engage in daily activities with reduced discomfort. Lastly, ESIs can often help patients avoid the necessity of surgery by providing sufficient relief, offering a less invasive alternative for managing conditions like herniated discs, spinal stenosis, and radiculopathy.

The effectiveness of ESIs varies depending on factors such as the underlying condition, patient characteristics, and precise placement of the injection. While some patients experience significant and long-lasting pain relief, others may only experience temporary or partial improvement. ESIs are generally safe when performed by experienced healthcare providers. However, like any medical procedure, they carry some risks, including infection, bleeding, nerve damage, or allergic reactions to the medications. Careful patient selection, proper technique, and adherence to sterile protocols help minimize these risks.

JOINT INJECTION IN MUSCULOSKELETAL PAIN MANAGEMENT

Joint injection is a medical procedure involving the delivery of medications directly into a joint space to alleviate pain, reduce inflammation, and improve joint function. This technique is commonly used in managing various musculoskeletal conditions, offering both diagnostic and therapeutic benefits.

Joint injections typically involve corticosteroids, hyaluronic acid, local anesthetics, or regenerative substances in the joint space.

Corticosteroids, such as triamcinolone and methylprednisolone, are potent anti-inflammatory agents that help reduce swelling and pain by suppressing the immune response. In osteoarthritis, they are administered in weight-bearing joints like knees and hips, offering significant short-term relief and improved function by reducing pain and inflammation. Similarly, in rheumatoid arthritis (RA), these injections help preserve joint function and slow down further damage by alleviating inflammation and pain in affected joints. Conditions such as bursitis and tendinitis respond well to corticosteroid injections, providing significant pain relief and improved range of motion. Moreover, in managing acute gout attacks characterized by severe pain and inflammation, these injections play a crucial role in rapidly alleviating symptoms and offering relief during acute episodes.

Intra-articular regenerative therapy involves injecting regenerative substances, such as platelet-rich plasma (PRP), mesenchymal stem cells (MSCs), or hyaluronic acid derivatives, directly into the affected joint.

Intra-articular regenerative therapy aims to not only alleviate pain but also promote healing and tissue regeneration, offering a potential alternative to more invasive treatments like joint replacement surgery. While research on its effectiveness is ongoing, preliminary studies have shown promising results in reducing pain and improving function for patients with osteoarthritis and other joint conditions. As with any medical intervention, proper patient selection, technique, and monitoring are essential to ensure safety and optimize outcomes.

While generally safe, joint injections carry some risks, including infection, bleeding, and allergic reactions. Repeated corticosteroid injections can potentially weaken tendons and ligaments or lead to joint cartilage damage. Long-term effects and optimal dosing of regenerative substances are still under research. Close monitoring post-treatment is crucial for detecting and managing any adverse reactions promptly.

TRIGGER POINT INJECTIONS IN MUSCULOSKELETAL PAIN MANAGEMENT

Trigger point injections (TPIs) are a common and effective treatment for managing musculoskeletal pain, particularly in patients with myofascial pain syndrome. This procedure targets trigger points, which are hyperirritable spots within tight bands of muscle that can cause localized and referred pain.

Trigger points are often palpable as knots or tight bands within the muscle, which can cause significant pain and limit function. TPIs involve injecting a small amount of anesthetic, saline, or corticosteroid directly into the trigger point. The injection works by inactivating the trigger point, reducing inflammation, and interrupting the pain cycle.

Trigger point injections are indicated for several conditions, including myofascial pain syndrome, characterized by chronic pain due to trigger points in muscles, where TPIs can significantly reduce pain and improve function. Tension headaches, often caused by trigger points in the neck and shoulder muscles, can also be alleviated by TPIs, leading to a reduction in headache frequency. While fibromyalgia is a more complex condition, some patients may find relief from specific muscle pain with TPIs, although their efficacy in this context may vary.

The effectiveness of TPIs varies, but many patients experience significant and rapid pain relief. TPIs can also enhance the effectiveness of physical therapy by reducing pain, allowing patients to participate more fully in rehabilitation exercises. They are generally safe when performed by trained healthcare providers. Risks are minimal but can include infection, bleeding, or temporary soreness at the injection site. Proper technique and sterile conditions minimize these risks.

RADIOFREQUENCY ABLATION IN MUSCULOSKELETAL PAIN MANAGEMENT

Radiofrequency ablation is a minimally invasive procedure used to manage chronic musculoskeletal pain, particularly in cases where other treatments have failed. It involves using radiofrequency energy to heat and destroy specific nerve tissues, thereby interrupting pain signals to the brain.

Radiofrequency ablation works by targeting the nerves responsible for transmitting pain signals. During the procedure, a needle-like probe is inserted into the affected area under imaging guidance, such as fluoroscopy or ultrasound. Once in place, the probe delivers radiofrequency energy, generating heat that ablates the nerve tissue. This process effectively stops the nerve from sending pain signals, providing relief to the patient.

Radiofrequency ablation is notably advantageous for individuals grappling with chronic pain conditions, including facet joint pain, a frequent source of chronic back and neck pain, and sacroiliac joint pain, effectively addressing discomfort originating from the lower back's sacroiliac joints. Moreover, RFA proves beneficial for individuals with knee osteoarthritis, particularly those experiencing severe knee pain unresponsive to conservative treatments. By precisely targeting nerves responsible for transmitting pain signals, RFA offers these patients significant relief, enhancing their quality of life and functional mobility.

Radiofrequency ablation can provide significant pain relief, often lasting from several months to more than a year. The procedure can be repeated if necessary. Patients usually experience improvement in pain and function within a few weeks post procedure.

Safety is a major advantage of RFA. The risks are relatively low, including minor complications such as temporary discomfort, swelling, or bruising at the treatment site. Serious complications are rare but can include infection or nerve damage if not performed correctly.

CONCLUSION

Various interventional techniques, including epidural and joint corticosteroid injections, trigger point injections, PRP therapy, RFA among many others play a key role in musculoskeletal pain management. These techniques target inflammation, enhance tissue repair, and provide localized pain relief, offering effective, minimally invasive treatment options for a range of musculoskeletal conditions. Proper technique and patient selection are crucial for optimal outcomes.

BIBLIOGRAPHY

1. Benyamin RM, Wang VC, Vallejo R, Singh V, Helm Ii S. A systematic evaluation of thoracic interlaminar epidural injections. Pain Physician. 2012;15(4):E497-514.
2. Diwan S, Manchikanti L, Benyamin RM, Bryce DA, Geffert S, Hameed H, et al. Effectiveness of cervical epidural injections in the management of chronic neck and upper extremity pain. Pain Physician. 2012;15(4):E405-34.
3. El-Tallawy SN, Nalamasu R, Salem GI, LeQuang JAK, Pergolizzi JV, Christo PJ. Management of musculoskeletal pain: an update with emphasis on chronic musculoskeletal pain. Pain Ther. 2021;10(1):181-209.
4. Manchikanti L, Knezevic E, Latchaw RE, Knezevic NN, Abdi S, Sanapati MR, et al. Comparative systematic review and meta-analysis of Cochrane Review of epidural injections for lumbar radiculopathy or sciatica. Pain Physician. 2022;25(7):E889-916.
5. Patel K, Chopra P, Upadhyayula S. Epidural steroid injections. In: StatPearls. Treasure Island, FL: StatPearls Publishing; 2024 [Updated July, 2023].
6. Patel CB, Patel AA, Diwan S. The role of neuromodulation in chronic pelvic pain: a review article. Pain Physician. 2022;25(4):E531-42.
7. Smith E, Hoy DG, Cross M, Vos T, Naghavi M, Buchbinder R, et al. The global burden of other musculoskeletal disorders: estimates from the Global Burden of Disease 2010 study. Ann Rheum Dis. 2014;73:1462-9.
8. World Health Organization. (2022). Musculoskeletal conditions. World Health Organization. [online] Available from https://www.who.int/newsroom/fact/detail/musculoskeletalconditions [Last accessed September, 2024].

CHAPTER 41

Joint Injection Techniques

Siddhartha Sharma, Tanveer Ahmed Bhat

INTRODUCTION

Pain and joint effusion can be the presenting symptoms in a variety of musculoskeletal disorders. Pain is a protective response to a noxious stimulus, and very often, the orthopedic surgeon may need to identify accurately which anatomical structure is contributing to pain generation. In such cases, a diagnostic injection of a local anesthetic may clinch the diagnosis. Furthermore, injection techniques may also be used to alleviate pain in chronic conditions.

This chapter will look at some of the common injection techniques in orthopedics. It is intended to be a quick and handy review of common techniques and is by no means intended to cover this subject exhaustively.

JOINT INJECTION INDICATIONS

- As a part of the diagnostic workup of painful pathologies—diagnostic injections.
- As a part of the treatment protocol for painful pathologies—therapeutic injections.

PREREQUISITES

As is the case with any surgical procedure, informed written consent must be obtained from the patient. Whether the injection is being performed as a diagnostic or a therapeutic modality must be clarified to the patient. Explaining the procedure to patients often allays any apprehensions that they may have and makes the procedure comfortable for the patient as well as for the surgeon. Aseptic skin preparation and draping techniques should be followed. For injections, the choice of local anesthetic or corticosteroid rests with the surgeon and depends on the nature of pathology and is beyond the scope of discussion of this chapter. For joints such as the hip and shoulder, ultrasonography/image intensifier guidance may improve the accuracy of injection or aspiration, and this may be planned in conjunction with radiology services.

INJECTION TECHNIQUES

Shoulder

It is indicated for subacromial bursitis, periarthritis of the shoulder (frozen shoulder), rotator cuff tendinopathies, and subacromial space, and can be approached via the posterior or lateral approach.

- *Posterior subacromial approach*:
  - *Position*: The patient sits on a stool; the arm is slightly externally rotated; the surgeon stands behind the shoulder.
  - *Needle position*: 1 cm inferior and 1 cm medial to the tip of the posterolateral part of the acromion, as given in **Figure 1**
  - *Needle direction*: Medially and anteriorly, aiming for the coracoid process. Insert to a depth of 2–3 cm.
- *Lateral approach*:
  - *Position*: The patient sits on a stool; the arm is in the neutral position; the surgeon stands by the side of the shoulder.
  - *Needle position*: 0.5 cm inferior to the tip of the lateral border of the acromion, as demonstrated in **Figure 2**
  - *Needle direction*: Medially and slightly posteriorly, to a depth of 1.5–2.5 cm

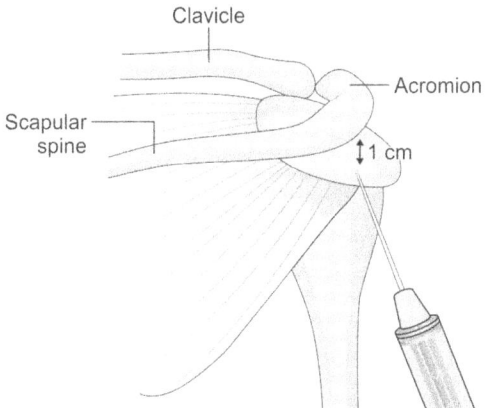

FIG. 1: Posterior subacromial approach.

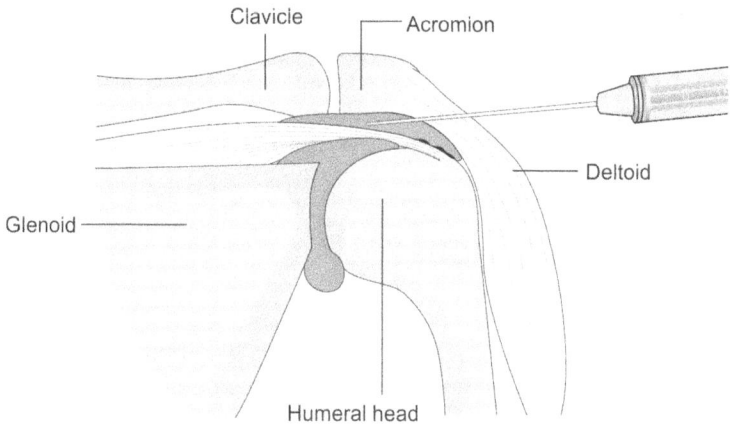

FIG. 2: Lateral subacromial approach.

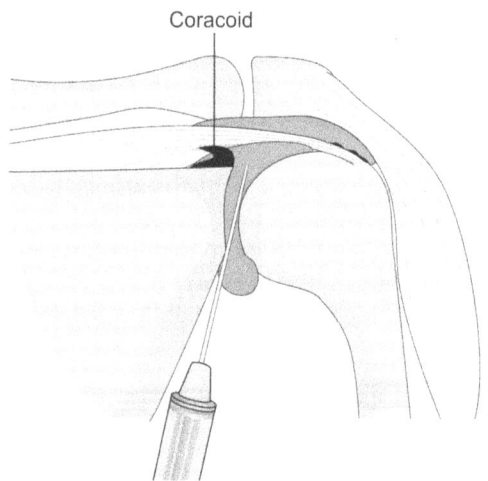

FIG. 3: Anterior approach to glenohumeral joint.

Glenohumeral Joint

The glenohumeral joint can be approached via anterior or posterior approaches. Note that for periarthritis, subacromial injection, rather than glenohumeral joint injection, is preferred, although either or both injections may be performed.

- *Anterior approach*:
  - *Position*: The patient sits on a stool; the arm is in slight internal rotation; the surgeon stands in front of the patient.
  - *Needle position*: Lateral and inferior to the coracoid process, as demonstrated in **Figure 3**
  - *Needle direction*: Slightly laterally and superiorly and posteriorly, to a depth of 1.5–2.5 cm

CHAPTER 41: Joint Injection Techniques

- *Posterior approach to glenohumeral joint*:
  - *Procedure steps*:
    a. Palpate the posterior aspect of the acromion and locate the soft spot just below the acromion (posterior glenohumeral joint line). This area is typically just lateral to the posterior angle of the acromion.
    b. Needle insertion
       - Using a 22- to 25-gauge needle, the needle is inserted approximately 2-3 cm inferior and medial to the posterolateral corner of the acromion.
       - The needle is directed anteriorly, slightly medially, and slightly superiorly toward the coracoid process. The angle is approximately 45° to the coronal and sagittal planes.
    c. Advancing the needle: Advance the needle gently while maintaining the angle until it enters the joint space. Resistance should decrease, and if aspirated, synovial fluid may be obtained, confirming the intra-articular placement.
    d. Injection: Once the needle is correctly positioned in the joint space, aspirate to ensure that there is no blood or synovial fluid, and then slowly inject the medication. The patient may feel a pressure sensation but should not feel significant pain.

Elbow

- *Lateral approach to elbow joint*: The elbow joint can be aspirated via the lateral approach.
  - *Position*: The patient sits or lies down; the elbow is flexed to 90°.
  - *Needle position*: An imaginary triangle is drawn, connecting the lateral epicondyle, the tip of the olecranon, and the radial head. The middle of this triangle is the entry point of the needle, as demonstrated in **Figure 4**.
  - *Needle direction*: It is parallel to the plane of the imaginary triangle described above.
- *Injection for lateral epicondylitis (tennis elbow)*:
  - *Position*: The patient sits or lies down; the elbow is flexed to 90°.
  - *Needle position*: 2 cm below and distal to the lateral epicondyle, at the point of maximum tenderness along the extensor carpi radialis brevis (ECRB) tendon, as delineated in **Figure 5**
  - *Needle direction*: Perpendicular, into the ECRB, for a depth of 1.5-2 cm
- *Injection for carpal tunnel syndrome*:
  - *Position*: The patient sits or lies down; the elbow is fully extended; the wrist is in a neutral position and the forearm is fully supinated.
  - *Needle position*: Just proximal to the distal wrist crease and ulnar to the palmaris longus tendon, as displayed in **Figure 6**
  - *Needle direction*: Toward the palm and slightly medially. Do not pierce the palmaris longus tendon as the median nerve lies beneath this. Insert for a depth of approximately 1 cm till the needle pierces the transverse carpal ligament, and a "give" is felt.

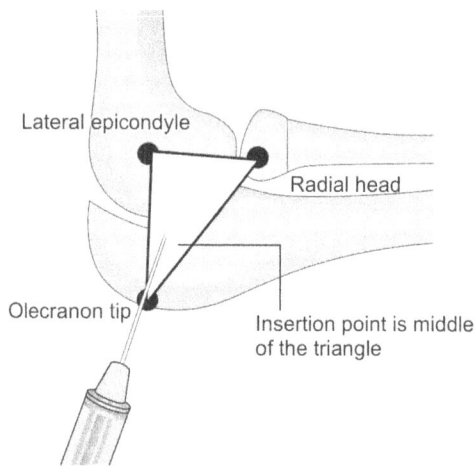

FIG. 4: Aspiration technique for elbow joint: Lateral approach.

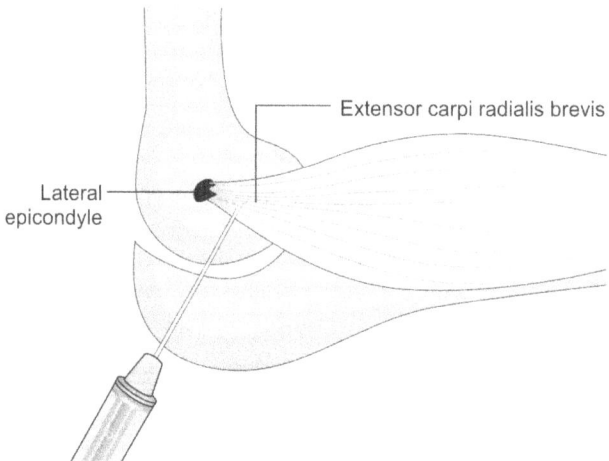

FIG. 5: Injection technique for tennis elbow.

Hip Joint

The hip joint can be aspirated via the anterolateral or the anterior approach. Ultrasonographic or radiographic guidance can improve the efficacy of the aspiration technique.
- *Anterolateral approach for hip joint aspiration:*
  - *Position*: The patient is supine; the limb is in a neutral position.
  - *Needle position*: Just distal and anterior to the tip of the greater trochanter
  - *Needle direction*: Along the femoral neck, aim for the femoral head. Insert for a depth of approximately 5–10 cm, till the needle pierces the hip joint capsule, and a "give" is felt.

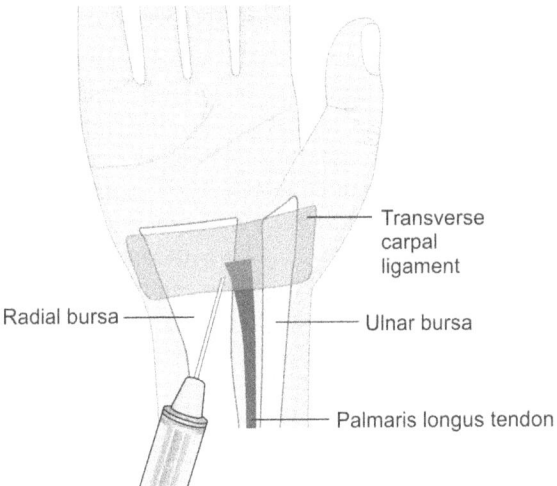

FIG. 6: Injection technique for carpal tunnel syndrome.

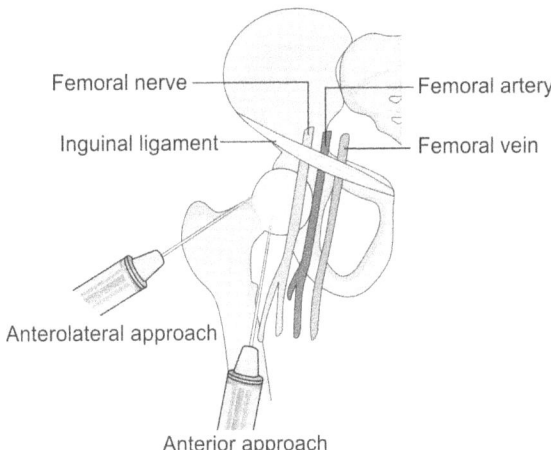

FIG. 7: Aspiration techniques for the hip joint.

- *Anterior approach for hip joint aspiration*:
  - *Position*: The patient is supine; the limb is in a neutral position.
  - *Needle position*: Palpate the femoral artery. The entry point is 2.5 cm lateral to the femoral artery pulse and 2.5 cm distal to the inguinal ligament, as displayed in **Figure 7**.
  - *Needle direction*: The needle is directed slightly medially, for a depth of approximately 5–8 cm, till it pierces the hip joint capsule, and a "give" is felt. This is best done under ultrasonographic or radiographic guidance.

Knee Joint: Lateral Retropatellar Approach

The knee joint can be aspirated via the lateral and medial retropatellar approaches, suprapatellar approach, or anterior approach. The medial retropatellar approach involves needle passage through the vastus medialis muscle and can therefore be painful. The suprapatellar approach can be used only if there is a significant collection in the suprapatellar pouch. The anterior approach to the tibiofemoral joint demands expertise on the part of the surgeon and is preferred for patients with knee flexion deformity. The lateral retropatellar approach is the workhorse approach for knee aspiration and injections. It does not involve any muscular planes and avoids damage to important neurovascular structures around the knee. This approach is described as follows:

- *Position*: Supine with the knee flexed to 10-15°. Place a small, folded towel under the knee to achieve this.
- *Needle position*: At the junction of the upper and middle thirds of the lateral border of the patella, and midway between the patella and the femoral condyle, as displayed in **Figure 8**.
- *Needle direction*: The needle is directed behind (posterior) to the patella and angled slightly inferiorly. The needle may need to be repositioned if bone is encountered. Care should be taken not to injure the cartilage or menisci.

Ankle

- *Position*: Sitting or supine, with the knee extended fully and the ankle plantarflexed to 10-15°
- *Needle position*: At the level of the ankle joint line, just medial to the tibialis anterior tendon; this is the medial-most tendon on the dorsal aspect of

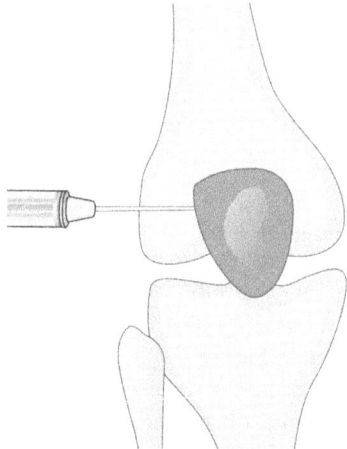

FIG. 8: Lateral retropatellar injection technique for the knee joint.

the ankle and can be readily visualized and marked by asking the patient to dorsiflex the ankle against resistance, as displayed in **Figure 9**.
- *Needle direction*: The needle is directed laterally and posteriorly.

Injection for Plantar Fasciitis
- *Position*: Sitting or supine, with the knee extended fully and the ankle in a neutral position. The surgeon stands on the caudal end of the couch and faces toward the patient's sole.
- *Needle position*: The plantar medial surface of the heel, at the site of maximal tenderness. The insertion point should be as close to the plantar medial surface of the calcaneus, as displayed in **Figure 10**.
- *Needle direction*: The needle is directed upward and posteriorly.

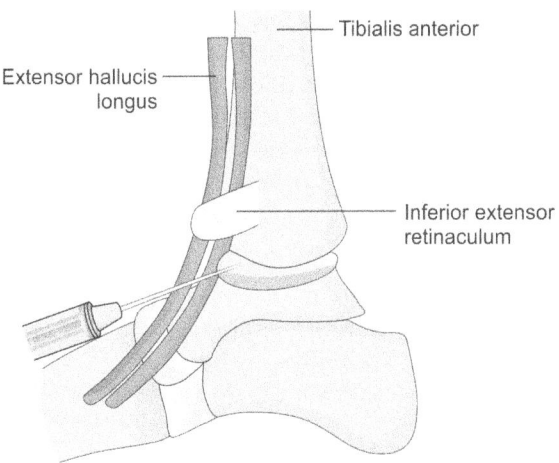

FIG. 9: Aspiration technique for ankle joint.

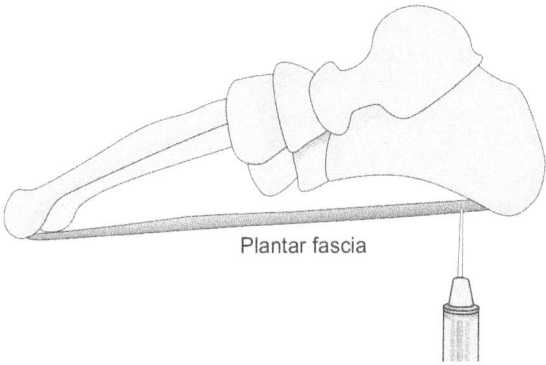

FIG. 10: Injection technique for plantar fasciitis.

AFTERCARE

Although these procedures can be performed on an outpatient basis, the patient must be monitored for some length of time after the injection, depending on the hospital or clinic protocols. If the patient is diabetic or has comorbid conditions that could predispose to infection, a short course of broad-spectrum antibiotics may be given. With injections such as corticosteroids or orthobiological agents, the patient may experience an initial increase in pain after the injection. This must be discussed before the injection, and a short course of analgesics may be prescribed. Icing can also be used to relieve pain in superficial joints such as the knee, ankle, elbow, and wrist.

CONCLUSION

Various injection techniques, including corticosteroid injections, platelet-rich plasma (PRP) therapy, and hyaluronic acid injections, play a key role in musculoskeletal pain management. These techniques target inflammation, enhance tissue repair, and provide localized pain relief, offering effective, minimally invasive treatment options for a range of musculoskeletal conditions. Proper technique and patient selection are crucial for optimal outcomes.

BIBLIOGRAPHY

1. Berkoff DJ, Miller LE, Block JE. Clinical utility of ultrasound guidance for intra-articular knee injections: a review. Clin Interv Aging. 2012;7:89-95.
2. Gado K, Elnady B, Said HG. Comparison between ultrasound-guided versus blind steroid injection in shoulder impingement syndrome. Alexandria J Med. 2016;52(4):327-33.
3. McCabe PS, Maricar N, Parkes MJ, Felson DT, O'Neill TW. The efficacy of intra-articular steroids in hip osteoarthritis: a systematic review. Osteoarthritis Cartilage. 2016;24(10):1509-17.
4. Skedros JG, Mears CS, Langston TH. Frequency of successful glenohumeral joint injections using specific anatomical guidelines. J Surg Orthop Adv. 2014;23(1):31-7.
5. Smith J, Wisniewski SJ, Mock BA, Creighton D, Koman LA, Smith TL. Anatomic study of the subacromial bursa in the shoulder: description of the bursal extension to the acromioclavicular joint region. J Shoulder Elbow Surg. 2015;24(8):e8-15.
6. Yu W, Fu X, Liu Y, Liu W, Sun Y, Zhu Y, et al. Efficacy and safety of ultrasound-guided intra-articular hyaluronic acid injection in knee osteoarthritis. Medicine (Baltimore). 2020;99(34):e21552.

CHAPTER 42

Role of Radiology in Managing Musculoskeletal Pain

Anchal Gupta

■ INTRODUCTION

The field of musculoskeletal (MSK) imaging has seen substantial growth over the past 20 years, with a remarkable increase of >500% in the utilization of magnetic resonance imaging (MRI), computed tomography (CT), and ultrasound (USG). While anatomical imaging remains a cornerstone of MSK radiology, significant advancements have been made in functional and molecular imaging, expanding the array of available technologies. This chapter aims to provide an overview of the most commonly used diagnostic and therapeutic modalities in managing MSK pain.

■ CONVENTIONAL RADIOGRAPHY

Radiographs are typically the initial investigation in assessing MSK disorders.

■ ULTRASOUND

Diagnostic USG serves as an alternative and complementary technique to MRI for evaluating soft tissues in the MSK system. USG offers advantages such as higher resolution, lower cost, portability, real-time and dynamic examination capabilities, and fewer contraindications. However, it is highly operator-dependent and limited by its inability to penetrate air and bone, restricting its use for structures deep within them. Despite these limitations, USG is often preferred over MRI for monitoring musculotendinous injuries due to its portability, lower cost, and real-time examination capability.

Key Points of Ultrasound Use
- *Point-of-care ultrasound (POCUS):* USG is increasingly used in various settings, including bedside, sports fields, and roadside, due to its flexibility, ease of operation, and portability.

- *Dynamic examination:* USG allows for dynamic evaluation of structures, useful for conditions like tendon instability and shoulder impingement, where abnormalities may not be apparent at rest.
- *Evaluation with metallic implants:* USG can effectively assess patients with metallic implants, which may not be suitable for MRI evaluation.
- *Doppler imaging:* Power Doppler provides critical information without intravenous contrast, aiding in the management of conditions like rheumatoid arthritis by indicating persistent disease activity.
- *Guidance for therapeutic interventions:* USG facilitates accurate needle placement for aspirations and therapeutic injections, making it ideal for real-time-guided procedures.

Common Indications for Ultrasound in Orthopedics
- *Acute conditions:* Tendon, muscle, and ligament injuries, foreign bodies, subtle fractures, and other soft-tissue traumas
- *Chronic conditions:* Infections, impingement, suspected nonunion, and nerve degeneration

Ultrasound-guided Interventional Pain Management
Types of Ultrasound-guided Interventions
- *Neuraxial:* Including intra-articular facet blocks, medial branch nerve blocks, and various types of epidural injections
- *Joint injections:* For knee, wrist, elbow, shoulder, hip, sacroiliac joint, and various nerves
- *Peripheral nerve blocks:* For nerves such as the stellate ganglion, greater occipital nerve, and branches of the brachial and lumbosacral plexus

Techniques
- *In-plane needle advancement:* The needle remains in view, maintaining an acute angle.
- *Out-of-plane needle advancement:* The needle tip enters the imaging plane, maintaining a perpendicular angle to the probe.

COMPUTED TOMOGRAPHY SCAN
Computed tomography imaging is utilized for both diagnostic and interventional purposes. It allows precise needle placement and identification of issues such as spinal stenosis prior to procedures, with minimal radiation exposure.

Common Procedures
- Transforaminal nerve blocks and facet joint blocks
- *Epidural steroid injections:* Performed using various techniques under fluoroscopic or CT guidance

- *Other guided procedures:* Including stellate ganglion and suprascapular nerve blocks, and barbotage for calcific tendinitis

ADVANCED INTERVENTIONAL TECHNIQUES

- *Vertebral augmentation:* Includes vertebroplasty and kyphoplasty, aimed at stabilizing osteoporotic compression fractures and reducing pain
- *Radiofrequency and cryoablation:* Used to treat conditions like osteoid osteoma, with applications expanding to metastatic lesions and benign tumors
- *Sacroplasty:* Performed to treat sacral insufficiency fractures, often using CT guidance
- *Transarterial embolization (TAE):* A minimally invasive procedure to control bleeding and reduce hypervascular tumors, now also applied to treat conditions like osteoarthritis and tendinopathy by targeting hypervascular tissues.

Indications for Transarterial Embolization
- Knee osteoarthritis
- Lateral epicondylitis
- Trapezius myalgia
- Adhesive capsulitis
- Tendinopathy and enthesopathy

CONCLUSION

Radiological imaging plays a crucial role in the management of MSK pain, offering a range of diagnostic and therapeutic options. From conventional radiography to advanced techniques like TAE, these modalities enhance the ability to diagnose, monitor, and treat various MSK conditions effectively.

BIBLIOGRAPHY

1. Babatunde OO, Jordan JL, Windt DA, Hill JC, Foster NE, Protheroe J. Effective treatment options for musculoskeletal pain in primary care: a systematic overview of current evidence. PLoS One. 2017;12:e0178621.
2. Breivik H, Collett B, Ventafridda V, Cohen R, Gallacher D. Survey of chronic pain in Europe: prevalence, impact on daily life, and treatment. Eur J Pain. 2006;10(4):287-333.
3. Cimmino MA, Ferrone C, Cutolo M. Epidemiology of chronic musculoskeletal pain. Best Pract Res Clin Rheumatol. 2011;25:173-218.
4. Ernstzen DV, Louw QA, Hillier SL. Clinical practice guidelines for the management of chronic musculoskeletal pain in primary healthcare: a systematic review. Implement Sci. 2017;12:1.
5. Merskey H, Fessard D, Bonica JJ, et al. Pain terms: a list with definitions and notes on usage. Recommended by the IASP subcommittee on taxonomy. Pain. 1979;6:249-52.
6. Saxena AK, Jain PN, Bhatnagar S. The prevalence of chronic pain among adults in India. Indian J Palliat Care. 2018;24(4):472-7.

7. Smith E, Hoy DG, Cross M, Vos T, Naghavi M, Buchbinder R, et al. The global burden of other musculoskeletal disorders: estimates from the Global Burden of Disease 2010 study. Ann Rheum Dis. 2014;73:1462-9.
8. Vos T, Abajobir AA, Abate KH, Abbafati C, Abbas KM, Abd-Allah F, et al. Global, regional, and national incidence, prevalence, and years lived with disability for 328 diseases and injuries for 195 countries, 1990–2016: a systematic analysis for the Global Burden of Disease Study 2016. Lancet. 2017;390:1211-59.
9. World Health Organization. (2019). Musculoskeletal conditions. Available from https://www.who.int/news-room/fact-sheets/detail/musculoskeletal-conditions [Last accessed September, 2024].

CHAPTER 43

Local Anesthesia in Musculoskeletal Pain Management

Zubair Ahmad Lone, Shubam Surmal

INTRODUCTION

Local anesthetics as part of multimodal analgesia, injection at the surgical site with a solution of bupivacaine or ropivacaine, or mixtures with the addition of nonsteroidal anti-inflammatory drugs (NSAIDs) are used. This is done in case of total knee prosthesis or spine surgery to reduce operating pain and opioid consumption without showing adverse effects. Infusion of locally anesthetic drugs directly to the wound proves to be an effective and safe method.

Local infiltration is done at the end of surgical procedures like:
- Intra-articular
- Incisional
- Subcuticular

It helps in decreasing immediate postoperative pain and the requirement of opioids.

Local anesthesia is also used very commonly for minor surgical procedures and for wound care. Apart from the humanitarian considerations, providing adequate analgesia and anesthesia will make it easy to do any small surgical procedure or any wound easier to treat. Without adequate pain relief:
- Wounds cannot be properly cleaned.
- Suturing becomes hurried and inappropriate.
- Abscesses may not be adequately drained.
- Muscle spasms prevent easy reduction of fractures and dislocations.

However, it is not always without risks, as local anesthesia can induce severe and life-threatening adverse effects such as convulsions, respiratory depression, hypotension, bradycardia, and cardiac arrest.

Therefore, before giving local anesthesia, always:
- Check history for previous sensitivity reactions.
- Have resuscitation equipment on hand.
- Avoid inadvertent intravenous (IV) administration.
- Do not exceed recommended safe doses.
- Have IV access by securing a cannula beforehand.

MAXIMUM SAFE DOSES

The maximum safe dose of commonly used local anesthetic (lidocaine or lignocaine) is shown in **Table 1**.

Lidocaine (lignocaine) with epinephrine (adrenaline) is contraindicated for injection around end arteries like: Fingers, toes, and if the patient is receiving tricycle antidepressants.

ANESTHETIC TECHNIQUES

Infiltration Around the Wound

The anesthetic will be most effective if injected immediately under the skin rather than into the subcutaneous fat layer. Therefore, injections should produce a visible "bleb."

Unless there is gross contamination or there is established infection, insert the needle through the cut edge of the wound and then work outward from the initial injection site.

Using 0.5% or 1% rather than 2% allows a larger area to be anesthetized and therefore usually is more suitable.

Once the injection is complete:
- Check the area for anesthetic effects (can take 15-20 minutes for anesthetic effects to occur).
- If adequate anesthesia is present, begin the procedure.
- Never "press on regardless" with a procedure unless there are exceptional reasons.
- Never exceed the maximum recommended dose of local anesthetic.

Nerve blockade is also used for analgesia and anesthesia like:
- *Peripheral nerve blocks*
    - Paravertebral blocks
    - Brachial plexus block

Table 1: Maximum safe dose and concentration of local anesthetic.	
Maximum total dose: 200 mg	
Concentration	Maximum safe volume
2%	25 mL
1%	50 mL

CHAPTER 43: Local Anesthesia in Musculoskeletal Pain Management

- Lumbar plexus block
- Femoral nerve block
- Fascia iliaca nerve block
- Adductor canal block
- Sciatic nerve blocks

A nerve block is a more elegant technique than wound infiltration and requires much smaller doses of local anesthetic.

- *Ring block—useful for fingers and toes*
  - Use 1-2 mL 2% of plain lidocaine (lignocaine) on either side of the digit, i.e., dorsally and ventrally, but preferably not distal to the interdigital web.
  - Use a rubber tourniquet held with forceps (more effective than a knot) to increase the duration of the block and stop bleeding.
  - The tourniquet must be released after a maximum duration of 30 minutes.
  - Always record the following in patients' notes:
    - The circulation returned on the release of the tourniquet
    - The time of application and release of the tourniquet

ANESTHESIA IN CHILDREN

Local anesthesia in children is fine if it can be effective and if the child is old enough to understand what is happening. *Do not* tell a child that he or she will "not feel anything" as the initial injection of anesthetic can be quite painful.

For simple, quick procedures in children too young to understand an explanation of the procedure (<4 years):
- Give alimemazine (trimeprazine) syrup according to the child's weight (**Table 2** for dose).
- Allow 30-60 minutes for the full sedative effect to occur.
- Explain to the parents that it is not a complete anesthetic.

Table 2: Dose of alimemazine as per body weight and age (for a dosage of 2 mg/kg).

Body weight		Approximate age (years)	Volume of 30 mg/5 mL alimemazine (trimeprazine) syrup
kg	Pounds		
12	26	2	3 mL
14	31	3	4 mL
16	35	4	4.5 mL
19	42	5	6 mL
21	46	6	7 mL
24	53	7	8 mL

Alimemazine (Trimeprazine)

Alimemazine (trimeprazine) can be given as a premedication for children aged between 2 and 7 years at a dose of 2 mg/kg with a maximum dosage of 60 mg. A detailed description of dosage is given in **Table 2**.

CONCLUSION

Local anesthesia plays a critical role in the effective management of musculoskeletal pain by providing targeted pain relief, minimizing systemic side effects, and enhancing patient comfort during diagnostic and therapeutic procedures. Its precise application in regional blocks or infiltrations offers a minimally invasive solution, improving recovery and overall outcomes.

BIBLIOGRAPHY

1. Chou R, Gordon DB, de Leon-Casasola OA, Rosenberg JM, Bickler S, Brennan T, et al. Management of postoperative pain: a clinical practice guideline from the American Pain Society, the American Society of Regional Anesthesia and Pain Medicine, and the American Society of Anesthesiologists' Committee on Regional Anesthesia, Executive Committee, and Administrative Council. J Pain. 2016;17(2):131-57.
2. Hadzic A, Vloka JD. Peripheral Nerve Blocks: Principles and Practice. New York: McGraw-Hill; 2004.
3. Horlocker TT, Wedel DJ, Rowlingson JC, Enneking FK, Kopp SL, Benzon HT, et al. Regional anesthesia in the patient receiving antithrombotic or thrombolytic therapy: American Society of Regional Anesthesia and Pain Medicine evidence-based guidelines (third edition). Reg Anesth Pain Med. 2010;35(1):64-101.
4. Ilfeld BM, Mariano ER, Williams BA. Local anesthetic infusion pumps. In: Brown DL (Ed). Atlas of Regional Anesthesia, 4th edition. Philadelphia: Elsevier Saunders; 2010. pp. 316-26.
5. Winnie AP. Plexus Anesthesia: Perivascular Techniques of Regional Anesthesia. Philadelphia: WB Saunders; 1983.

CHAPTER 44

Surgical Management of Musculoskeletal Pain

Sumeet Singh Charak

■ INTRODUCTION

Surgical management of musculoskeletal pain is typically considered when conservative treatments like medication, physical therapy, and injections have not provided relief, and the pain significantly impacts daily life or poses a risk of further damage. However, surgery is usually the last resort.

Indications for surgery in musculoskeletal pain vary depending on the specific condition, but some common indications include:
- Severe joint damage (e.g., advanced osteoarthritis)
- Persistent nerve compression (e.g., herniated disc causing radiculopathy)
- Traumatic injuries requiring surgical intervention (e.g., fractures not amenable to conservative management)
- Occasionally in inflammatory conditions, when resistant to medical treatment (e.g., rheumatoid arthritis)
- Progressive deterioration despite conservative management
- Loss of function or mobility impacting quality of life
- Overuse injuries, also known as cumulative trauma disorders (CTDs) or repetitive strain injuries, may occur due to repetitive work-related activities (e.g., carpel tunnel syndrome, tennis elbow).
- Infections of bone and joints (e.g., acute and chronic osteomyelitis, septic arthritis)
- Benign and musculoskeletal tumors (e.g., osteosarcoma, glomus tumor, bone cysts)
- Ischemic gangrene
- Structural deformities (e.g., scoliosis, kyphosis)
- Patients depending on regular use of analgesics
- Night sleep disturbed because of pain
- Activity of daily living being affected by pain
- Patient not able to cope

Ultimately, the decision for surgery should be made after careful consideration of the individual's specific circumstances, risks, and potential benefits of surgery.

Common surgical procedures for pain relief in musculoskeletal conditions include:
- Joint replacement surgery (e.g., knee replacement, and hip replacement) for severe osteoarthritis or joint damage
- Arthroscopic surgery to repair or remove damaged tissue in joints [e.g., meniscus repair, anterior cruciate ligament (ACL), posterior cruciate ligament (PCL) ligaments, repair in the knee, repairing of Bankart and rotator cuff tear in the shoulder]
- Spinal decompression surgery to relieve pressure on nerves caused by conditions like herniated discs or spinal stenosis in the cervical and lumbar spine
- Spinal fusion surgery to stabilize the spine in cases of instability or severe degenerative disc disease
- Laminectomy to remove part of the vertebral bone to relieve pressure on the spinal cord or nerves
- Osteotomy to correct bone deformities or realign joints (e.g., in cubitus varus, medial compartment osteoarthritis of the knee, malunion of the diaphysis of long bones in the lower limb, genu varum and valgus)
- Tendon or ligament repair surgery for injuries or chronic conditions affecting these structures
- Surgeries of CTDs or repetitive strain injuries (e.g., carpel tunnel release, lateral epicondylitis release for tennis elbow)
- Removing infection source by doing arthroscopic or open arthrotomy for septic arthritis, drainage and sequestrectomy for osteomyelitis, and debridement of infected soft tissues
- Surgical resection and curettage of tumors
- Amputation at different levels in nonsalvageable limbs or part of a limb (e.g., malignant tumors, ischemic gangrene)

These procedures aim to alleviate pain, restore function, and improve the quality of life for individuals with musculoskeletal pain that has not responded to conservative treatments.

CONCLUSION

Surgical management of musculoskeletal pain is essential when conservative treatments fail. By addressing underlying structural issues, surgery can provide lasting pain relief and restore function. While it carries risks, advancements in minimally invasive techniques have improved outcomes and recovery times, making surgery a viable option for many patients with chronic or severe musculoskeletal conditions.

BIBLIOGRAPHY

1. Bădilă AE, Rădulescu DM, Niculescu AG, Grumezescu AM, Rădulescu M, Rădulescu AR. Recent advances in the treatment of bone metastases and primary bone tumors: an up-to-date review. Cancers (Basel). 2021;13:4229.
2. Claes L, Kirschner S, Perka C, Rudert M. AE Manual of Endoprosthetics—Hip and Hip Revision. Heidelberg: Springer; 2012.
3. Iqbal ZA, Alghadir AH. Cumulative trauma disorders: a review. J Back Musculoskelet Rehabil. 2017;30(4):663-6.
4. Martin BI, Lurie JD, Tosteson AN, Deyo RA, Tosteson TD, Weinstein JN, et al. Indications for spine surgery: validation of an administrative coding algorithm to classify degenerative diagnoses. Spine. 2014;39(9):769-79.
5. Treuting R. Minimally invasive orthopedic surgery: arthroscopy. Ochsner J. 2000;2:158-63.
6. Wallace GF. Indications for amputations. Clin Podiatr Med Surg. 2005;22(3):315-28.
7. Wirtz DC. AE-Manual of Endoprosthetics—Knee. Heidelberg: Springer; 2011.

CHAPTER 45

Preemptive Analgesia

Yassir Mehmood

INTRODUCTION

Preemptive analgesia is defined as antinociceptive treatment given before a surgical incision. Amplification of postoperative pain is reduced by preventing the development of altered central processing of afferent input.

Pathophysiologically, surgical pain includes peripheral and central sensitization. The former is based on inflammatory meditators which are released locally at the wound site, enhancing the nociceptive pain, whereas the latter results from the hyperexcitability of neurons in the dorsal horn of the spinal cord in response to afferent generated at the site of injury.

OBJECTIVES

- To minimize the pain triggered by inflammatory mechanism post surgical incision
- To block the central nervous system's memory of pain
- To effectively manage the postoperative pain and development of the chronic pain

PHARMACOLOGICAL AND NONPHARMACOLOGICAL APPROACHES TO PREEMPTIVE ANALGESIA

Pharmacological Approaches

Nonsteroidal Anti-inflammatory Drugs Especially COX-2 Inhibitors

The use of selective cyclooxygenase-2 (COX-2) inhibitor nonsteroidal anti-inflammatory drugs (NSAIDs) reduces both postoperative pain and dependence on opioid consumption and their side effects. The most common

COX-2 inhibitors used as preemptive analgesia are celecoxib, valdecoxib, etoricoxib, and lumiracoxib.

Gabapentinoids
Gabapentinoids (gabapentin and pregabalin) are the mainstay of preemptive analgesia for significant reduction of postoperative pain and chronic neuropathic pain. Many studies have indicated that the use of gabapentin as a single dose preoperatively has significant beneficial effects on both pain scores and opioid dependence.

Marked inhibitory effect of gabapentin on preexisting allodynia and hyperalgesia is also seen.

Opioids
These are potent analgesics used in perioperative pain management. However, continuous patient assessment and monitoring of vital signs in the perioperative window are very important.

N-methyl-D-aspartate Receptor Antagonists
These analgesics are mainly used for patients undergoing major surgeries. Additional benefits like reduced opioid consumption and prevention of chronic pain are associated with these drugs.

Alpha-2-adrenergic Agonists
These drugs reduce the transmission of pain signals by inhibiting the release of norepinephrine.

These also offer a stable hemodynamic response by reducing sympathetic outflow.

Timing and Administration of Preemptive Analgesic Interventions
The effect of preemptive analgesia should last throughout the entire surgery and postoperative period as well.

Therefore, the timings of preemptive analgesia are very important for its overall effectiveness as mentioned in **Table 1**.

When administered at an appropriate time, it can significantly diminish the postoperative pain and development of chronic pain as well.

Nonpharmacological Approaches
Nonpharmacological approaches use physical and the psychological basis of pain management. They complement the pharmacological approaches and reduce the dependence on drugs and their side effects. *Various modalities include*:
- *Transcutaneous electrical nerve stimulation (TENS)*: It is an easy and noninvasive technique which reduces the perception of pain by delivering the electrical impulses to the skin surface. It provides anxiety relief and enhanced recovery.

CHAPTER 45: Preemptive Analgesia

Table 1: Commonly used medications for preemptive analgesia.

Drugs	Timing	Example
NSAIDs	30 minutes to 1 hour (*before incision*)	• Ketorolac 30 mg IV/IM • Ibuprofen, oral 400–80 mg • Celecoxib, oral 200–400 mg
Opioids	30 minutes to 1 hour (*before incision*)	Morphine 5–10 mg IV
NMDA receptor antagonists	30 minutes to 1 hour (*before incision*)	Ketamine 0.5 mg/kg IV
Gabapentinoids	One night before surgery and in the morning	• Gabapentin, oral 300–600 mg • Pregabalin, oral 150–300 mg
Local anesthetics	Before surgical incision	Lidocaine
Alpha-2-adrenergic agonist	30 minutes to 1 hour (*before incision*)	Dexmedetomidine 0.5–1 µg/kg IV

(IM: intramuscular; IV: intravenous; NMDA: *N*-methyl-D-aspartate; NSAID: nonsteroidal anti-inflammatory drug)

- *Psychological interventions*: These involve cognitive-behavioral therapy (CBT), relaxation techniques, and mindfulness meditation which encourage the patient for pain coping mechanism.
- *Physical therapy and exercise*: These include preoperative exercise programs which are tailored to an individual patient to improve the overall physical condition and enhanced recovery.

ROLE OF PREOPERATIVE EDUCATION AND PREPARATION IN OPTIMIZING PAIN

Patient education prior to the surgery potentially improves the pain postoperatively.

It includes preoperative teaching by using simple language to interact with patients and families.

Modalities like the use of multiple educational tools including videos and interactive sessions, tailored individualized educational plans, and the use of technology (mobile apps, online portals) to deliver preoperative education enhance overall patient satisfaction and help in effective pain management and efficient recovery as well. These approaches are cost-effective and patient centered and reduce the side effects of pharmacological interventions.

It improves patient satisfaction with decreased postoperative complications and shorter hospital stays.

CONCLUSION

Preemptive analgesia is a key strategy in pain management aimed at preventing central sensitization and reducing postoperative pain by administering analgesia before the onset of pain. By disrupting the pain pathways early, this approach can lead to improved patient outcomes, reduced analgesic requirements, and enhanced recovery after surgery.

BIBLIOGRAPHY

1. Campiglia L, Consales G, De Gaudio AR. Pre-emptive analgesia for postoperative pain control: a review. Clin Drug Investig. 2010;30 Suppl 2:15-26.
2. Katz J. Timing of treatment and pre-emptive analgesia. Pain. 1993;53: 243-5.
3. Patil JD, Sefen JAN, Fredericks S. Exploring non-pharmacological methods for pre-operative pain management. Front Surg. 2022;9:801742.
4. Penprase B, Brunetto E, Dahmani E, Forthoffer JJ, Kapoor S. The efficacy of preemptive analgesia for postoperative pain control: a systematic review of the literature. AORN J. 2015;101:94-105.e8.
5. Rosero EB, Joshi GP. Preemptive, preventive, multimodal analgesia: what do they mean? Plast Reconstr Surg. 2014;134(4 Suppl 2):85S-93S.

CHAPTER 46

Intraoperative Measures to Reduce Postoperative Pain

Heena Saini

INTRODUCTION

Musculoskeletal pain following orthopedic surgery is a common occurrence that causes soreness and discomfort leading to functional limitation, delayed recovery, and decreased patient satisfaction. Postoperative musculoskeletal pain results from tissue damage during surgery and the release of inflammatory mediators with activation of nociceptive receptors present in terminal nerve fibers. Adequate postoperative pain control is required for early postoperative recovery and rehabilitation of orthopedic surgery patients and prevent the chronicity of pain.

With the introduction of the concept of early recovery after surgery (ERAS), multimodal analgesia has become the preferred method for adequate pain control. Multimodal analgesia combines various classes of analgesics with different mechanisms of action to improve pain control and reduce drug-related side effects. Advantages of multimodal analgesia include better functional recovery, increased patient satisfaction, reduced length of stay in hospital, and reduced hospital cost.

Intraoperative measures should start with preemptive analgesia, which involves the administration of pain medication before the painful stimulus, i.e., surgical incision to decrease pain response. It prevents peripheral and central sensitization, reduces hyperalgesia, decreases postoperative pain intensity, and decreases the risk of developing postoperative chronic pain. Drugs commonly used for preemptive analgesia include low-dose ketamine, acetaminophen, pregabalin, and cyclooxygenase-2 (COX-2) inhibitors like celecoxib.

Intraoperative analgesic techniques can be broadly divided into pharmacological and nonpharmacological techniques. Pharmacological techniques include systemic analgesics and regional anesthesia.

REGIONAL ANESTHESIA

Regional anesthesia can be used as the primary anesthetic technique or can be given in addition to general anesthesia for postoperative pain control. It can be broadly classified into central neuraxial technique and peripheral nerve blocks. Regional anesthesia is preferably used for intraoperative anesthetic management wherever possible avoiding the need for general anesthesia and hence decreasing the incidence of general anesthesia-related side effects. It also helps to reduce immediate postoperative pain.

Central Neuraxial Technique

Central neuraxial blockade includes spinal anesthesia, epidural anesthesia, and combined spinal-epidural technique. It is commonly used for providing anesthesia for lower limb and pelvic surgeries. Its advantages include a reduced opioid requirement, better postoperative pain control, decreased surgical stress response and thromboembolic event with reduced pulmonary complications, decreased intraoperative blood loss, faster recovery, and early return of bowel function. These are part of the multimodal analgesia technique provided for orthopedic procedures. Adjuvants added to local anesthetic (bupivacaine) like clonidine, fentanyl, and morphine can further prolong the duration of postoperative analgesia. Intrathecal morphine 0.1 mg has also been advocated for analgesia after total hip and knee arthroplasty.

Peripheral Nerve Blocks

Peripheral nerve blocks provide site-specific anesthesia and analgesia. As part of multimodal analgesia for postoperative pain management, peripheral nerve blockade with local anesthetic can provide adequate pain relief. Adjuvants like dexamethasone, clonidine, or dexmedetomidine are added to local anesthetics to increase the duration of blockade. Various nerve blocks are available according to the site of injury. **Table 1** provides details of various nerve blocks with their indication and block-specific complications. Besides peripheral nerve blocks, *periarticular injections* are also used for providing postoperative pain control by injecting drugs directly into the operative site. Drugs used for periarticular infiltration include bupivacaine, ropivacaine, ketorolac, etc.

Infiltration of skin with long-acting local anesthetic, at the time of wound closure especially in surgeries like total knee replacement (TKR) and spine surgery, is helpful in decreasing the immediate postoperative pain.

SYSTEMIC ANALGESICS

Systemic analgesics are included in multimodal analgesic techniques. These are broadly classified as opioid and nonopioid analgesics. Opioid analgesics commonly used intraoperatively include morphine, fentanyl, and

CHAPTER 46: Intraoperative Measures to Reduce Postoperative Pain

Table 1: Peripheral nerve blocks for upper and lower limb orthopedic surgery.

Name of block	Nerves blocked	Site of providing analgesia	Complication, if any
Upper limb blocks			
Interscalene block	C5, C6, C7 nerve roots of brachial plexus	Upper arm surgery involving shoulder	• Ipsilateral phrenic nerve block • Severe hypotension and bradycardia • Horner's syndrome • Inadvertent epidural and intrathecal injection
Supraclavicular block	At level of trunk and division of brachial plexus	Surgery of elbow, forearm, and hand	• Pneumothorax • Phrenic nerve block • Horner's syndrome
Infraclavicular block	At level of cord of brachial plexus	Surgery of hand, forearm, elbow, and lateral upper arm	• Pneumothorax • Inadvertent intravascular injection
Axillary block	Branches of brachial plexus	Surgery of forearm and hand	• Nerve injury • Hematoma
Lower limb blocks			
Femoral nerve block	Femoral nerve	Surgeries involving anterior aspect of thigh and medial aspect of leg below knee	• Intravascular injection • Hematoma
Fascia iliaca block	• Femoral nerve • Lateral femoral cutaneous nerve	Analgesia for hip surgeries	Hematoma formation
Adductor canal block	• Saphenous nerve • Nerve to vastus medialis	Surgeries involving medial aspect of knee, total knee replacement, foot, and ankle	• Nerve injury • Bleeding
Sciatic nerve block	Sciatic nerve	Foot, ankle, and posterior knee surgery	• Muscle trauma • Residual dysesthesias
Popliteal fossa block	Sciatic nerve branch	Foot and ankle surgery	• Neuropathy • Intravascular injection
Ankle block	Terminal branches of sciatic nerve	Foot surgery	• Persisting paresthesia • Intravascular injection

CHAPTER 46: Intraoperative Measures to Reduce Postoperative Pain

tramadol. They provide effective analgesia but have abuse potential and are associated with significant side effects classified as opioid-related adverse effects (ORAEs) like nausea, vomiting, pruritus, ileus, urinary retention, and respiratory depression. Nonopioid analgesics include acetaminophen, nonsteroidal anti-inflammatory drugs (NSAIDs), *N*-methyl-D-aspartate (NMDA) antagonists like ketamine, anticonvulsants like pregabalin, beta-blockers, alpha-2 agonists, lignocaine infusions, and glucocorticoids like dexamethasone. **Table 2** depicts various systemic analgesics with their mechanism of action and dose.

Nonpharmacological techniques of postoperative pain control include acupuncture, music therapy, transcutaneous electrical nerve stimulation (TENS), and hypnosis. They are believed to decrease pain by stimulating large-diameter fibers activating opioid receptors through endogenous pathways.

Hence, for adequate postoperative pain control, *multimodal analgesia* should be employed that combines regional anesthesia with systemic analgesics with different mechanisms of action. The technique of providing adequate pain control depends on the type and duration of surgery and involves a multidisciplinary approach between patients, surgeons, anesthesiologists, and nursing staff.

Table 2: Commonly used systemic analgesics as part of multimodal analgesia for orthopedic surgery.

	Drug name	Mechanism of action	Dose	Duration	Additional remarks
Opioids	Morphine	Opioid receptor agonists—mu, delta, kappa	0.1 mg/kg IV	3–4 hours	• Can cause respiratory depression, nausea, vomiting • Dose adjustment required in renal failure
	Fentanyl	Opioid receptors	1–2 µg/kg IV	0.5–1 hour	More potent than morphine
	Tramadol	Mu receptor agonist and SNRI	1–2 mg/kg IV	2–3 hours	
	Acetaminophen	COX inhibition	15 mg/kg IV	4–6 hours	• Maximum dose 4 g/day • Dose modification in liver disease

Continued

Continued

	Drug name	Mechanism of action	Dose	Duration	Additional remarks
NSAIDs	Diclofenac	COX inhibition	1.5 mg/kg IV	8 hours	Increased risk of platelet dysfunction, gastrointestinal ulceration, and nephrotoxicity
	Celecoxib	Selective COX-2 inhibitor	200 mg PO	12 hours	Avoid in coronary artery disease and renal impairment
Local anesthetic infusion	Lignocaine infusion	Na channel blocker	0.5 mg/kg loading followed by 1–1.5 mg/kg/h	30–90 minutes	Avoid in patients with seizures
	Ketamine	NMDA antagonist	0.5–1 mg/kg/h	30–60 minutes	Avoid in hypertension
	Dexmedetomidine	Alpha-2 agonist	1 µg/kg over 10 minutes followed by 0.2–0.7 µg/kg/h IV	2–3 hours	Causes hypotension and bradycardia
	Esmolol	Beta-blocker	0.5 mg/kg	10–30 minutes	Avoid in asthmatics and in patients with severe bradycardia
	Dexamethasone	Glucocorticoids—inhibit arachidonic acid production	8–10 mg IV	48 hours	Additional benefit of decreased postoperative nausea, vomiting

(COX: cyclooxygenase; NMDA: N-methyl-D-aspartate; NSAID: nonsteroidal anti-inflammatory drug; SNRI: serotonin–norepinephrine reuptake inhibitor)

CONCLUSION

Intraoperative pain management is essential for improving patient outcomes and recovery. A multimodal approach, combining pharmacological methods like local anesthetics and opioids with techniques such as nerve blocks and proper positioning, effectively reduces pain during surgery. Collaboration between surgeons and anesthesiologists ensures tailored care, preventing both immediate and long-term pain. Continued integration of evidence-based strategies will enhance patient comfort and surgical success.

BIBLIOGRAPHY

1. Aldanyowi SN. Novel techniques for musculoskeletal pain management after orthopaedic surgical procedures: a systematic review. Life. 2023;13(12):2351.
2. Anger M, Valovska T, Beloeil H, Lirk P, Joshi GP, Van de Velde M, et al. PROSPECT guideline for total hip arthroplasty: a systematic review and procedure-specific postoperative pain management recommendations. Anaesthesia. 2021;76(8):1082-97.
3. Chunduri A, Aggarwal AK. Multimodal pain management in orthopaedic surgery. J Clin Med. 2022;11(21):6386.
4. Kamel I, Ahmed MF, Sethi A. Regional anaesthesia for orthopaedic procedures: what orthopaedic surgeons need to know. World J Orthop. 2022;13(1):11-35.
5. Miller RD, Eriksson LI, Fleisher LA, Wiener-Kronish JP, Cohen NH, Young WL. Miller's Anaesthesia. Amsterdam: Elsevier Health Sciences; 2014 [E-book].
6. Schwenk ES, Mariano ER. Designing the ideal perioperative pain management plan starts with multimodal analgesia. Korean J Anesthesiol. 2018;71(5):345.

CHAPTER 47

Postoperative Pain Management Strategies

Madan Lal Katoch

▌ INTRODUCTION

The experience of pain involves not just the physical sensation but also the emotional and psychological response.

Effective management of postoperative pain is crucial, not only for patient comfort but also for reducing the risk of complications and promoting faster recovery.

▌ POSTOPERATIVE PAIN CONTROL MULTIMODAL ANALGESIA APPROACHES

Multimodal analgesia is the most important and recommended, because it is a comprehensive approach to pain management that utilizes a combination of pharmacological and nonpharmacological methods to target different mechanisms and pathways involved in pain perception. This strategy aims to provide superior pain relief while minimizing the reliance on opioids, thus reducing the potential for side effects and promoting a quicker recovery. Multimodal analgesia represents a sophisticated and tailored approach to postoperative pain management. This strategy not only improves pain relief but also enhances the overall recovery process, facilitating a quicker return to normal activities and reducing the likelihood of chronic pain development.

Multimodal analgesia starts with the use of nonopioid analgesics such as *acetaminophen and nonsteroidal anti-inflammatory drugs (NSAIDs)* and then combines with the use of opioids if and when required depending on the severity of pain and other patient-related factors. Acetaminophen is effective for mild-to-moderate pain. By combining opioids with nonopioids, the overall opioid requirement is decreased, which reduces the risk of opioid-related adverse effects such as respiratory depression, nausea, and constipation.

CHAPTER 47: Postoperative Pain Management Strategies

Local anesthetics are another crucial component. Techniques such as local infiltration at the surgical site, nerve blocks, and epidural or spinal anesthesia can provide targeted pain relief. Local anesthetics block the transmission of pain signals from peripheral nerves to the central nervous system, offering effective pain control without systemic side effects.

Adjuvant medications like gabapentinoids (e.g., gabapentin and pregabalin) are increasingly incorporated into multimodal protocols and are particularly useful in managing neuropathic pain, often reducing the incidence of chronic postsurgical pain.

PATIENT-CONTROLLED ANALGESIA AND OTHER ANALGESIC DELIVERY SYSTEMS

Patient-controlled analgesia (PCA) represents a significant advancement in pain management, particularly in the postoperative setting. It allows patients to self-administer a predetermined dose of analgesics, usually opioids, through a programmable pump. This method provides patients with unique control over their pain management, aiming to maintain a consistent plasma level of analgesics by allowing the self-administration of small doses at frequent intervals.

The fundamental principle behind PCA is based on the understanding that patients can individually titrate the amount of analgesics they require to manage their pain effectively. By pressing a button, the patient activates the pump to deliver a small, controlled dose of the drug from an intravenous or epidural line. This approach not only ensures immediate pain relief but also reduces the peaks and troughs in drug levels associated with traditional analgesic administration schedules. PCA devices are equipped with safety features, such as lockout intervals (a minimum time interval between doses), to prevent overdose.

Aside from opioids, *PCA can be used to administer nonopioid medications such as ketamine or lidocaine,* providing alternatives for patients who may not tolerate opioids well. The adaptability of PCA systems also allows for combinations of drugs, potentially enhancing the efficacy of pain management while minimizing side effects.

Another significant advancement in analgesic delivery systems is the development of *continuous regional analgesia,* which involves the continuous infusion of local anesthetics through a catheter placed near a nerve or into the epidural space. This technique is particularly effective for surgeries involving limbs or specific body areas. Continuous regional analgesia offers excellent pain control and can significantly reduce the need for systemic analgesics, thereby decreasing the risk of systemic side effects and promoting faster recovery.

Transdermal patches represent another method of analgesic delivery. These patches deliver medication through the skin directly into the bloodstream over an extended period. Commonly used drugs in transdermal systems include *fentanyl and buprenorphine.* This method is advantageous for providing consistent drug levels and improving patient compliance and is particularly useful for patients who have difficulty with oral intake or those who require long-term pain management.

Recent developments have also seen the introduction of smart technology into analgesic delivery systems. *Smart pumps* equipped with monitoring systems can now adjust doses based on feedback from sensors that assess physiological parameters indicative of pain level or drug concentration in the blood. This technology represents a move toward more personalized pain management, potentially improving outcomes and patient satisfaction.

The use of these varied delivery systems is not without challenges. Issues such as device malfunctions, infections at the catheter or implant site, and complications related to drug dosing require vigilant monitoring. Education for healthcare providers and patients on the use and maintenance of these systems is essential to mitigate risks and improve efficacy.

By providing more control to patients and delivering medication more efficiently and safely, these systems help improve pain control, enhance patient satisfaction, and potentially shorten hospital stays. As technology advances, future developments are likely to offer even more effective and personalized solutions to pain management.

STRATEGIES FOR MINIMIZING OPIOID-RELATED ADVERSE EFFECTS AND PROMOTING EARLY RECOVERY

The management of postoperative pain often involves opioids due to their effective analgesic properties. However, the adverse effects associated with opioids, such as nausea, vomiting, constipation, respiratory depression, and the risk of dependency, necessitate strategies to minimize these effects while promoting early recovery. Effective management strategies are essential to optimize patient outcomes, enhance recovery, and reduce the length of hospital stays.

The implementation of multimodal analgesia not only limits opioid exposure and its associated risks but also often results in better pain control and patient satisfaction.

Another critical component is the *optimization of opioid dosing*. Personalized pain management plans, which consider factors such as the patient's age, body weight, renal and hepatic function, and previous opioid use, can significantly improve outcomes. Using the lowest effective dose for the shortest duration necessary can reduce the incidence and severity of adverse effects.

The use of *opioid-sparing protocols* is an effective method to enhance early recovery. Techniques such as regional anesthesia (nerve blocks, epidurals) can provide excellent pain relief and reduce the need for systemic opioids. For instance, peripheral nerve blocks are particularly effective for surgeries involving limbs, where they can provide targeted pain relief and allow earlier mobilization.

Enhanced recovery after surgery (ERAS) protocols incorporate various strategies, including the proactive management of nausea and vomiting, encouragement of early oral intake, and early mobilization. These protocols aim to reduce the stress response to surgery and the reliance on opioids, which can help decrease the risk of opioid-related adverse effects and promote quicker recovery.

Corticosteroids (though very rarely and briefly only) can be used for their strong anti-inflammatory and analgesic benefits in the postoperative setting. By reducing inflammation, steroids indirectly alleviate pain and are especially beneficial in orthopedic surgeries.

In addition to pharmacological treatments, *nonpharmacological approaches* play a significant role in multimodal analgesia. Techniques such as physical therapy, massage, and cold therapy help reduce pain and inflammation while promoting mobility and faster healing. *Psychological interventions,* including cognitive–behavioral therapy and relaxation techniques, can also significantly impact pain management by addressing the emotional and cognitive aspects of pain.

Recent advancements in technology have also introduced innovative methods like transcutaneous electrical nerve stimulation *(TENS),* which uses low-voltage electrical currents to relieve pain. Similarly, acupuncture has gained acceptance as a viable method for postoperative pain control, potentially influencing pain modulation mechanisms at both local and central levels.

The integration of these diverse techniques addresses pain at various points in its transmission and perception, leading to more effective pain control, reduced side effects, and enhanced patient outcomes. By reducing the severity of pain experienced postoperatively, patients are likely to experience fewer pain-related complications, such as thromboembolic disease from prolonged immobility or respiratory issues from inadequate pain control.

Educating patients on the effective use of nonopioid techniques and setting realistic expectations for postoperative pain can enhance their coping strategies and reduce anxiety, which is often a component that exacerbates the perception of pain.

Monitoring and managing the potential side effects of opioids actively are crucial. Protocols for the prophylactic use of antiemetics can reduce the incidence of nausea and vomiting. Similarly, implementing regular bowel regimens can prevent constipation, a common and often debilitating side effect of opioid use.

Finally, *ongoing assessment and adjustment* of pain management strategies are essential. Regular pain assessments and adjustments to the pain management plan, including *stepping down opioid* use as pain decreases, can prevent prolonged opioid use and reduce the risk of developing chronic pain or opioid dependence.

All in all, it requires a comprehensive approach that includes the use of multimodal analgesia, personalized dosing strategies, opioid-sparing techniques, implementation of ERAS protocols, and nonpharmacological interventions. Such strategies not only improve the safety and efficacy of postoperative pain management but also enhance overall patient outcomes and satisfaction.

CONCLUSION

Effective postoperative pain management is essential for recovery and reducing complications. A multimodal approach, combining medications and non-pharmacological techniques, ensures comprehensive pain control. Tailored strategies and continuous assessment help minimize side effects, speed up recovery, and improve overall patient outcomes.

BIBLIOGRAPHY

1. Chou R, Gordon DB, de Leon-Casasola OA, Rosenberg JM, Bickler S, Brennan T, et al. Management of postoperative pain: a clinical practice guideline from the American Pain Society, the American Society of Regional Anesthesia and Pain Medicine, and the American Society of Anesthesiologists' Committee on Regional Anesthesia, Executive Committee, and Administrative Council. J Pain. 2016;17(2):131-57.
2. Dahl JB, Kehlet H. The value of multimodal or balanced analgesia in postoperative pain treatment. Anesth Analg. 2011;93(5):1125-35.
3. Joshi GP, Ogunnaike BO. Consequences of inadequate postoperative pain relief and chronic persistent postoperative pain. Anesthesiol Clin N Am. 2005;23(1):21-36.
4. Kehlet H, Jensen TS, Woolf CJ. Persistent postsurgical pain: risk factors and prevention. Lancet. 2006;367(9522):1618-25.
5. McMahon SB, Koltzenburg M. Wall and Melzack's Textbook of Pain, 5th edition. Amsterdam: Elsevier Churchill Livingstone; 2005.
6. Raja SN, Carr DB, Cohen M, Finnerup NB, Flor H, Gibson S, et al. The revised International Association for the Study of Pain definition of pain: concepts, challenges, and compromises. Pain. 2020;161(9):1976-82.
7. Tracey I, Mantyh PW. The cerebral signature for pain perception and its modulation. Neuron. 2007;55(3):377-91.
8. White PF, Kehlet H. Improving postoperative pain management: what are the unresolved issues? Anesthesiology. 2007;110(2):220-5.
9. Woolf CJ. Central sensitization: implications for the diagnosis and treatment of pain. Pain. 2011;152(3 Suppl):S2-15.

CHAPTER 48

Enhanced Recovery after Surgery Protocols

Anita Vig Kohli

INTRODUCTION

In the 1990s, a multimodal approach to perioperative management of surgical patients was popularized by Henrik Kehlet and the word "fast-track surgery" was coined by him. This later developed into the enhanced recovery after surgery (ERAS) program which comprises the entire spectrum of preoperative, intraoperative, and postoperative care. The ERAS protocol is now becoming the standard of care for many surgeries including orthopedic as they reduce hospitalization, lower complication rate, and promote faster recovery so that the patient resumes his or her preoperative functional status early.

WHY NEEDED?

With ever-increasing population and increasing longevity, the number of orthopedic surgical procedures and patients opting for surgery are always on the rise. Therefore, there is a lot of pressure on healthcare facilities and the target is to shorten the length of hospital stay. Emphasis is now given on daycare surgeries even for major orthopedic surgeries like arthroplasties and spine surgery. Meanwhile, there is significant variation across institutions related to surgery leading to varied perioperative surgical outcomes. This has led to the adoption of ERAS protocols with evidence-based standardization of perioperative management and improved outcomes, especially in pain management.

PREOPERATIVE RECOMMENDATIONS FOR ENHANCED RECOVERY AFTER SURGERY

Preoperative Patient Assessment and Risk Stratification

Preoperatively, a multidisciplinary evaluation of the patient is done through a proper history, examination, and investigations to assess and optimize functional capacity and comorbid status.

The American Society of Anesthesiologists (ASA) physical status classification system is used for this assessment, but the final assessment is done on the day of surgery. The ASA helps to grade along with the type of surgery, frailty, and level of deconditioning in predicting perioperative risks and surgical outcomes.

The existence of preoperative neuropathic pain is a significant risk factor for higher postoperative pain scores. This has to be documented in preanesthetic checkups as patients with preoperative chronic pain can be associated with psychological conditions like anxiety, depression, and pain leading to increased postoperative pain. Preoperative psychological counseling may help to reduce the severity of postsurgical pain and improve the quality of recovery.

Preoperative Education and Counseling

Current ERAS protocols emphasize the importance of preoperative patient education and counseling as they can influence patient expectations and set the stage for patient empowerment and improved outcomes. Orthopedic surgeries like joint replacement and spine surgeries might have uncertain postoperative pain outcomes and long recovery periods. This can contribute to preoperative fear and anxiety which can affect recovery after surgery. Allaying the patient's fear and conveying clearly about pain management, early ambulation, and resuming oral intake can help in accelerated recovery.

Preoperative nutritional supplementation, cessation of smoking and alcohol intake, preoperative fasting, carbohydrate treatment, and correction of anemia also come under the ERAS protocol and can reduce postoperative complications. For all this, the patient has to be properly educated.

Prehabilitation

Prehabilitation is enhancing functional capacity before surgery. This speeds up the function following surgery and includes exercise and physiotherapy along with nutrition and psychological preparation.

Preanesthetic Medication

Preoperative anxiety can lead to increased perioperative analgesic requirements. Sedative or anxiolytic drugs like benzodiazepine may be used for patients' comfort and to facilitate technical procedures. However, the use of benzodiazepines has been associated with an increased risk of adverse events postoperatively.

Preemptive analgesia is also a part of the ERAS protocol and multimodal opioid-sparing analgesics like acetaminophen, nonsteroidal anti-inflammatory drugs (NSAIDs), and gabapentinoids can be given.

Gabapentinoids have been shown to reduce pain scores leading to less consumption of opioids, hence leading to decreased opioid-related side effects like postoperative nausea and vomiting (PONV), pruritus, and urinary retention. However, dizziness and sedation due to gabapentinoids can occur so the dose should be adjusted according to age, renal functions, and other comorbidities, especially in elderly and frail patients.

INTRAOPERATIVE RECOMMENDATIONS

Anesthetic care of patients involves the delivery of anesthetics and postoperative analgesia. ERAS protocols for the intraoperative period are directed to lower the effect of anesthetic techniques on organs, hemodynamic stability, blood loss, and pain control. Also, antimicrobial prophylaxis, skin preparation, prevention of hypothermia, perioperative fluid management, and prevention of perioperative blood loss are included in the ERAS protocol for early discharge of the patient.

Standardized Anesthetic Protocol

This is the core component of the ERAS protocol in orthopedic surgery. It is seen that hip and knee replacement surgeries are mostly taken up under neuraxial block. Large epidemiological studies have shown that central neuraxial anesthesia is a better option for these patients. Although epidural anesthesia helps in improved hemodynamic stability, less blood loss, better pain control, and early initiation of normal activity in established ERAS setups, no clinically important differences have been seen in functional recovery, length of hospital stay, urinary complications, and mobilization when compared with general anesthesia. Thus, both may be used as part of a multimodal anesthetic regimen in the ERAS protocol.

Using general anesthesia for orthopedic patients, the choice of agents that leads to a decrease in postoperative pain is preferred. The use of neuromuscular agents leading to skeletal muscle relaxation improves the pain score as it leads to reduced airway pressure and muscle damage associated with prolonged retraction, especially in spine surgeries. The use of sevoflurane is also seen to decrease pain scores postoperatively for 1 day. Dexmedetomidine and ketamine show good pain control postoperatively and are used as a part of the ERAS protocol.

Surgical Techniques

Surgical techniques can affect the length of stay of patients and pain scores by optimizing the approach, controlling pain, both intraoperative and postoperative, and reducing bleeding. Various techniques regarding approach, minimally invasive techniques, endoscopy, specific implants, navigation, robotics, and biologics have not been shown to affect the pain and discharge criteria. However, minimally invasive techniques have an edge in the ERAS protocol.

Regional Blocks

Of the multimodal techniques for intraoperative and postoperative analgesia, the use of regional blocks is a good option in orthopedic surgery. Epidural analgesia is seen to reduce postoperative pain after lumbar fusion without significant side effects. Use of long-acting local anesthetics (LAs) like bupivacaine, levobupivacaine, or ropivacaine, either alone or with adjuncts, can be used in these patients as a single-shot or continuous infusion. Patient-controlled analgesia (PCA) with an epidural catheter is better than intravenous analgesia. Intrathecal single-shot anesthesia with adjuvants or opioids is also used.

Nerve Blocks

Several nerve block techniques may be used like femoral nerve block in knee and hip replacement surgeries for intraoperative and postoperative pain relief. It reduces the risk of hypotension and the use of opioids. However, it may delay recovery due to late mobilization. Hunter canal block is an attractive alternative with better preservation of muscle strength. Sciatic nerve block on the other hand does not seem to have substantial benefit in hip surgery. Brachial plexus block for upper limb surgeries is a good option with or without continuous catheter infusion.

Various blocks like erector spinae plane block, quadratus lumborum block, and thoracolumbar interfacial plane (TLIP) block have been described for spine surgery and they have good results like decreased analgesic drug consumption postoperatively.

Local Infiltration

Local infiltration analgesia allows for earlier ambulation and thus has an advantage over nerve blocks and regional anesthesia. Hypotension and urinary retention with delayed recovery can lead to an increase in the length of stay in regional anesthesia. However, there are concerns regarding delayed wound healing, infection, and LA toxicity, especially where wound infusion techniques are used. However, in spine surgery, continuous infiltration using a wound catheter provides good pain relief postoperatively, especially with adjuvants like dexmedetomidine.

Thus, the use of a multimodal approach for analgesia by combining the use of acetaminophen infusion, NSAIDs, alpha-2 agonists, *N*-methyl-D-aspartate (NMDA) antagonists like ketamine, and locoregional blocks leads to good intraoperative analgesia. This regimen has the added advantage of limiting intraoperative opioid administration for pain relief, thus decreasing the risk factors for chronic opioid use among opioid-naïve patients in the postoperative period.

POSTOPERATIVE RECOMMENDATIONS

Poor postoperative pain control is seen in about 50% of operated patients. Inadequate acute pain control can lead to chronic pain and systemic inflammatory response leading to organ dysfunction. Thus, a standardized ERAS protocol for pain results in better pain relief and improved outcomes for patients.

The ERAS protocol includes multimodal analgesia in the postoperative period. Here, analgesia from various categories is employed along with nerve blocks for regional and local infiltration leading to optimal pain management.

Multimodal analgesia uses nonopioid analgesia like NSAIDs, gabapentinoids, acetaminophen, alpha-2 agonists, and ketamine.

Acetaminophen

Acetaminophen is a regularly prescribed drug and is known to reduce acute postoperative pain and PONV, and has a favorable side effect profile. Thus, it is a core component of the ERAS protocol, both intraoperatively and postoperatively.

Nonsteroidal Anti-inflammatory Drugs

Nonsteroidal anti-inflammatory drugs have been known to decrease pain and reduce supplemental analgesics. However, there is a debate about their side effects like the potential for bleeding complications, gastroduodenal ulcers, cardiovascular morbidity, aspirin-sensitive asthma, renal and hepatic dysfunction, and impaired osteogenesis. Since there is no conclusive evidence for the negative impact of NSAIDs on bone healing and there is Level I evidence of postoperative analgesia following orthopedic surgeries, NSAIDs are recommended in the ERAS protocol. However, individual patient risk should be assessed.

Gabapentinoids

Their use in acute postoperative pain is on the increase as several meta-analyses have suggested their positive results. There is also a decreased incidence of PONV with them. They are included in the ERAS protocol as their use leads to less consumption of opioids, but there is an increase in dizziness, diplopia, and ataxia with it. Some cases of respiratory depression during Phase I recovery are also noted, especially in patients who are elderly and have received intrathecal opioids or large doses of opioids intraoperatively.

Supplemental Opioid Analgesia

The ERAS program aims to minimize the use of opioids postoperatively but they can be used when required as their efficacy is well established. They can be used as a step down from peripheral techniques to nonopioid analgesia. Controlled-release oxycodone has been associated with shorter hospital stays and better tolerance than PCA regimens which require intravenous access and a PCA pump. Oral regimen makes patients more independent and with early discharge criteria.

In addition, catering to the analgesic needs of the patients in the postoperative period and taking care of nutrition also come in the ERAS protocol as early feeding and good nutritional supplementation lead to early discharge and better satisfaction.

Another important aspect of the ERAS protocol is early mobilization with patients being discharged on the first or second day.

CONCLUSION

Although the focus of ERAS is "pain- and risk-free" surgery, a better understanding of the physiological mechanism of recovery is needed. More studies are needed to understand how to reduce the inflammatory response, pain, and impairment of physical activity and thus improve function quickly.

BIBLIOGRAPHY

1. Adogwa O, Elsamadicy AA, Mehta AI, Cheng J, Begley CA, Karikar IO. Pre-operative nutritional status an independent predictor of 30-day hospital re-admission after elective spine surgery. Spine. 2016:41:1400-4.
2. Brady MC, Kinn S, Stuart P, Ness V. Pre-operative fasting for adults to prevent peri-operative complications. Cochrane Database Syst Rev. 2003;(4):CD004423.
3. Clevenger B, Richards T. Pre-operative anaemia. Anaesthesia. 2015;70(Suppl 1):20-8, e6-8.
4. Dilmen OK, Yentor E, Tunali Y, Balchi H, Behar M. Does preoperative oral carbohydrate treatment reduce the post-operative surgical stress response in lumbar disc surgery? Clin Neural Neurosurg. 2017;153:82-6.
5. Eldawlatly A. Is enhanced recovery after anaesthesia a synonym for enhanced recovery after Surgery? Sardi J Anaesth. 2016;10(2):119-20.
6. Gan TJM, Thacker JK, Miller TM, Scot MJM, Holubar SDM. Enhanced Recovery for Major Abdominopelvic Surgery, 1st edition. New York: Professional Communication, Inc; 2016.
7. Gronkjaer M, Eliasen M, Skov-Ettrup LS, Tolstrup JS, Christernisen AH, Mikkelsen SS, et al. Pre-operative smoking status and post-operative complications: a systematic review and meta-analysis. Ann Surg. 2014:259:52-71.
8. Helhten EK, Henbidge MA, Manos AN, Lewis SJ, Massicotte EM, Fewhling MG, et al. An economic evaluation of peri-operative adverse events associated with spinal surgery. Spine J. 2013;13:44-53.
9. Horosz B, Nawrocka K, Milweska MM. Anaesthetic pre-operative management according to ERAS protocol. Anaesthesiol Intensive Ther. 2016;48(1):49-54.
10. Hurley RW, Cohen SP, Wilhaim KA, Rowlingson AJ, Wu CL. The analgesic effects of preoperative gabapentine on post-operative pain: a meta-analysis. Reg Anaesth Pain Med. 2006;31:237-47.
11. Kehlet H. Multimodal approach to control post-operative patho-physiology and rehabilitation. Br J Anaesth. 1997;78:606-17.
12. Lee YJ, Koch EM, Breidebach JB, Bornemann R, Wirtz DC, Pflugmacher R. Diagnosis of neuropathic components in patients with back pain before and after surgery. Z Orthop Unfall. 2016;154:571-7.

13. Mckee MD. Efficacy and safety of steroid use for post-operative pain relief. J Bone Joint Surg Am. 2007;89:1134.
14. Minto G, Biccard B. Assessment of the high-risk pre-operative patient. Contin Educ Anaesth Crit Care Pain. 2014;14:12-7.
15. Oppendal K, Moller AM, Pederson B, Tonnesen H. Pre-operative alcohol cessation prior to elective surgery. Cochrane Database Syst Rev. 2012;(7):CD008343.
16. Sorensen LT. Wound healing and infection in surgery. The clinical impact of smoking and cessation: a systematic review and meta-analysis. Arch Surg. 2012;147:373-83.
17. Starkweather A, Perry M. Enhanced recovery programs and pain management. Top Pain Manage. 2017;32:1-9.
18. Theunissen M, Peter ML, Bruer J, Gramke HF, Marcus MA. Preoperative anxiety and catastrophizing: a systematic review and meta-analysis of the association with chronic postsurgical pain. Clin J Pain. 2012;28:819-41.
19. Thomas K, Wong KH, Steelman SC, Rodriguez A. Surgical risk assessment and prevention in elderly spinal deformity patients. Geriatr Orthop Surg Rehabil. 2019:10:2151459319851681.
20. Wood TJ, Thornley P, Petrualli D, Kabali C, Winemaker M, de Beer J. Preoperative predictions of pain catastrophizing anxiety and depression in patients undergoing total joint arthroplasty. J Arthroplasty. 2016;31:2750-6.

CHAPTER 49

Role of Steroid in Musculoskeletal Pain Management

Abhai Singh Bhadwal

INTRODUCTION

Steroids play a significant role in musculoskeletal ailments because of their anti-inflammatory properties. The use of steroids in orthopedics is indicated for specific conditions characterized by inflammation or pain. Some specific indications for the use of steroids in orthopedics are given in the following text.

INFLAMMATORY JOINT CONDITIONS

Steroids may be used to alleviate pain associated with inflammatory conditions, providing both anti-inflammatory and analgesic effects.
- *Rheumatoid arthritis, psoriatic arthritis, gout, systemic lupus erythematosus (SLE)*: Steroids can be used to manage acute flares or as a bridge therapy until disease-modifying antirheumatic drugs (DMARDs) take effect.
- *Osteoarthritis*: Intra-articular steroid injections may provide short-term relief for pain and inflammation in osteoarthritic joints. However, they should be rarely used.
- *Ankylosing spondylitis*: Steroids may be prescribed to manage inflammation in the spine and other joints.
- *Soft-tissue injuries*: Very rarely, steroids may be used in acute soft-tissue injuries to control inflammation and facilitate healing.

POSTOPERATIVE CARE

Postoperative inflammation: Steroids may be prescribed after orthopedic surgeries to control postoperative inflammation and pain, though rarely only.

SPINAL CONDITIONS

- *Disc herniation*: Oral steroids may be used in the management of acute disc herniation to reduce inflammation around the affected nerve roots.
- *Spinal stenosis*: Steroid injections may be considered to reduce inflammation in the spinal canal.
- *Joint inflammation due to allergies*: Steroids can be used to manage acute joint inflammation caused by allergic reactions or hypersensitivity.
- *Localized injections*:
  - *Intra-articular injections*: Steroid injections directly into joints are indicated for localized anti-inflammatory effects. Intra-articular injections are effective in controlling synovitis and can be repeated as necessary—a maximum of every 3 months.
  - *Tendonitis and bursitis*: Steroid injections can be used to reduce inflammation in tendons and bursae, providing relief from pain and swelling.
  - *Epidural steroid injections/nerve root block or facet joint injection*: These injections can be used for managing pain and inflammation related to spinal conditions.

IMPORTANT CONSIDERATIONS AND SIDE EFFECT

Steroids are contraindicated in any suspicion of infection or uncontrolled diabetes.

VARIOUS ROUTES OF ADMINISTRATION OF STEROIDS

- *Oral corticosteroids*: These should be used very rarely and cautiously. Oral steroids provide good symptom relief in moderate to low dosages.
- *Parenteral corticosteroids:* Intramuscular methylprednisolone is suitable for short-term symptom control, e.g., in disease flares and for disease control during initiation of DMARD treatment. 120 mg Depo-Medrol is effective for 3–4 weeks and can be repeated once or twice but not often.
- *High-dose IV corticosteroids*, like methylprednisolone 1 g, are seldom indicated but can be useful in combination with cyclophosphamide for rheumatoid vasculitis.

SOME GENERAL PRECAUTIONS AND CONSIDERATIONS WHILE USING STEROIDS

- *Patient assessment*:
  - Thoroughly review the patient's medical history, including any history of infections, diabetes, osteoporosis, or previous adverse reactions to steroids.

- Assess the patient's current medications, including over-the-counter drugs and supplements, to identify potential interactions.
- *Dose and duration*:
    - Prescribe the lowest effective dose for the shortest duration possible to minimize the risk of side effects.
    - *Avoid prolonged use*: Long-term or high-dose steroid use is associated with an increased risk of adverse effects, including osteoporosis, cardiovascular issues, and immunosuppression.
- *Monitoring*:
    - Patients on long-term steroid therapy should be regularly monitored for potential side effects such as weight gain, blood pressure changes, and blood glucose levels.
    - Consider bone density testing for patients at risk of osteoporosis due to prolonged steroid use.
- *Infection risk*:
    - Steroids can suppress the immune system, thereby increasing the risk of infections. Evaluate the patient for existing infections before initiating treatment.
    - Consider prophylactic measures such as vaccinations for patients at an increased risk of infections.
- *Glucose monitoring*: Monitor blood glucose levels closely in patients with diabetes, as steroids can lead to elevated blood sugar levels.
- *Osteoporosis risk*: Assess the patient's baseline bone health and consider preventive measures such as calcium and vitamin D supplementation to reduce the risk of osteoporosis.
- *Psychiatric effects*: Steroids may cause mood swings or psychiatric effects. Monitor patients for changes in mood or behavior.
- *Pregnancy and breastfeeding*:
    - Discuss the potential risks and benefits of steroid use during pregnancy. In some cases, the benefits may outweigh the risks.
    - Consider the impact of steroids on breastfeeding and discuss alternatives if necessary.
- *Gradual tapering*: When discontinuing steroid therapy, it is often necessary to taper the dose gradually to prevent withdrawal symptoms and adrenal insufficiency.
- *Patient education*:
    - Ensure that patients are informed about the potential risks and benefits of steroid therapy and provide them with an opportunity to ask questions.
    - *Adherence to treatment plan*: Emphasize the importance of following the prescribed dose and duration, as well as attending follow-up appointments for monitoring.

FREQUENCY OF LOCAL STEROID INJECTIONS

It depends on various factors, including the specific condition being treated, the type of steroid used, the response to previous injections, and individual patient characteristics. Some general considerations are as follows:
- *Acute inflammation*: For acute inflammatory conditions, such as acute tendonitis or bursitis, a local steroid injection may be given as a one-time treatment or as part of a short-term treatment plan.
- *Chronic conditions*: In chronic conditions like osteoarthritis or chronic tendinopathies, the frequency of local steroid injections may be limited due to the potential for side effects with repeated use.
- *Response to previous injections*: If a patient experiences prolonged relief from a single injection, there may be less need for frequent repeat injections.
- *Limitations on repeat injections*:
  - *Tendons*: In certain tendons, such as the Achilles tendon, repeated injections may be limited due to concerns about tendon weakening or rupture.
  - *Joints*: The frequency of intra-articular injections into joints is often limited to prevent potential joint damage or infection.
- *Consideration of alternatives*: Explore alternative treatments, such as physical therapy, nonsteroidal anti-inflammatory drugs (NSAIDs), or other interventions, to reduce the need for frequent steroid injections
- *Risk of side effects*: Repeated use of steroids can increase the risk of side effects, including skin atrophy, depigmentation, and the potential for systemic effects. Hence, one must balance the benefits of symptom relief with the potential risks.
- *Patient-specific factors*: Consider individual patient factors such as age, overall health, and comorbidities when determining the frequency of steroid injections.

TYPES OF STEROIDS

Different steroids have different durations of action. Short-acting steroids may necessitate more frequent injections, while longer-acting steroids may provide a more prolonged effect.

The choice of the "safest and better" steroid in orthopedics depends on the specific clinical scenario, the nature of the condition being treated, and individual patient factors. Different steroids have varying potencies, durations of action, and side effect profiles. A few commonly used steroids in orthopedics are as follows:
- *Prednisone*: It is often used for systemic anti-inflammatory effects. It is available in the oral form and may be used in conditions like rheumatoid arthritis or SLE.

- *Methylprednisolone*: It is commonly used for short-term systemic treatment. It is available in oral and injectable forms. In orthopedics, it may be administered as an intramuscular injection or as an intravenous infusion.

Intra-articular Steroids
- *Triamcinolone*: It is frequently used in intra-articular injections for joint inflammation associated with conditions like osteoarthritis or rheumatoid arthritis. It has intermediate- to long-acting effects.
- *Betamethasone*: It is another steroid commonly used in intra-articular injections. It has a longer duration of action compared with some other options.

Soft-tissue Injections
Dexamethasone: It is used in soft-tissue injections, such as for tendonitis or bursitis. It has potent anti-inflammatory effects and is available in various formulations.

Spinal Injections
Dexamethasone or betamethasone, triamcinolone: These steroids are commonly used in epidural or intrathecal injections to reduce inflammation around spinal nerves.

When considering the "safest" steroid, it is crucial to note that all steroids have potential side effects, and the goal is often to use the lowest effective dose for the shortest duration possible.

The newly licensed preparation deflazacort may have a lower toxicity. It could be considered for children, the elderly, and those especially at risk of side effects, e.g., patients with diabetes.

■ SIDE EFFECTS ASSOCIATED WITH STEROIDS
Prolonged or high-dose steroid use can have side effects, including:
- Osteoporosis
- Immunosuppression with increased susceptibility to infections
- Hyperglycemia
- Fluid retention, weight gain, and increased blood pressure
- Increased incidence of hypertension, cataracts, and gastrointestinal (GI) disease
- Psychiatric effects including mood changes and insomnia

Because of steroids' side effects, they should be reserved for diseases uncontrolled by DMARDs and disease flares.

Toxicity is proportional to the daily dose and duration of therapy.

CONCLUSION

Steroids play a significant role in managing musculoskeletal pain by reducing inflammation and providing rapid symptom relief. When used judiciously, they can improve function and mobility in conditions such as arthritis, tendinitis, and bursitis. However, careful consideration of dosage, duration, and potential side effects is essential to maximize benefits and minimize risks. A balanced, individualized approach incorporating steroids as part of a broader pain management plan can lead to improved patient outcomes.

BIBLIOGRAPHY

1. Arroll B, Goodyear-Smith F. Corticosteroid injections for osteoarthritis of the knee: meta-analysis. BMJ. 2004;328(7444):869.
2. Conaghan PG, Dickson J, Grant RL. Care and management of osteoarthritis in adults: summary of NICE guidance. BMJ. 2008;336(7642):502-3.
3. Coombes BK, Bisset L, Vicenzino B. Efficacy and safety of corticosteroid injections and other injections for management of tendinopathy: a systematic review of randomised controlled trials. Lancet. 2010;376(9754):1751-67.
4. Cummings MH, Dunning CE, Russell ML, Johnson JA, Boughner DR, King GJ. Intra-articular corticosteroids in the treatment of adhesive capsulitis. A randomized double-blind trial. Arthritis Rheum. 1999;42(6):1132-41.
5. Evans CH. Biochemistry of cortisone and hydrocortisone. Clin Orthop Relat Res. 1976;(123):53-7.
6. Galer BS, Rosenquist RW, Narouze S, Deer TR. Perioperative corticosteroids for total joint arthroplasty. J Am Acad Orthop Surg. 2010;18(2):87-93.
7. Hollander JL. The local effects of corticosteroids on periarticular tissues. Bull Rheum Dis. 1970;20(3):622-5.
8. Hsu ES. Injectable agents other than corticosteroids for intra-articular and soft-tissue injections. Clin J Pain. 2008;24(6):529-38.
9. Khan KM, Cook JL, Bonar F, Harcourt P, Astrom M. Histopathology of common tendinopathies. Update and implications for clinical management. Sports Med. 1999;27(6):393-408.
10. Peterson ME, Hodler J. Evidence-based radiology (part 2): strategies for improving study quality and relevance in musculoskeletal imaging. Skeletal Radiol. 2010;39(5):449-55.

CHAPTER 50

Role of Physiotherapy in the Management of Musculoskeletal Pain

Deepika Saroj, Deepali Gupta

■ INTRODUCTION

Physiotherapy, or physical therapy, plays a pivotal role in the multidisciplinary approach to managing musculoskeletal pain, employing a variety of modalities to alleviate pain, restore function, and improve overall well-being. The various aspects of treatment in physiotherapy include manual therapy, exercise therapy, electrotherapy, and other modalities.

■ MANUAL THERAPY

Manual therapy includes a range of hands-on techniques such as mobilization, manipulation, and massage. These techniques aim to improve joint mobility, reduce pain, and enhance muscle function.

Evidence and Applications
- *Spinal manipulation and mobilization*: Spinal manipulation is effective for acute lower back pain. A systematic review by the American College of Physicians supports its use for short-term pain relief.
- *Myofascial release*: Techniques targeting myofascial trigger points can significantly reduce pain and improve function in patients with chronic pain conditions like fibromyalgia.
- *Massage therapy*: Regular massage therapy can reduce pain and improve mobility in conditions like osteoarthritis and chronic lower back pain.

■ EXERCISE THERAPY

Exercise therapy is a cornerstone of physiotherapy, tailored to individual patient needs to enhance strength, flexibility, and endurance.

Evidence and Applications
- *Strengthening exercises*: A Cochrane review found that strengthening exercises are effective in reducing pain and improving function in patients with knee osteoarthritis.
- *Aerobic exercise*: Regular aerobic exercise, such as walking or cycling, has been shown to reduce pain and improve function in chronic low back pain.
- *Flexibility and stretching*: Stretching exercises are beneficial in managing musculoskeletal pain by improving range of motion and reducing stiffness, particularly in conditions like ankylosing spondylitis.

ELECTROTHERAPY

Electrotherapy encompasses various modalities like transcutaneous electrical nerve stimulation (TENS), ultrasound therapy, and laser therapy.

Evidence and Applications
- *TENS*: This has been widely studied and found to be effective for short-term pain relief in chronic musculoskeletal conditions.
- *Ultrasound therapy*: While the evidence is mixed, some studies suggest that ultrasound therapy can be beneficial for conditions like tendinitis and bursitis by promoting tissue healing.
- *Laser therapy*: Low-level laser therapy has shown promise in reducing pain and inflammation in conditions such as rheumatoid arthritis and chronic neck pain.

OTHER MODALITIES

In addition to the aforementioned techniques, physiotherapists employ other modalities such as thermotherapy, cryotherapy, and hydrotherapy.

Evidence and Applications
- *Thermotherapy (heat therapy)*: Applying heat can reduce pain and stiffness in conditions like chronic lower back pain and osteoarthritis.
- *Cryotherapy (cold therapy)*: Cold therapy is effective in reducing acute pain and inflammation, particularly after injury or surgery.
- *Hydrotherapy*: Water exercise provides resistance and support, making it an excellent modality for patients with arthritis and those undergoing rehabilitation post surgery.

INDICATIONS AND CONTRAINDICATIONS OF VARIOUS MODALITIES

Transcutaneous Electrical Nerve Stimulation

Indications
- Chronic pain (e.g., low back pain, osteoarthritis)
- Postoperative pain

- Neuropathic pain
- Musculoskeletal pain

Contraindications
- Pacemakers or other electronic implants
- Pregnancy (especially over the abdomen or lower back)
- Epilepsy
- Malignancy in the treatment area
- Infection or open wounds in the treatment area

Interferential Current (IFC)

Indications
- Pain relief (chronic and acute)
- Muscle spasm reduction
- Improvement of local blood flow
- Edema reduction

Contraindications
- Pacemakers or other implanted electronic devices
- Pregnancy
- Infection or malignancy in the treatment area
- Recent fractures
- Hemorrhagic conditions

Ultrasound Therapy

Indications
- Soft-tissue injuries (e.g., ligament sprains, tendonitis)
- Chronic inflammatory conditions (e.g., bursitis, osteoarthritis)
- Muscle spasm and tightness
- Promotion of tissue healing and scar tissue management

Contraindications
- Malignancy
- Pregnancy (over the abdomen, pelvis, or lower back)
- Epiphyseal plates in children
- Areas of impaired circulation or sensation
- Over fractures or acute infections

Electrical Muscle Stimulation (EMS)

Indications
- Muscle re-education and strengthening
- Prevention of muscle atrophy
- Enhancing muscle endurance
- Postoperative rehabilitation

CHAPTER 50: Role of Physiotherapy in the Management of Musculoskeletal Pain

Contraindications
- Pacemakers or other electronic implants
- Pregnancy
- Malignancy
- Areas of thrombosis or thrombophlebitis
- Infection or open wounds in the treatment area

Shortwave Diathermy (SWD)
Indications
- Deep heating for muscle relaxation
- Joint stiffness (e.g., osteoarthritis, rheumatoid arthritis)
- Muscle spasms
- Pain relief

Contraindications
- Pacemakers or other implanted electronic devices
- Pregnancy
- Malignancy
- Acute inflammation
- Metallic implants in the treatment area

Laser Therapy
Indications
- Pain relief (acute and chronic)
- Reduction of inflammation
- Promotion of wound healing
- Soft-tissue injuries (e.g., sprains, strains)
- Osteoarthritis and rheumatoid arthritis

Contraindications
- Pregnancy (especially over the abdomen and lower back)
- Malignancy
- Over the thyroid gland
- Areas with recent hemorrhage
- Direct exposure to the eye

Combining multiple physiotherapy modalities often yields better outcomes than single-modality treatments. An integrative approach tailored to individual patient needs, considering both the physical and the psychological aspects of pain, is crucial for effective management.

Evidence
- *Multimodal therapy*: A study on patients with chronic lower back pain showed that a combination of manual therapy, exercise, and education

resulted in better pain relief and functional improvement compared with single interventions.
- *Patient education*: Educating patients about pain, proper posture, and ergonomics is essential for long-term management and prevention of recurrence.

CONCLUSION

Physiotherapy, with its diverse range of modalities, plays an indispensable role in the management of musculoskeletal pain. The integration of manual therapy, exercise, electrotherapy, and other techniques, underpinned by strong scientific evidence, offers a comprehensive approach to pain management. As research continues to evolve, physiotherapists must stay abreast of the latest evidence to provide optimal care for their patients.

BIBLIOGRAPHY

1. Bennett R. Myofascial pain syndromes and their evaluation. Best Pract Res Clin Rheumatol. 2002;16(5):707-20.
2. Dagfinrud H, Hagen KB. Physiotherapy interventions for ankylosing spondylitis. Cochrane Database Syst Rev. 2008; 2008(1):CD002822.
3. Field T. Massage therapy research review. Complement Ther Clin Pract. 2014;20(4):224-9.
4. Fransen M, McConnell S, Harmer AR, Van der Esch M, Simic M, Bennell KL. Exercise for osteoarthritis of the knee. Cochrane Database Syst Rev. 2015;(1):CD004376.
5. Qaseem A, Wilt TJ, McLean RM, Forciea MA. Noninvasive treatments for acute, subacute, and chronic low back pain: a clinical practice guideline from the American College of Physicians. Ann Intern Med. 2017;166(7):514-30.
6. Shnayderman I, Katz-Leurer M. An aerobic walking programme versus muscle strengthening programme for chronic low back pain: a randomized controlled trial. Clin Rehabil. 2013;27(3):207-14.

CHAPTER 51

Role of Integrated Medicine Including Alternative Medicine in Pain Management

Harsh Chauhan

INTRODUCTION

There are various types of integrative medical therapies including Ayurveda, homoeopathic medicine, and naturopathic medicine. *Natural therapies* use substances derived from nature, like herbs, foods, and vitamins. Mind–body practices employ different techniques to enhance the mind's influence on bodily functions, such as yoga, biofeedback, cognitive-behavioral therapy (CBT), hypnosis, relaxation therapy, meditation, prayer, mental healing, and music therapy. *Manual techniques* focus on the movement of various body parts, including chiropractic, osteopathic, and massage therapies. *Bioenergetic therapies* focus on the use of energy fields and encompass methods like acupuncture, therapeutic touch, and electromagnetic field therapy.

AYURVEDA AND BOTANICAL THERAPIES

Ayurveda is an ancient Indian system of medicine that emphasizes the importance of maintaining balance and harmony within the body, mind, and spirit. This holistic approach to health and wellness has gained increasing attention in the West, particularly for its potential benefits in managing chronic pain.

For example, *turmeric*, a common Ayurvedic spice, has been extensively studied for its anti-inflammatory and analgesic properties. *Numerous studies* have shown that curcumin, the active compound in turmeric, can be effective in reducing pain and improving function in individuals with conditions such as osteoarthritis, rheumatoid arthritis, and chronic low back pain. Likewise, *Boswellia serrata*, a herb used in Ayurvedic medicine, has strong anti-inflammatory properties and may aid in alleviating joint pain and stiffness. In addition to these well-known Ayurvedic botanicals, a wealth of other herbal

and natural remedies has been traditionally used for pain management. These include:
- *Ginger (Zingiber officinale):* Known for its anti-inflammatory and analgesic properties, ginger has been used to alleviate various types of pain, including headaches, menstrual cramps, and muscle soreness.
- *Ashwagandha (Withania somnifera):* This adaptogenic herb is thought to assist the body in coping with stress and has been employed in Ayurveda to treat chronic pain, especially in cases of fibromyalgia and rheumatoid arthritis.
- *Valerian (Valeriana officinalis):* Traditionally used as a sedative and relaxant, valerian may be helpful in reducing muscle tension and improving sleep quality, which can be important for pain management.
- *Arnica (Arnica montana):* This herb is widely used for its topical application for treating bruises, sprains, and muscle soreness because of its anti-inflammatory and analgesic properties.

By incorporating these and other Ayurvedic botanicals into a comprehensive pain management plan, individuals may be able to find natural and effective relief for their chronic pain conditions.

NUTRITIONAL AND DIETARY SUPPLEMENTS

Nutrition and dietary supplements have long been explored as potential therapies for chronic pain management. There is growing recognition of the role that certain nutrients and supplements may play in reducing inflammation, improving pain perception, and supporting overall physical and emotional well-being.

One of the most well-studied areas in this regard is the use of *omega-3 fatty acids,* such as those found in fish oil, for the management of chronic pain. Numerous studies have demonstrated the anti-inflammatory properties of omega-3 fatty acids and their potential to alleviate pain associated with rheumatoid arthritis, osteoarthritis, and neuropathic pain. By reducing inflammation and modulating the body's pain response, omega-3 fatty acid supplements may provide a natural and complementary approach to pain management.

Another area of interest is the use of *vitamin D* for treating chronic pain. Vitamin D plays a crucial role in various physiological processes, including bone health and immune function. Low levels of vitamin D have been associated with increased pain sensitivity and a higher risk of developing chronic pain conditions, such as musculoskeletal pain and fibromyalgia. Supplementation with vitamin D may help address deficiencies and potentially improve pain management.

The effectiveness and safety of dietary supplements can vary greatly. Proper dosage, quality, and potential interactions with other medications or health conditions should be carefully considered.

CHAPTER 51: Role of Integrated Medicine Including Alternative...

By integrating nutritional and dietary approaches into a comprehensive pain management strategy, individuals may find additional relief and support their overall health and well-being.

MANIPULATIVE THERAPIES

Manipulative therapies, such as chiropractic and massage therapy, have long been used to address various types of pain, including headaches, neck pain, lower back pain, and joint discomfort. These approaches focus on the manipulation and adjustment of the musculoskeletal system to improve function, reduce pain, and promote overall well-being.

Chiropractic care is a form of manipulative therapy that emphasizes the relationship between the spine and the nervous system. Chiropractors use a variety of techniques, including spinal adjustments, to realign the spine and improve the body's natural ability to heal itself. Numerous studies have shown the effectiveness of chiropractic care in the management of low back pain, neck pain, and headaches, with many patients reporting significant improvements in their symptoms and reduced reliance on pain medication.

Massage therapy, on the other hand, involves the manipulation of the soft tissues of the body, such as muscles, tendons, and ligaments. Massage can help reduce muscle tension, improve blood circulation, and promote relaxation, all of which can contribute to pain relief.

Massage therapy has been found to be particularly beneficial for individuals with chronic low back pain, neck pain, and myofascial pain syndrome, a condition characterized by localized muscle pain and tenderness.

In addition to these well-established manipulative therapies, other approaches, such as *osteopathic manipulation and myofascial release,* have been used to address various types of pain. These techniques focus on the restoration of normal structure and function within the musculoskeletal system, with the goal of reducing pain and improving overall physical well-being.

The effectiveness of manipulative therapies may vary depending on the individual, the underlying cause of the pain, and the skill and experience of the practitioner. As with any healthcare intervention, it is essential to consult a qualified and licensed professional to ensure the safe and effective implementation of these therapies.

MIND-BODY PRACTICES

Mind-body practices such as yoga, meditation, and CBT have gained increasing recognition for their potential to manage chronic pain. These approaches harness the power of the mind to influence the body's physical and emotional responses, thereby reducing pain and improving overall well-being.

Yoga, a centuries-old practice that combines physical postures, breathing exercises, and meditation, has been shown to be effective in the management of various types of chronic pain, including low back pain, neck pain, and osteoarthritis. Physical postures and stretches can help to improve flexibility, strength, and posture, while breathing and meditation practices can promote relaxation, reduce stress, and enhance pain coping strategies.

Meditation, on the other hand, focuses on the cultivation of mindfulness and present-moment awareness. By learning to observe and accept their thoughts and sensations without judgment, individuals with chronic pain can develop more effective coping mechanisms and potentially reduce the intensity and frequency of their pain episodes. Numerous studies have demonstrated the benefits of mindfulness-based interventions in the management of chronic pain conditions, such as fibromyalgia, headaches, and neuropathic pain.

Cognitive-behavioral therapy is a type of psychotherapy designed to assist individuals in recognizing and changing negative thoughts and behaviors that may influence their experience of pain. By teaching coping strategies and stress management techniques, CBT can empower individuals to take a more active role in managing their pain and improving their overall quality of life. Research has shown that CBT can be effective in reducing pain intensity, improving physical function, and reducing reliance on pain medication in individuals with chronic pain conditions.

Other mind–body practices, such as *hypnosis, biofeedback, and relaxation therapy,* have also been used to address chronic pain. These approaches focus on the mind's ability to influence physiological processes, such as muscle tension, blood flow, and pain perception, intending to reduce pain and improve overall well-being.

Incorporating mind–body practices into a comprehensive pain management plan can be a potent strategy for those aiming to adopt a more holistic approach to their health and well-being.

CONCLUSION

To navigate the complex landscape of pain management, it is clear that a *multifaceted approach* that combines the best of conventional and alternative therapies is the key to unlocking lasting relief and improving quality of life.

BIBLIOGRAPHY

1. Berman BM. Integrative approaches to pain management: how to get the best of both worlds. BMJ. 2003;326(7402):1320-1.
2. Lin YC, Wan L, Jamison RN. Using integrative medicine in pain management: an evaluation of current evidence. Anesth Analg. 2017;125(6):2081-93.
3. Trivedi H, Avrit TA, Chan L, Burchette M, Rathore R. The benefits of integrative medicine in the management of chronic pain: a review. Cureus. 2022;14(10):e2996.

CHAPTER 52

Role of Acupuncture in the Management of Musculoskeletal Pain

Nusrat Jabeen

■ INTRODUCTION

Acupuncture, an ancient therapeutic technique originating from traditional Chinese medicine (TCM), has gained substantial traction in modern clinical practice and is very well used in treating musculoskeletal pain.

■ HOW DOES IT WORK?

According to Chinese theory, human beings have two energy channels (yin and yang) flowing through the whole body and diseases occur because of an imbalance between yin and yang energy, so by doing acupuncture, we restore the energy balance.

■ MECHANISMS OF ACUPUNCTURE

Acupuncture involves inserting fine needles into specific points on the body, known as acupoints. The proposed mechanisms through which acupuncture alleviates pain include:
- *Neurotransmitter modulation*: Acupuncture stimulates the release of endogenous opioids, serotonin, and norepinephrine, which modulate pain perception and induce analgesia.
- *Neuroplastic changes*: Functional MRI studies indicate that acupuncture can alter brain activity patterns, particularly in regions associated with pain processing, suggesting a central modulation of pain.
- *Anti-inflammatory effects*: Acupuncture has been shown to reduce proinflammatory cytokines and increase anti-inflammatory cytokines, aiding in the reduction of inflammation-associated pain.
- *Peripheral mechanisms*: Needle insertion induces local effects, such as increased blood flow and the release of adenosine, which contributes to pain relief.

EFFICACY OF ACUPUNCTURE FOR MUSCULOSKELETAL PAIN

Chronic Low Back Pain

Numerous randomized controlled trials (RCTs) and systematic reviews support acupuncture's efficacy in reducing chronic low back pain. A landmark study by Vickers et al. concluded that acupuncture provides significant pain relief and improves function in patients with chronic low back pain compared with sham acupuncture and conventional treatments.

Osteoarthritis

Acupuncture has demonstrated benefits in managing osteoarthritis, particularly of the knee. A meta-analysis by Liu et al. found that acupuncture significantly reduces pain and improves physical function in patients with osteoarthritis, with effects lasting up to 6 months post-treatment.

Neck Pain

Evidence supports acupuncture's role in alleviating chronic neck pain. A systematic review by Yuan et al. highlighted that acupuncture significantly improves pain and disability in patients with chronic neck pain, with minimal adverse effects.

PREREQUISITES, PROCEDURE, AND PRECAUTIONS

Proper patient selection and assessment are critical for optimizing acupuncture outcomes. Clinicians should evaluate the patient's medical history, pain characteristics, and previous treatment responses.

Acupuncture can be particularly beneficial for patients who have not achieved adequate pain relief from conventional therapies.

- *Frequency and duration*: Typically, acupuncture treatments are administered once or twice weekly for 6-8 weeks. Chronic conditions may require maintenance sessions.
- *Technique*: Practitioners may employ various techniques, including manual needle manipulation, electroacupuncture (application of electrical current to needles), and auricular acupuncture (acupoints on the ear).

SAFETY AND CONTRAINDICATIONS

Acupuncture is generally safe when performed by trained professionals. Common side effects include minor bleeding, bruising, and transient pain at needle sites.

Contraindications include severe coagulopathies, local infections, and certain skin conditions.

CONCLUSION

Acupuncture is a valuable adjunct in the management of musculoskeletal pain, offering a complementary approach to conventional therapies. Its efficacy in conditions such as chronic low back pain, osteoarthritis, and neck pain is well supported by evidence, making it a viable option for integrated pain management strategies.

BIBLIOGRAPHY

1. Liu F, You J, Li Q, Fang T, Chen M, Tang N, et al. Acupuncture for chronic pain-related insomnia: a systematic review and meta-analysis. Evid Based Complement Alternat Med. 2019;2019:5381028.
2. Vickers AJ, Vertosick EA, Lewith G, MacPherson H, Foster NE, Sherman KJ, et al. Acupuncture for chronic pain: update of an individual patient data meta-analysis. J Pain. 2018;19(5):455-74.
3. Yuan QL, Wang P, Liu L, Sun F, Cai YS, Wu WT, et al. Acupuncture for musculoskeletal pain: a meta-analysis and meta-regression of sham-controlled randomized clinical trials. Sci Rep. 2016;6:30675.

CHAPTER 53

Musculoskeletal Pain and Mental Health

Ankita Khajuria

INTRODUCTION

Mental health and musculoskeletal pain are interlinked. Mental stress can worsen physical pain, while chronic pain impacts emotional well-being. Effective management combines physical therapies with mental health support, improving both pain and overall quality of life.

CHRONIC PAIN AND MENTAL HEALTH DISORDERS: AN INTERCONNECTED RELATIONSHIP

Chronic pain and mental health disorders frequently co-occur, with research indicating that each can exacerbate the other. The link between chronic pain and increased rates of major depressive disorder, suicidal thoughts, and attempts is well documented. Psychopathological disorders affect 33–46% of individuals with chronic pain, compared with just 10% in those without pain or with shorter pain durations. A study on acute and chronic back pain revealed that 8% of patients with pain lasting <6 months suffered from major depression, whereas this figure rose significantly to 46% among those with longer-lasting pain.

BIOPSYCHOSOCIAL MODEL OF PAIN

First proposed by George Engel in 1977, the biopsychosocial model posits that understanding a person's medical condition requires considering not only biological factors but also psychological and social aspects. This comprehensive model is particularly relevant in chronic pain management, emphasizing the interplay between physiological pathology, psychological elements (such as distress and coping mechanisms), and social influences

CHAPTER 53: Musculoskeletal Pain and Mental Health

(including socioeconomic and cultural factors). Integrating psychological treatments with physical therapy can address all dimensions of chronic pain.

PSYCHOLOGICAL INTERVENTIONS IN PAIN MANAGEMENT

- *Cognitive-behavioral therapy (CBT)*: Recognized as a leading treatment for chronic pain, CBT focuses on modifying negative thought patterns and behaviors. Recent "third-wave" CBT therapies incorporate mindfulness and acceptance strategies, significantly reducing pain intensity and enhancing quality of life.
- *Acceptance and commitment therapy (ACT)*: ACT, a form of third-wave CBT, encourages acceptance of pain while committing to personal values. It has been shown to effectively reduce pain interference, disability, and depression, offering a cost-effective clinical option.
- *Mindfulness-based stress reduction (MBSR)*: MBSR uses mindfulness meditation to foster present-moment awareness and nonjudgmental acceptance of pain, reducing pain-related distress and improving psychological well-being.

CENTRAL SENSITIZATION AND PAIN MANAGEMENT

Central sensitization, in which the central nervous system's response to stimuli is amplified, plays a crucial role in chronic musculoskeletal pain. Addressing psychological factors like anxiety and depression can mitigate central sensitization's impact on pain and disability.

PSYCHOLOGICALLY INFORMED PHYSICAL THERAPY

Psychologically informed physical therapy (PIPT) combines psychological techniques with physical therapy to improve outcomes for patients with chronic pain. By integrating pain education, cognitive restructuring, and stress management into physical therapy, this holistic approach enhances pain management and functional recovery.

ADDITIONAL PAIN MANAGEMENT STRATEGIES

- *Pharmacological interventions*: Medications, particularly antidepressants and anticonvulsants, can be effective in managing neuropathic pain and reducing central sensitization.
- *Exercise and physical activity*: Regular exercise improves physical function and reduces pain while also providing psychological benefits like decreased depression and anxiety. Tailored exercise programs enhance adherence and outcomes.

- *Relaxation techniques*: Techniques such as progressive muscle relaxation, guided imagery, and deep breathing exercises reduce muscle tension, lower stress, and improve pain control.
- *Biofeedback*: This method uses electronic devices to help patients control physiological functions, reducing pain and enhancing relaxation.
- *Social support and group therapy*: Support groups and group therapy provide emotional support, reduce isolation, and improve coping skills and psychological well-being.

CONCLUSION

Effective musculoskeletal pain management requires a holistic approach integrating psychological, physical, and pharmacological interventions. Addressing pain's multifaceted nature can significantly enhance a patient's outcomes and quality of life, offering a comprehensive framework for managing chronic pain.

Various therapeutic approaches address both the physical and the psychological dimensions of pain.

BIBLIOGRAPHY

1. Cherkin DC, Sherman KJ, Balderson BH, Cook AJ, Anderson ML, Hawkes RJ, et al. Effect of mindfulness-based stress reduction vs cognitive behavioural therapy or usual care on back pain and functional limitations in adults with chronic low back pain: a randomized clinical trial. JAMA. 2016;315(12):1240-9.
2. McCracken LM, Yu L, Vowles KE. New generation psychological treatments in chronic pain. BMJ. 2022;376:e057212.
3. Nijs J, Van Houdenhove B, Oostendorp RA. Recognition of central sensitization in patients with musculoskeletal pain: application of pain neurophysiology in manual therapy practice. Man Ther. 2013;18(2):135-40.
4. Zhou F, Wang Y, Luo W. Impact of central sensitization on pain, disability and psychological distress in patients with knee osteoarthritis and chronic low back pain. BMC Musculoskelet Disord. 2023;24:47.

CHAPTER 54

Essentials of Regenerative Medicine in Pain Management

Rashid Anjum

■ INTRODUCTION

Traditional pain management strategies, such as pharmacotherapy and invasive surgeries, often provide limited relief and come with substantial side effects. Regenerative medicine, an emerging field, offers a novel approach to pain management by harnessing the body's intrinsic healing capabilities to repair and regenerate damaged tissues.

■ PRINCIPLES OF REGENERATIVE MEDICINE

Regenerative medicine aims to restore function and structure to damaged tissues or organs through mechanisms such as cellular therapy, tissue engineering, and molecular therapy. Its primary components include the following:
- *Stem cells:* These undifferentiated cells have the potential to differentiate into various cell types. Mesenchymal stem cells (MSCs), derived from the bone marrow, adipose tissue, or umbilical cord, are particularly noted for their anti-inflammatory and regenerative properties. They can be home to sites of injury, where they can differentiate into the required cell types, such as osteocytes, chondrocytes, and tenocytes. They also secrete bioactive molecules that modulate the immune response and stimulate endogenous repair processes.
- *Growth factors and cytokine:* These are proteins that regulate cellular processes such as proliferation, differentiation, and migration. Examples include platelet-derived growth factor (PDGF) and transforming growth factor-beta (TGF-β). Growth factors can be delivered directly or via gene therapy to enhance tissue repair and regeneration.
- *Scaffolds:* Three-dimensional structures that provide a framework for cell attachment and tissue formation. Scaffolds can be composed of synthetic materials like polylactic acid or natural materials such as collagen and

hyaluronic acid. They support cell proliferation, differentiation, and organization into functional tissues.
- *Biomaterials:* Materials that interact with biological systems to promote healing. Biomaterials can deliver cells and bioactive molecules to the target site, providing mechanical support and enhancing the regenerative process. Examples include hydrogels, which can encapsulate cells and growth factors, and bioactive glass, which can stimulate bone regeneration.

TECHNIQUES IN REGENERATIVE MEDICINE FOR PAIN MANAGEMENT

Several regenerative medicine techniques have shown promise in managing chronic pain, including the following:
- *Platelet-rich plasma (PRP) therapy:* PRP is an autologous blood product enriched with platelets, which release growth factors and cytokines that promote tissue repair and modulate inflammation. It is used in treating conditions such as osteoarthritis, tendinopathies, and muscle injuries. The preparation involves centrifuging the patient's blood to concentrate platelets, which are then injected into the affected area. Clinical studies have demonstrated PRP's effectiveness in enhancing tendon and cartilage healing and reducing pain.
- *Stem cell therapy:* This involves the injection of stem cells into damaged tissues to stimulate regeneration and reduce inflammation. Commonly used stem cells include MSCs and adipose-derived stem cells (ASCs). For instance, MSCs can be harvested from one marrow or adipose tissue, expanded in culture, and injected into areas of injury such as intervertebral discs or osteoarthritic joints. Stem cell therapy has shown promise in reducing pain and improving function in various musculoskeletal conditions.
- *Prolotherapy:* This involves injecting irritant solutions (e.g., hypertonic dextrose) into the affected area to induce a localized inflammatory response, stimulating the body's healing mechanisms. Prolotherapy is used for chronic ligament and tendon injuries, where it promotes the repair of degenerative tissues by triggering the body's natural healing processes.
- *Exosome therapy:* Exosomes are extracellular vesicles released by cells that carry proteins, lipids, and genetic material. They facilitate intercellular communication and have anti-inflammatory and regenerative effects. Exosome therapy is being explored for conditions like osteoarthritis and neuropathic pain. MSC-derived exosomes, e.g., can reduce inflammation, promote tissue regeneration, and protect against further damage.
- *Tissue engineering:* This combines scaffolds, cells, and bioactive molecules to create functional tissues. Tissue engineering is particularly relevant for repairing large tissue defects. For instance, bioengineered cartilage constructs can be created by seeding chondrocytes or stem cells onto scaffolds, which are then implanted into the damaged joint to promote cartilage regeneration.

APPLICATIONS OF REGENERATIVE MEDICINE IN PAIN MANAGEMENT

- *Osteoarthritis:* Role of PRP therapy and stem cell therapy can be used.
- *Tendinopathies:* Role of PRP therapy and prolotherapy
- *Intervertebral disc degeneration:* Role of stem cell therapy and role of tissue engineering
- *Neuropathic pain:* Role of exosome therapy and stem cell therapy

CLINICAL EVIDENCE AND CHALLENGES

The clinical application of regenerative medicine in pain management is supported by growing evidence from preclinical studies and clinical trials. However, several challenges remain which are as follows:
- *Standardization:* Variability in cell sources, preparation methods, and administration protocols can affect outcomes. Standardized protocols are needed to ensure consistency and efficacy. Differences in stem cell isolation, expansion, and delivery methods can lead to inconsistent results across studies.
- *Regulation:* Regulatory frameworks for regenerative therapies are still evolving. Ensuring the safety and efficacy of these treatments while facilitating innovation is a complex task. Regulatory agencies must balance the need for rigorous clinical trials with the desire to accelerate the availability of promising therapies.
- *Long-term outcomes:* While short-term benefits are evident, the long-term efficacy and safety of regenerative therapies need further investigation through large-scale, long-term studies. There is a need for robust clinical trials that follow patients over several years to assess the durability of the therapeutic effects.
- *Cost and accessibility:* High costs and limited accessibility can restrict the widespread adoption of regenerative therapies. Efforts are needed to make these treatments more affordable and available. Strategies to reduce costs include optimizing manufacturing processes and developing scalable production methods for cells and biomaterials.

FUTURE DIRECTIONS

The future of regenerative medicine in pain management is promising, with ongoing research focusing on the following:
- *Combination therapies:* Integrating multiple regenerative approaches (e.g., combining PRP with stem cells) to achieve synergistic effects. Combination therapies can enhance the regenerative potential and improve clinical outcomes by targeting multiple aspects of the healing process.
- *Personalized medicine:* Tailoring regenerative treatments based on individual patient characteristics, such as genetic profile and disease

phenotype. Artificial intelligence (AI) can be utilized to optimize treatment protocols, predict outcomes, and personalize therapies. AI can analyze large datasets to identify patterns and predict which patients will respond best to certain treatments, improving the efficiency and effectiveness of regenerative medicine.

CONCLUSION

Regenerative medicine represents a paradigm shift in pain management, offering potential disease-modifying therapies that go beyond symptom relief. By harnessing the body's intrinsic healing capabilities, regenerative approaches hold promise for effectively treating chronic pain conditions that have been refractory to traditional treatments. Continued research, standardization, and innovation will be crucial in realizing the full potential of regenerative medicine in alleviating chronic pain and improving patients' quality of life.

BIBLIOGRAPHY

1. Ankrum J, Karp JM. Mesenchymal stem cell therapy: two steps forward, one step back. Trends Mol Med. 2010;16(5):203-9.
2. Barry FP, Murphy JM. Mesenchymal stem cells: clinical applications and biological characterization. Int J Biochem Cell Biol. 2004;36(4):568-84.
3. Caplan AI. Adult mesenchymal stem cells for tissue engineering versus regenerative medicine. J Cell Physiol. 2007;213(2):341-7.
4. Centeno CJ, Schultz JR, Cheever M, Robinson B, Freeman M, Marasco W. Safety and complications reporting on the re-implantation of culture-expanded mesenchymal stem cells using autologous platelet lysate technique. Curr Stem Cell Res Ther. 2010;5(1):81-93.
5. Chen RR, Mooney DJ. Polymeric growth factor delivery strategies for tissue engineering. Pharm Res. 2003;20(8):1103-12.
6. Griffith LG, Naughton G. Tissue engineering—current challenges and expanding opportunities. Science. 2002;295(5557):1009-14.
7. Lai RC, Yeo RW, Tan KH, Lim SK. Exosomes for drug delivery—a novel application for the mesenchymal stem cell. Biotechnol Adv. 2013;31(5):543-51.
8. Patel S, Dhillon MS, Aggarwal S, Marwaha N, Jain A. Treatment with platelet-rich plasma is more effective than placebo for knee osteoarthritis: a prospective, double-blind, randomized trial. Am J Sports Med. 2013;41(2):356-64.
9. Rabago D, Best TM, Zgierska AE, Zeisig E, Ryan M, Crane D. A systematic review of four injection therapies for lateral epicondylitis: prolotherapy, polidocanol, whole blood and platelet-rich plasma. Br J Sports Med. 2009;43(7):471-81.
10. Ratner BD, Bryant SJ. Biomaterials: where we have been and where we are going. Annu Rev Biomed Eng. 2004;6:41-75.
11. Sampson S, Gerhardt M, Mandelbaum B. Platelet rich plasma injection grafts for musculoskeletal injuries: a review. Curr Rev Musculoskelet Med. 2008;1(3-4):165-74.
12. Vivek S, Rashid A, Ravish, Ravinder S. Efficacy and outcome of platelet-rich plasma in the management of primary osteoarthritis knee; a prospective study. Indian J Orthopaed Surg. 2019;2019:9390.

CHAPTER 55

Multidisciplinary Approaches to Pain Management

John Mohd, Parul Raina

■ INTRODUCTION

As chronic pain persists, the link between pain and associated factors becomes less clear. Additionally, pain behaviors and social factors related to pain can become more complex. Consequently, treatment from a single department may not suffice for chronic pain sufferers. The International Association for the Study of Pain (IASP) suggests a multidisciplinary approach to pain management, distinguishing between acute and chronic pain and considering various types of pain. This approach has been used in Europe and the United States since Bonica emphasized its importance in the 1950s.

■ MULTIDISCIPLINARY AND INTERDISCIPLINARY APPROACHES

Relying solely on one discipline, such as pharmacological treatment, is inadequate for managing chronic pain. The complexity of chronic pain and its comorbidities necessitates integrative pain management, evolving from monodisciplinary to multidisciplinary treatments, and further to interdisciplinary programs based on a biopsychosocial model.

■ BIOPSYCHOSOCIAL MODEL

This model highlights the interaction among physiological, psychological, and social factors contributing to pain. Among these elements, the psychological aspect is particularly challenging to address, underscoring the need to tackle both sensory and psychological drivers of chronic pain. An integrated treatment approach that considers physiological, psychological, and social components is essential for managing chronic pain effectively.

COMPONENTS OF MULTIDISCIPLINARY PAIN MANAGEMENT

- Pharmacological treatment
- *Nonpharmacological treatment*: Physical therapy/occupational therapy
- *Psychological therapy*: Acceptance and commitment therapy (ACT), cognitive–behavioral therapy (CBT)
- Interventional treatment
- *Complementary treatments*: Acupuncture, chiropractic, tai chi, etc.

ADVANTAGES OF INTERDISCIPLINARY PAIN MANAGEMENT

- Strong recommendations with high-quality evidence, especially for lower back pain
- Improved outcomes across various domains, including pain severity and functional interference, with gains maintained at 1-year follow-up
- Cost-effective long-term treatment option
- Individualized treatment plans
- Better treatment adherence

CHALLENGES

- Often short-term
- Difficulty in establishing all disciplines under one roof
- Lack of awareness among healthcare providers

COLLABORATION AND COORDINATION

Interdisciplinary pain management involves greater coordination of services within a comprehensive program and frequent communication among healthcare professionals at the same facility. Key components include a common rehabilitation philosophy, regular communication, and active patient involvement, resulting in effective, comprehensive treatment.

CASE STUDIES

Case Study 1

A 72-year-old male with carcinoma of the esophagus and bony metastasis to L1, L2, and L3 was unable to undergo positron emission tomography-computed tomography/magnetic resonance imaging (PET-CT/MRI) scans due to severe pain. After various pharmacological pain relief methods, including oral morphine and IV dexamethasone, an epidural catheter was inserted at T5. This allowed the patient to lie supine for radiotherapy, which significantly improved his condition.

Case Study 2

A 31-year-old female with fibromyalgia for 9 years experienced severe pain flare-ups triggered by a COVID-19 infection. Initially managed with duloxetine, her condition worsened over time. A pain physician prescribed pregabalin and amitriptyline, and she was referred to a psychologist for CBT. Along with graded exercises from a physiotherapist, her daily functions were restored, highlighting the effectiveness of a multidisciplinary approach.

CONCLUSION

Chronic pain is a significant and costly global issue. For optimal patient outcomes, an interdisciplinary team should collaborate to assess and treat the patients, addressing their pain while providing education and support. This approach enables patients to set and achieve meaningful functional goals, improving their quality of life. More awareness and resources are needed to bring all disciplines together under one roof, especially in developing countries. Elevating the conversation around chronic musculoskeletal pain management to include functional outcomes and quality of life benefits is crucial.

BIBLIOGRAPHY

1. Eklund K, Stålnacke BM, Sundberg A, Eklund F, Eklund M. Introduction of a multimodal pain rehabilitation intervention in primary care: a pilot study. J Rehabil Med Clin Commun. 2023;6:3712.
2. Nahin RL. Use of multimodal multidisciplinary pain management in the US. JAMA Netw Open. 2022;5(11):e2240620.
3. Takahashi N, Takatsuki K, Kasahara S, Yabuki S. Multidisciplinary pain management program for patients with chronic musculoskeletal pain in Japan: a cohort study. J Pain Res. 2019;12:2563-76.
4. World Health Organization. (2022). Musculoskeletal health. Fact sheet. Available from https://www.who.int/news-room/fact-sheets/detail/musculoskeletal-conditions [Last accessed September, 2024].

CHAPTER 56

Palliative Care and End-of-Life Pain Management in Musculoskeletal Pain

Rajesh Mahajan, Sunana Gupta

■ INTRODUCTION

Research indicates that up to 70–90% of individuals with advanced malignancies experience pain, which often includes musculoskeletal pain (MSP) as a significant component.

■ ETIOLOGY

Many terminal diseases can cause MSP in pediatric, young, and adult patients. These diseases may be malignant or nonmalignant.
- *Malignant*: Pediatric cancers such as leukemia and osteosarcoma can involve the bones, leading to MSP. This includes bone metastases from cancers like breast, lung, or prostate cancer, as well as primary bone cancers such as osteosarcoma.
- *Nonmalignant causes*: Conditions like juvenile idiopathic arthritis (JIA) and Duchenne muscular dystrophy (DMD) can also cause MSP in pediatric patients. Other noncancerous conditions can lead to disabling MSP in adults like rheumatoid arthritis, osteoarthritis, fibromyalgia, and various other autoimmune or degenerative diseases.

■ PALLIATIVE CARE IN MUSCULOSKELETAL PAIN MANAGEMENT

Pain management in palliative care, particularly for MSP, focuses on improving quality of life by alleviating pain and other distressing symptoms. Effective pain management requires a holistic approach, incorporating pharmacological and nonpharmacological interventions tailored to the individual needs of the patient. Regular assessment and a patient-centered approach ensure that pain management strategies are both effective and responsive to the evolving needs of the patient.

- *Assessment*: Thorough assessment of pain, including its intensity, quality, duration, and impact on the patient's life. Tools like the Visual Analog Scale (VAS) or the Numeric Rating Scale (NRS) are commonly used.
- *Individualized treatment plan*: Tailoring treatment plans to the specific needs, preferences, and medical conditions of the patient. This may involve combining different pharmacological and nonpharmacological strategies.
- *Regular monitoring and adjustment*: Continuous evaluation of pain levels and treatment effectiveness. Adjustments to the pain management plan are made based on ongoing assessments.
- *Interdisciplinary approach*: Collaboration among healthcare professionals, including doctors, nurses, physical therapists, psychologists, and social workers, to address all aspects of the patient's well-being

PHARMACOLOGICAL INTERVENTIONS

Nonopioid Analgesics

- *Acetaminophen*: Often used as a first-line treatment for mild-to-moderate pain
- *Nonsteroidal anti-inflammatory drugs (NSAIDs)*: However, they must be used cautiously due to potential side effects like gastrointestinal bleeding and renal impairment.

Opioids

- *Mild opioids*: Codeine or tramadol for moderate pain
- *Strong opioids*: Morphine, oxycodone, hydromorphone, and fentanyl for severe pain. Dosage and administration must be carefully monitored to manage side effects and avoid dependence.

Adjuvant Medications

- *Antidepressants*: Such as amitriptyline and duloxetine, for neuropathic pain or when pain is associated with depression
- *Anticonvulsants*: Gabapentin and pregabalin for neuropathic pain
- *Muscle relaxants*: Baclofen or tizanidine for muscle spasms
- *Topical agents*: Lidocaine patches, capsaicin cream, and NSAID gels can be effective for localized MSP with fewer systemic side effects.

NONPHARMACOLOGICAL INTERVENTIONS

- *Physical therapy*: Techniques include massage, heat/cold therapy, and exercise programs designed to improve strength and flexibility, and reduce pain.
- *Occupational therapy*: Helps patients adapt their daily activities to reduce strain on painful areas

- *Cognitive-behavioral therapy (CBT)*: Assists patients in managing the psychological aspects of chronic pain
- *Acupuncture and acupressure*: Can provide relief for some patients by stimulating certain points on the body to alleviate pain
- *Transcutaneous electrical nerve stimulation (TENS)*: Uses low-voltage electrical current to provide pain relief
- *Complementary therapies*: Techniques such as meditation, mindfulness, and relaxation exercises can help manage pain by reducing stress and improving coping mechanisms.

GOALS OF CARE AND MANAGEMENT IN "END-OF-LIFE IN MUSCULOSKELETAL PAIN MANAGEMENT"

Primary Goals
- Pain relief
- Enhancing quality of life
- Maintaining functional ability
- Emotional and psychosocial support

Supportive Measures
- *Psychosocial support*: Providing counseling and emotional support to address anxiety, depression, and existential distress
- Spiritual care
- Family support

ETHICAL CONSIDERATIONS IN MANAGEMENT FOR TERMINALLY ILL PATIENTS WITH MUSCULOSKELETAL PAIN

- Respect for the autonomy of the patient
- *Shared decision-making*: Engaging in shared decision-making with patients and their families is crucial. This entails clear communication regarding the prognosis, the potential benefits and risks of pain management options, and consideration of the patient's values and preferences.
- *Advance directives*: Encouraging patients to prepare advance directives can ensure that their wishes regarding pain management and other aspects of end-of-life care are respected, even if they become unable to communicate them later.

BENEFICENCE AND NONMALEFICENCE

- *Respecting cultural sensitivity*: Adapt pain management strategies to align with the patient's cultural and personal values.

- *Legal and regulatory compliance*: Adherence to laws
- Regular reassessment

PALLIATIVE SEDATION

In cases where pain and suffering cannot be adequately controlled, palliative sedation may be considered. This involves sedating the patient to relieve intractable pain or distress, with the ethical justification being the principle of double effect: The intent is to alleviate suffering, not to hasten death.

COMMUNICATION AND COORDINATION

Interdisciplinary Approach and Holistic Care

An interdisciplinary approach involving physicians, nurses, social workers, and chaplains can offer comprehensive care, catering to the physical, emotional, social, and spiritual needs of terminally ill patients. This collaborative approach ensures that pain management is integrated into a broader palliative care plan.

CONCLUSION

Provide with compassionate, patient-centered care that respects the dignity and wishes of terminally ill patients with MSP while also ensuring the effective management of their symptoms.

BIBLIOGRAPHY

1. Caravaca F, Gonzales B, Bayo MÁ, Luna E. Musculoskeletal pain in patients with chronic kidney disease. Nefrologia. 2016;36(4):433-40.
2. Hashem M, AlMohaini RA, Alharbi TM, Aljurfi MM, Alzmamy SA, Alhussainan FS. Impact of musculoskeletal pain on health-related quality of life among adults in Saudi Arabia. Cureus. 2024;27:16(3):e57053.
3. Platt M. Pain challenges at the end of life—pain and palliative care collaboration. Rev Pain. 2010;4(2):18-23.
4. Rao CM, Singh P, Maikap D, Padhan P. Musculoskeletal disorders in chronic obstructive airway diseases: a neglected clinical entity. Mediterr J Rheumatol. 2021;32(2):118-23.
5. Sentandreu-Mañó T, Deka P, Almenar L, Tomás JM, Alguacil-Sancho L, López-Vilella R, et al. Correlates of musculoskeletal pain and kinesiophobia in older adults with heart failure: a structural equation model. Geriatr Nurs. 2023;53:72-7.

CHAPTER 57

Preventive Strategies for Musculoskeletal Pain

Abhishek Mahajan

INTRODUCTION

With advancing age, musculoskeletal pain significantly contributes to morbidity and illness among individuals. Conditions such as low back pain, osteoarthritis (OA), rheumatoid arthritis, and gouty arthritis are prevalent. Various strategies can be employed to prevent musculoskeletal pain.

PHYSICAL EXERCISE

Incorporating physical activity and optimizing exercise are essential for improving musculoskeletal health. The World Health Organization (WHO) recommends around 2 hours of moderate physical activity per week, equating to roughly 20 minutes a day of activities such as brisk walking or running. For individuals with knee OA, enhancements in locomotor function, balance, and strength, as well as pain reduction, have been observed following a home exercise regimen supplemented by an 8-week class-based program. Patients with chronic low back pain who engaged in a combined exercise program focusing on muscle strength and aerobic fitness reported reduced stiffness, thereby alleviating back pain. Sedentary lifestyles contribute to the increase in obesity and type 2 diabetes, both of which are major factors in the development and progression of OA. Epidemiological studies have confirmed the link between obesity and musculoskeletal degeneration.

PROPER NUTRITION

The European Society for Clinical and Economic Aspects of Osteoporosis, Osteoarthritis, and Musculoskeletal Conditions (ESCEO) Task Force has highlighted the importance of dietary protein, vitamin D, and calcium supplementation. They recommend increased protein intake in combination with physical exercise, especially for postmenopausal women who are more susceptible to musculoskeletal conditions. Previously, high-protein diets in older individuals were thought to harm the renal system. However, it is now understood that protein supplementation should not be reduced, as the effects of metabolic acidosis on the renal system can be mitigated by increased consumption of fruits and vegetables, which decrease renal acid load. Many health organizations advocate for a varied diet rich in fresh fruits and vegetables. Vitamin D, calcium, and protein optimize muscle, bone, and functional health in older adults, reducing metabolic imbalances and the risk of fractures. Calcium and protein together enhance bone health. Patients with OA should ensure that they meet the recommended intake of micronutrients such as vitamin K, which is crucial for bone and cartilage mineralization. A diet high in antioxidants may aid athletes by improving tissue repair. Although glucosamine and chondroitin are popular supplements suggested for promoting healthy joint function, there is limited evidence supporting their efficacy.

WEIGHT REDUCTION

There is a direct correlation between obesity and musculoskeletal pain. OA is more prevalent among obese individuals, and low back pain is a common complaint among those with sedentary lifestyles and obesity. Combining exercise with a healthy diet helps maintain a better physique, boosts confidence, and prevents multiple health issues, including musculoskeletal pain. Addressing obesity in childhood can also prevent musculoskeletal problems later in life.

ADEQUATE SLEEP

Sleep deprivation is positively correlated with low back pain and shoulder pain. Improper sleeping posture can also cause neck pain. Therefore, obtaining adequate, healthy sleep with proper neck alignment and posture is crucial for preventing musculoskeletal pain. Additionally, the mattress should be comfortable, neither too soft nor too hard, and the pillow should be appropriately sized, not too large.

PROPER POSTURE

- *Extended sitting:* Prolonged sedentary positions, particularly among office workers, increase the risk of developing musculoskeletal pain. There is a dose-response relationship between sedentary behavior and adverse outcomes.
- *Excessive weight bearing:* Excessive weight bearing, especially in gym-goers, is associated with back pain. It is important to work out within one's physical limits.

MENTAL HEALTH/PSYCHOSOCIAL FACTORS

Depression, anxiety, and stress are significant factors in adolescent musculoskeletal pain. Reducing stress through yoga, meditation, and other relaxation techniques can help manage and prevent pain related to these factors.

ERGONOMICS

Using ergonomic equipment, such as specially designed chairs, desks, and computer accessories, in addition to ergonomic training, has positive effects. These practices, combined with physical interventions, promote a safe and healthy work environment, thereby preventing stress and musculoskeletal issues.

PREVENTION OF WORKPLACE INJURIES

Education on occupational safety and health skills is vital for strengthening workplace safety. Regular seminars and training sessions on occupational safety should be conducted to promote a safer work environment.

PREVENTION OF SPORTS INJURIES

Many sports-related injuries are preventable. Factors such as muscle performance, strength, coordination, and endurance can be targeted in injury prevention programs. Developing a fitness plan that includes cardiovascular exercise, strength training, and flexibility can reduce injury risk. Stretching exercises can also improve muscle function and reduce injury likelihood.

Preventing falls in elderly patients requires multiple strategies. Early recognition, diagnosis, and treatment, along with aggressive management of acute pain to prevent chronic pain, are essential since chronic pain is more challenging to treat than acute pain.

CONCLUSION

Implementing a multifaceted approach is key to preventing musculoskeletal pain. By integrating ergonomic adjustments, regular physical activity, proper posture, and early intervention, individuals can significantly reduce their risk. Education on body mechanics, strengthening exercises, and fostering workplace wellness are essential components of a proactive strategy. These preventive measures not only mitigate the onset of pain but also enhance overall physical well-being, promoting long-term health and productivity.

BIBLIOGRAPHY

1. Ekelund U, Steene-Johannessen J, Brown WJ, Fagerland MW, Owen N, Powell KE, et al. Does physical activity attenuate, or even eliminate, the detrimental association of sitting time with mortality? A harmonised meta-analysis of data from more than 1 million men and women. Lancet. 2016;388(10051):1302-10.
2. Felson DT, Anderson JJ, Naimark A, Walker AM, Meenan RF. Obesity and knee osteoarthritis. The Framingham Study. Ann Intern Med. 1988;109(1):18-24.
3. Gordon R, Bloxham S. A systematic review of the effects of exercise and physical activity on non-specific chronic low back pain. Healthcare (Basel). 2016;4(2):22.
4. Hardcastle AC, Aucott L, Reid DM, Macdonald HM. Associations between dietary flavonoid intakes and bone health in a Scottish population. J Bone Miner Res. 2011;26(5):941-7.
5. McCarthy CJ, Mills PM, Pullen R, Richardson G, Hawkins N, Roberts CR, et al. Supplementation of a home-based exercise programme with a class-based programme for people with osteoarthritis of the knees: a randomised controlled trial and health economic analysis. Health Technol Assess. 2004;8(46):iii-v, 1-61.

CHAPTER 58

Occupational and Ergonomics Considerations in Musculoskeletal Pain Management

Shubham Pandoh

INTRODUCTION

Persons working in their workplace may seem relatively safe, but they can still be at risk for developing musculoskeletal pain (MSP).

Bad posture or unfavorable work settings can cause disruptive sprains, strains, and tears in the body.

Work-related injuries are painful, exhausting, and costly, whether caused by a one-time accident or from repetitive actions or movements over time.

Primary risk factors include:
- Lifting heavy objects
- Routine exposure to vibration
- Overhead work
- Forceful repetitive tasks
- Improper or prolonged postures
- Mechanical compression
- Temperature extremes
- Inadequate lighting
- Material handling
- Activities involving regular gripping, carrying, pushing, or pulling

The most prevalent forms of MSP are low backache (most common), neck pain, wrist pain, knee pain, and pain associated with osteoarthritis.

A multidisciplinary and holistic approach should be used to prevent work-related MSP. Appropriate work *ergonomics* can play a vital role in the prevention of and decreasing such pain.

Ergonomics is the study of people's interaction with their work environment, especially when concerned with making that environment physically, mentally, and organizationally safe, comfortable, and efficient.

The Occupational Safety and Health Administration (OSHA) defines ergonomics as the science of "designing the job to fit the worker, instead of forcing the worker to fit the job."

ADVANTAGES OF ERGONOMICS

- Improvement in worker's health and safety
- Reduction in risk of injuries
- Better job satisfaction
- Increased productivity
- High morale
- Absenteeism reduction
- Decreased drug consumption

STRATEGIES TO PREVENT WORK-RELATED INJURIES

- *Identification of groups at risk of being most vulnerable* like:
  - Individuals who manually move freight, stock, luggage
  - Heavy motor vehicle drivers
  - Production workers
  - Janitors and cleaners
  - Recyclable material collectors
  - Plumbers, pipe and steamfitters
  - Maintenance and repair workers
  - Housekeeping cleaners
  - Telecom line installers and repairers
  - Air conditioning and refrigeration mechanics and installers
  - Firefighters
  - Nursing assistants and psychiatric aides
- *Implementation of the ergonomic process* including:
  - *Management commitment*:
    - Involvement of workers
    - Proper training
    - Problem identification
    - Encourage early reporting of musculoskeletal disorder symptoms.
    - Progress evaluation
- *Implementation of workplace controls* which includes:
  - Engineering controls
  - Administrative controls
  - Use of personal protective equipment

The aims of these workplace controls are to reduce, eliminate, or control workplace hazards.

- *Use of engineering controls (preferred approach) like*:
  - Mechanical assist devices should be used for transportation of materials
  - Sliding objects instead of carrying or lifting

- Height-adjustable chairs or benches should be used
- Knee pads for kneeling tasks
- Footrests, wrist supports, anti-fatigue mats, etc., should be used in the offices
- *Administrative control strategies and policies should be framed and followed including*:
  - Reduction in shift length or overtime limit
  - Breaks to allow for rest and recovery
  - Rotation of workers in case of highly exhausting jobs
  - Change tasks often within the job
  - Break each job up into smaller or different tasks
  - Employers should also consider their employees' capabilities and limitations
- *Use of personal protective equipment which includes*:
  - Respirators, earplugs, safety googles, chemical aprons, safety shoes
  - Hard hats, etc.

VARIOUS MEASURES IN THE OFFICE TO DECREASE MUSCULOSKELETAL AILMENTS AND MUSCULOSKELETAL PAIN

- Maintain an erect position of the back and neck with the shoulders relaxed. Minimize twisting and bending motions. Position equipment and work tasks so that the body is directly in front of and close to the major work tasks.
- Use proper positioning during all activities. Keep the upper arms close to the body, elbows at 100°, forearms neutral (thumb toward ceiling), and wrist straight. Keep the feet flat on the floor when seated by proper adjustment of your chair, or use of a footrest.
- Keep the wrists as neutral as possible. Avoid extreme motions. There is a safe zone of movement for your wrist. This zone is about 15° in all directions.
- Avoid bending the neck forward for prolonged periods. If typing from a manuscript, place the document on a holder beside or below the computer screen.
- Avoid static positions for prolonged periods. Muscles fatigue faster when they are held in one position. Keep moving to increase blood circulation.

A *comprehensive rehabilitation program* is required for work-related injuries so that workers can recover faster and return to work earlier. This will also help to prevent or decrease further damage and recurrence of such injuries and work-related MSP.

It consists of three phases as describe in **Table 1**:
1. Acute phase
2. Recovery phase
3. Maintenance phase

Table 1: Describing different phases of rehabilitation for recovery from occupational injury.

Phases	Therapy focus
Acute	Education, relative rest, pain control
Recovery	Full or optimal range of motion, strength, balance, proprioception
Maintenance	Return to work and sport-specific activity, aerobic conditioning

THERAPEUTIC EXERCISES

The main goal is to improve flexibility, muscle strength, and aerobic capacity.

Flexibility exercises like stretching are necessary for maintaining or regaining muscle flexibility and range of motion.

Stretching should be maintained for 30 seconds with the patient perceiving a pulling sensation rather than pain.

Muscle strengthening is an important part of therapeutic rehabilitation. An appropriate balance should be maintained between agonist and antagonist muscle groups. Training is most effective when exercises focus on different muscle groups in rotating sessions.

The therapeutic rehabilitation plan also emphasizes re-establishing cardiovascular fitness.

To improve aerobic capacity, the oxidation metabolism of the muscle must be stressed. The duration of aerobic training is usually >15 minutes of continuous exercise. Frequency is usually three to six times a week.

PSYCHOLOGICAL THERAPY

Psychological therapy includes cognitive behavioral therapy, explanation, reassurance, stress reduction, and counseling.

CONCLUSION

Addressing occupational and ergonomic factors is crucial in the effective management of musculoskeletal pain. By understanding how workplace design, job demands, and ergonomic practices contribute to musculoskeletal disorders, healthcare providers and employers can implement targeted interventions that alleviate pain and prevent recurrence. Integrating ergonomic assessments, personalized adjustments, and education on proper body mechanics into treatment plans not only improves patient outcomes but also promotes a healthier work environment. Ultimately, a proactive approach to ergonomics in occupational settings can reduce the incidence and severity of musculoskeletal pain, supporting both employee well-being and productivity.

BIBLIOGRAPHY

1. Boström C, Dellve L, Carlsson L, Lagerström M. Effects of a workplace ergonomics intervention on neck-specific exercise and health promotion for office workers: A randomized trial. BMC Musculoskeletal Disord. 2022;23(1):65.
2. van Rijn RM, Huisstede BMA, Koes BW, Burdorf A. Associations between work-related factors and specific disorders of the shoulder – a systematic review of the literature. Scand J Work Environ Health. 2023;49(2):85-98.
3. Tullar JM, Brewer S, Amick BC III, Irvin E, Mahood Q, Pompeii LA, et al. Workplace interventions for neck pain in workers. Occup Environ Med. 2023;80(1):59-69.
4. Rasmussen CDN, Holtermann A, Jørgensen MB, Søgaard K, Aagaard P, Østergaard L. Rehabilitative interventions for musculoskeletal pain among employees with physically demanding work: A systematic review. J Occup Rehabil. 2023;33(2):216-28.

CHAPTER 59

Pain Education and Patient Empowerment

Sonakshi Gupta

"Each patient carries their doctor inside them."
—**Norman Cousins, Anatomy of an Illness**

INTRODUCTION

Patient education and empowerment in managing musculoskeletal pain involve providing individuals with knowledge about their condition, treatment options, and self-care strategies. By understanding pain triggers, exercise routines, and medication use, patients gain control over their symptoms, leading to better outcomes and improved quality of life. Empowered patients are more engaged in decision-making, adhere to treatment plans, and adopt healthier lifestyle choices for long-term pain management.

IMPORTANCE OF PATIENT EDUCATION IN PAIN MANAGEMENT

Several patient factors, such as underreporting, unrealistic expectations, and a lack of understanding of pain and treatment options, can lead to poor pain management outcomes. Therapeutic patient education is a technique developed to enable healthcare professionals to share their knowledge with patients, transforming them into partners in their care. This approach involves structured activities designed to help patients and their families gain a comprehensive understanding of the disease and treatment options. This knowledge can improve the quality of life and help manage pain more effectively.

At the 2011 UK Pain Summit, patient education was identified as a priority, and the Patient's Association has since launched a campaign focused on pain management. Information should be presented in an easily understandable way, tailored to the patient's language and comprehension level.

The effectiveness of patient education can be evaluated using attitude and knowledge assessments, treatment plan adherence, patient satisfaction, and pain-related measures. Educational interventions can include one-on-one counseling, group sessions, audio guides, books, DVDs/podcasts, telecare, or informational leaflets. The chosen method depends on available resources. Educated patients can take an active role in managing their pain, thereby increasing their sense of control.

A therapeutic patient education program can serve as the foundation of the analgesic ladder, complementing other acute and chronic pain management modalities. The revised three phase model of patient education includes:

1. *Acute and mild pain:* With increased knowledge, patients can adjust their attitudes, develop skills, and reinforce their aspirations to adapt to both acute and chronic pain.
2. *Chronic and moderate pain:* Consultation with a physiotherapist, psychiatrist, or psychologist can help maintain physical activity and function. Engaging in social activities can support the patient in accepting pain-related limitations.
3. *Chronic pain, severe pain, palliative care:* Successful treatment centers on a multidisciplinary approach that empowers patients to actively participate in their individualized care.

TEACHING PATIENTS SELF-MANAGEMENT TECHNIQUES

Self-management involves a person's ability to manage the consequences of living with a chronic condition, including treatment, and physical, social, and lifestyle changes. This approach leads to an individualized, patient-led strategy. An empowering approach to pain management ensures that patients are confident and well informed, enhancing their skills to manage their pain, recognize the need for additional support, and handle analgesics and their side effects. Self-management techniques include:

- Psychological training
- Pain education
- Lifestyle modifications (nutrition, mindful consumption, music, art, shifting focus)
- Physical activity
- Heat and ice compresses
- Complementary therapies
- Relaxation techniques (muscle relaxation, breathing techniques, guided imagery)

Other components include:
- Coping skills training
- Cognitive restructuring to replace negative self-talk with positive affirmations

- Cognitive-behavioral therapy to change thoughts, behaviors, and emotions related to pain
- Mindfulness and acceptance-based strategies
- Self-hypnosis and hypnotic techniques for pain relief

EMPOWERING PATIENTS TO ADVOCATE FOR THEIR PAIN MANAGEMENT NEEDS

Patient advocacy involves representing and protecting the rights and interests of patients within the healthcare system. Empowering patients to make informed choices about their pain management can lead to significant improvements. The practice of shared decision-making between patients and healthcare providers is increasingly common.

Patient advocacy in pain management helps in several ways:
- *Enhancing research:* Involving patients in research planning and prioritization ensures that the most important issues to them are addressed.
- *Improving treatment outcomes:* Patients provide valuable insights into the diverse manifestations of pain.
- *Fostering trust and transparency:* Building meaningful partnerships with patients
- *Promoting access to care:* Improving access to pain management resources and services. Advocates can influence policies and increase funding for pain research by amplifying patient voices.
- *Driving innovation:* Engaging patients in the research process can lead to better ideas and innovations.

CONCLUSION

Patient education and empowerment are key to effective musculoskeletal pain management. By fostering self-management through individualized care, communication, and holistic strategies, patients are better equipped to control their pain.

BIBLIOGRAPHY

1. Lin I, Wiles L, Waller R, Caneiro JP. Patient-centred care: the cornerstone for high-value musculoskeletal pain management. British Journal of Sports Medicine. 2022.
2. Fritz JM, Kongsted A. A new paradigm for musculoskeletal pain care: moving beyond structural impairments. Conclusion of a chiropractic and manual therapies thematic series. Man Therap. 2023;31:15.
3. Benzon H, Raja SN, Fishman SM, Liu SS, Cohen SP. Essentials of Pain Medicine, 4th edition. Amsterdam: Elsevier; 2018.
4. Briggs E. Evaluating the impact of pain education: how do we know we have made a difference? Br J Pain. 2012;6(2):85-91.

CHAPTER 60

Technology and Innovation in Pain Management

Shruti Gupta

INTRODUCTION

Healthcare is in the midst of a technological revolution with advances in mobile health (also known as mHealth) which is changing many areas of medical practice. Mobile health technologies include several methods and tools that collect both subjective data on individuals through mobile apps known as ecological momentary assessment (EMAs) and objective data, which can be collected by the use of variable or implantable devices.

Technology and innovation have significantly impacted musculoskeletal pain management.

Advanced imaging techniques like MRI and CT scans provide detailed insights into the root causes of pain, allowing for more precise diagnoses.

Robotics and minimally invasive surgical procedures have revolutionized the treatment, reducing recovery times and complications. Additionally, advancements in pharmaceuticals, such as targeted drug delivery systems and biologics, offer new avenues for pain relief with fewer side effects.

WEARABLE DEVICES FOR PAIN, MONITORING, AND MANAGEMENT

Wearable devices for pain monitoring and management of musculoskeletal pain are becoming increasingly sophisticated. These innovative devices have the potential to revolutionize the approach to pain management and empower individuals to take a more active role in their well-being and physical training.

Wearable sensors can track movement patterns, posture, and activity levels, providing valuable data for assessing pain triggers and monitoring progress. These devices are often integrated with mobile apps or online platforms to analyze data trends and provide personalized feedback or interventions.

Examples of variable devices include:
- *Wearable activity trackers:* Devices such as Fitbit or Apple Watch can monitor the patient's physical activity, sleep patterns, and heart rate. This can be useful in understanding how certain activities affect musculoskeletal pain.
- *Smart clothing:* Garments embedded with sensors can monitor posture, muscle activity, and movement patterns in real time, offering insights into biomechanics and potential pain triggers.
- *Electromyography (EMG) sensors:* EMG sensors measure electrical activity in muscles and identify areas of muscle imbalance or dysfunction contributing to pain.
- *Wearable pain relief devices:* Wearable transcutaneous electrical nerve stimulation (TENS) devices have been evaluated in chronic lower extremity pain, chronic low back pain, and chemotherapy-induced peripheral neuropathy (CIPN) with generally encouraging results.
- *Smartphone apps:* It is becoming an attractive tool to assist patient self-management, continuous symptoms and vital sign monitoring, and communication between patients and physicians.
- *Virtual reality (VR) and augmented reality (AR):* AR is emerging as a dynamic tool within the healthcare system. While the exact neurobiological mechanisms behind VR's action remain unclear, investigations are currently underway to examine the complex interplay of cortical activity associated with immersive neural VR. VR can help patients undergoing physical rehabilitation as they imagine themselves performing slow, simple movements while immersed. VR immersion, coupled with the patient's visualization, is believed to create brain patterns closer to actual motor skills than visualization alone. This gives the patient a huge advantage in healing.
- *Implantable devices:* Advanced neurostimulation implants, such as spinal cord stimulators or peripheral nerve stimulators, can modulate pain signals before they reach the brain, offering long-term relief for chronic musculoskeletal pain conditions.

These wearable devices not only assist in monitoring patients' movement for pain management and performance enhancement but also empower individuals to actively participate in their pain management strategies, leading to more personalized and effective treatment.

The evidence base for the efficacy of these wearable devices is expanding. Still, research is going on regarding their long-term certainty and efficacy. To advance our understanding of the use of these systems in rehabilitation, further research and development is needed to address issues like power consumption, standardization, privacy, and confidentiality.

As there are several approaches to monitoring movement, two approaches, in particular, have been proven to be effective in enhancing pain management and physical performance.

Movement Analysis

Analyzing movement data can help pinpoint specific movement patterns that contribute to pain, allowing for targeted interventions and corrective exercises. In sports activities, wearable sensors allow athletes to monitor performance and body movements objectively, going beyond the coach's subjective evaluation limits. They can also prevent injuries by identifying early signs of faulty movement patterns or muscle imbalances, thus preventing potential injuries for athletes and individuals who engage in physical activity.

Muscle Activity Monitoring

Electromyography sensors incorporated into variable devices can help to track muscle activities. Sport and rehabilitation scientists are increasingly using surface EMG as a research tool because it can be used to assess muscle function which can act as a guide to develop a targeted rehabilitation program aimed at improving muscle strength and coordination.

Monitoring muscle activity during exercise can help to improve exercise techniques. Real-time feedback on muscle fatigue levels can help individuals adjust their exercise intensity and prevent overexertion, potentially reducing pain and promoting faster recovery.

TELEMEDICINE AND DIGITAL HEALTH PLATFORM FOR REMOTE PAIN

By employing these telemedicine approaches, healthcare providers can effectively manage pain and improve the quality of life for individuals with musculoskeletal disorders, even in remote or underserved areas. Several telemedicine approaches can be utilized for remote pain management in musculoskeletal disorders.

Remote Monitoring

Wearable devices and mobile apps can track patients' activity levels, movement patterns, and pain levels over time. The ultimate goal with these devices and apps is to provide real-time feedback to patients so that they see data that illustrates how destructive behaviors impact them physically. Also, this data can be transmitted to the healthcare providers for ongoing assessment and interpretation to adjust the treatment plans.

Other areas where telemedicine is really helpful in pain management include:
- Virtual consultations
- Telerehabilitation

- Educational resources
- *Medication management:* Moderate-quality studies indicate the potential of online cognitive-behavioral therapy to improve pain in a mixed chronic pain population.
- *Behavioral health support:* Telemedicine platforms may include access to mental health professionals who can provide counseling and support for patients dealing with the psychological aspects of chronic pain

ADVANCEMENTS IN NEUROSTIMULATION AND NEUROMODULATION THERAPIES FOR PAIN RELIEF

Neuromodulation therapies for musculoskeletal disorders involve various methods of targeting the nervous system to alleviate pain. Some common approaches include the folllowing:

- *Spinal cord stimulation (SCS):* This technique involves implanting electrodes near the spinal cord to deliver electrical impulses, interrupting pain signals before they reach the brain. SCS can provide long-term pain relief with a concomitant improvement in the quality of life, daily function, and patient satisfaction, although the initial costs may be high.
- *Peripheral nerve stimulation (PNS):* Similar to SCS, PNS targets specific peripheral nerves responsible for transmitting pain signals, providing localized pain relief. It is effective in treating musculoskeletal disorders, such as knee pain and back pain, as well as other conditions like nerve injuries and complex regional pain syndromes.
- *Dorsal root ganglion (DRG) stimulation:* DRG stimulation is a neuromodulation therapy that targets the cell bodies of sensory neurons before they enter the spinal column, which is different from traditional SCS. It can help to relieve focal nerve pain and interrupt pain signals in areas that are difficult to treat with SCS.
- *Percutaneous electrical nerve stimulation (PENS):* PENS can be used in chronic mixed and refractory pain as multimodal rehabilitation management of chronic muscular disorder. To date, PENS efficacy and safety have been investigated in lower back pain and knee osteoarthritis only but research is still going on to determine its efficacy in the complex management of chronic and refractory pain conditions.

Continued research and innovation in the field of neuromodulation hold the potential to further enhance outcomes and improve the quality of life for individuals suffering from musculoskeletal pain.

KEY POINTS

- Technology has revolutionized pain management by offering novel approaches to assess, diagnose, and treat various types of pain.
- From wearable devices to VR, a wide range of technological solutions exists to address different aspects of pain management, providing both patients and healthcare providers with more options and flexibility.

- Despite the advancements, challenges remain, including accessibility, affordability, and ensuring the ethical use of technology in pain management.
- Continued research and collaboration between technology developers, healthcare professionals, and patients are essential to further harness the potential of technology in improving pain management outcomes.

CONCLUSION

Technology plays a transformative role in the management of musculoskeletal pain by enhancing diagnostic accuracy, treatment personalization, and patient engagement. Innovations such as digital health tools, wearable devices, and telemedicine have improved access to care and empowered patients in their pain management journey. While challenges remain, the integration of technology offers promising advancements that can further optimize outcomes and revolutionize musculoskeletal care.

BIBLIOGRAPHY

1. Ayyad MA, Owida HA, Fazio RD, Naami BA, Visconti P. Electromyography monitoring systems in rehabilitation: a review of clinical applications, wearable devices and signal acquisition methodologies. Electronics. 2023;12(7):1520.
2. Bohr A, Memarzadeh K. The rise of artificial intelligence in healthcare applications. Artificial Intelligence in Healthcare. Amsterdam: Elsevier; 2020. pp. 25-60.
3. Chander H, Burch RF, Talegaonkar P, Saucier D, Luczak T, Ball JE, et al. Wearable stretch sensors for human movement monitoring and fall detection in ergonomics. Int J Environ Res Public Health. 2020;17(10):3554.
4. Chapman KB, Tupper C, Vissers KC, van Helmand N, Yousef T. Dorsal root ganglion stimulation for the treatment of joint pain with predominantly nociceptive characteristics: a case series. Pain Pract. 2023;23(3):317-24.
5. Chehade MK, Yadav L, Kopansky-Giles D, Merolli M, Palmer E, Jayatilaka A, et al. Innovations to improve access to musculoskeletal care. Best Pract Res Clin Rheumatol. 2020;34(5):101559.
6. Chew MT, Chan C, Kobayashi S, Cheng HY, Wong TM, Nicholson LL. Online pain management programs for chronic, widespread musculoskeletal conditions: a systematic review with meta-analysis. Pain Pract. 2023;23(6):664-83.

CHAPTER 61

Emerging Trends and Future Directions in Musculoskeletal Pain Management

Nanie Bhadrala

INTRODUCTION

Traditional approaches to managing musculoskeletal pain, such as pharmacotherapy, physical therapy, and surgery, remain vital, but advances in technology are rapidly transforming the landscape of care. As healthcare systems evolve, new modalities are emerging, promising more precise, personalized, and efficient pain management strategies.

EMERGING TRENDS IN MUSCULOSKELETAL PAIN MANAGEMENT

Precision Medicine and Personalized Pain Management

Precision medicine, an approach that tailors treatment based on an individual's genetic, environmental, and lifestyle factors, is gaining traction in musculoskeletal pain management. Traditional "one-size-fits-all" approaches are being replaced by therapies designed for specific patient subgroups based on their biological profiles.

- *Genomic medicine*: Recent research is exploring the genetic predisposition to musculoskeletal disorders and the varying responses to pain treatment. Pharmacogenetics allows clinicians to prescribe medications more effectively, minimizing side effects and maximizing therapeutic outcomes by tailoring drug regimens to individual genetic profiles. For example, some genetic variations influence how patients metabolize opioids, nonsteroidal anti-inflammatory drugs (NSAIDs), and other analgesics, enabling clinicians to choose the most effective and safest options for each patient.
- *Biomarker development*: The identification of biomarkers, measurable indicators of biological states, is revolutionizing pain management.

Biomarkers can predict an individual's risk of developing chronic pain after injury, aiding early intervention. For instance, inflammatory biomarkers like C-reactive protein (CRP) levels can indicate the likelihood of persistent pain following acute musculoskeletal trauma, guiding early and personalized treatment plans.

Regenerative Medicine: Beyond Symptom Management

Regenerative medicine, which focuses on repairing or replacing damaged tissues, represents a paradigm shift from managing symptoms to addressing the root causes of musculoskeletal disorders. Rather than relying solely on pain relief, these approaches aim to restore function and promote tissue healing.

- *Stem cell therapy: Platelet-rich plasma (PRP)*—PRP therapy involves injecting a concentrated solution of a patient's platelets into injured tissues to promote healing. PRP has been widely used in orthopedic injuries. As technology advances, PRP formulations will become more refined, offering targeted treatment for specific musculoskeletal conditions.
- *Gene therapy*: It holds the potential to treat musculoskeletal pain by modifying the expression of pain-related genes.
- Artificial intelligence (AI) and machine learning (ML) in pain diagnosis and management

Artificial intelligence and ML are transforming healthcare, potentially revolutionizing how musculoskeletal pain is diagnosed, monitored, and treated. By analyzing large datasets, AI can provide predictive analytics and guide treatment decisions and personalized care.

- AI-assisted imaging
- *Predictive models for chronic pain*: ML models are being developed to predict which patients are at risk of developing chronic pain following an acute injury or surgery.
- *AI in treatment planning*: AI can optimize treatment protocols by analyzing patient data, including pain levels, functional outcomes, and responses to previous therapies.
- Wearable technologies for pain monitoring and rehabilitation

Wearable technology is playing an increasingly important role in musculoskeletal pain management, particularly in monitoring real-time physiological and biomechanical data.

Nonopioid Pharmacological Approaches

- Topical analgesics and patches
- *Liposomal and nanoparticle drug delivery systems*: Nanotechnology is enabling the development of drug delivery systems that provide sustained and controlled release of pain medications. Liposomal formulations of local anesthetics like bupivacaine offer prolonged pain relief, reducing

the need for repeated dosing. Nanoparticles can be engineered to deliver anti-inflammatory drugs directly to the site of injury, enhancing therapeutic effects while minimizing systemic toxicity.
- *Neuromodulation*: Neuromodulation techniques, such as spinal cord stimulation and peripheral nerve stimulation, are gaining popularity as nonpharmacological options for managing chronic musculoskeletal pain.

FUTURE DIRECTIONS IN MUSCULOSKELETAL PAIN MANAGEMENT

Integration of Artificial Intelligence and Robotics in Surgery and Rehabilitation

The integration of AI with robotic systems is set to revolutionize surgical interventions and postoperative rehabilitation for musculoskeletal conditions. Robotic-assisted surgeries offer greater precision, minimizing tissue damage and promoting faster recovery. In the future, AI-driven robots may autonomously perform certain aspects of surgery, improving outcomes and reducing the risk of complications.

In rehabilitation, robotic exoskeletons are being developed to assist patients with mobility impairments, such as those recovering from spinal injuries. These devices offer real-time feedback and adjust to the patient's movement patterns, promoting more effective rehabilitation.

Advances in Bioprinting for Musculoskeletal Tissue Engineering

Bioprinting, the process of creating three-dimensional biological structures using cells and biomaterials, is a promising future direction for musculoskeletal pain management. Researchers are exploring the use of bioprinting to create cartilage, bone, and muscle tissues for transplantation in patients with degenerative or traumatic musculoskeletal conditions. As bioprinting technologies advance, they could provide personalized, regenerative treatments that restore function and alleviate pain.

Global Access to Advanced Pain Management Techniques

One of the critical challenges in musculoskeletal pain management is ensuring that advanced technologies are accessible to all patients, regardless of geographic or socioeconomic barriers. Telemedicine and mobile health (mHealth) platforms are emerging as solutions to bridge this gap, allowing patients in underserved areas to access cutting-edge care. Future developments in telemedicine, combined with AI-driven diagnostic tools, will enable more widespread access to expert pain management, improving outcomes on a global scale.

CONCLUSION

Musculoskeletal pain management is undergoing a transformative shift, driven by technological innovations and emerging therapies. Precision medicine, regenerative treatments, AI, wearable technologies, and nonopioid pharmacological approaches are redefining how musculoskeletal pain is diagnosed, treated, and monitored. As these trends continue to evolve, the future of pain management will be more personalized, efficient, and effective, ultimately improving the quality of life for millions of individuals suffering from musculoskeletal conditions.

BIBLIOGRAPHY

1. Clarke H, Katz J, McCartney CJ. Emerging Pain Management Approaches: Non-opioid Analgesics and Neuromodulation. J Pain Res. 2022;15:123-35.
2. Hurley DA, McDonough SM. Advances in the Diagnosis and Management of Musculoskeletal Pain. Pain Manage Today. 2020;10(3):27-33.
3. Kwoh CK, O'Connell D. Innovation in Regenerative Medicine: Current Trends and Future Perspectives. J Regen Ther. 2014;9:17-24.
4. Loeser JD. The Evolution of Pain Medicine. Pain Med. 2021;22(6):1043-5.
5. Patel KV, Guralnik JM. Musculoskeletal Pain in Older Adults: Prevalence and Impact. J Gerontol 2019;74(4):591-8.

Index

Page numbers followed by *b* refer to box, *f* refer to figure, *fc* refer to flowchart, and *t* refer to table.

A

Abduction 128
Abductor pollicis longus 148
Acceptance therapy 251, 258
Aceclofenac 35
Acetaminophen 11, 16, 27, 28, 31-33, 65, 66, 76, 80, 82, 87, 90, 95, 113, 119, 133, 158, 173, 214, 217, 220, 227, 229, 261
Achilles
 tendinopathy 160, 165
 tendon 161, 164
Acromioclavicular
 disease 139
 joint arthritis 141, 142
Acupressure 27, 93, 113, 262
Acupuncture 17, 61, 93, 113, 217, 247, 248, 249, 258, 262
 efficacy of 248
 mechanism of 247
 role of 247
 use of 82, 83
Acute flare-ups, management of 24
Acute gout 106*fc*, 109
 attacks 107
 pain, management of 104
Acute musculoskeletal pain 10, 28, 50, 58
 management of 10
 pathophysiology of 10
Acute pain 20, 24, 29, 35, 113, 121, 274
 flares 25
 management 12
Acute painful musculoskeletal
 disorders 50
Adalimumab 120
Adductor canal block 205, 216
Adequate sleep 265
Adhesive capsulitis 141, 201
Adipose-derived stem cells 254
Adjunctive therapies 107
Adrenaline 204
Adrenocorticotropic hormone 108

Advanced interventional techniques 201
Advanced pain management
 techniques 283
Alcohol 32, 37, 45, 50
 abuse 99
Alfentanil 40
Algodystrophy 175
Alimemazine 205, 206
 dose of 205*t*
Allergy 49, 233
Allopurinol 106
Alpha-2-adrenergic agonists 45, 52, 53, 211, 212
Alpha-2-receptor agonist produces
 antinociception, stimulation of 59
American Academy of Family
 Physicians 27, 28
American College of Physicians 27, 28, 238
American College of Rheumatology 101, 104, 169, 170*b*
 and Arthritis Foundation 132
 criteria 169
American Society of Anesthesiologists 226
American Society of Regional
 Anesthesia and Pain Medicine 53
Amiodarone 33
Amitriptyline 16, 45, 54, 59, 99, 122, 172
Amputation 21
Amyotrophic lateral sclerosis 49
Analgesia 53, 87, 216
 continuous regional 221
 epidural 45, 95
 multimodal 2, 11, 22, 28, 52*t*, 214, 217, 217*t*, 220
 topical 56, 61
Analgesics 54, 80, 113, 119, 158, 173, 217*t*
 adjunct 52
 delivery systems 221
 drugs 178
 regular use of 207

safe use of 79
systemic 215
topical 11, 45, 56, 57, 81, 123
use 77
   general principles of 79
Anaphylactoid reactions 35
Anemia 128
Anesthesia 205
  epidural 12
  local 203, 205, 206
  regional 215
  spinal 12
Anesthetics
  techniques 204
  topical 58, 88
Angiectasis 177
Angiotensin-converting enzyme inhibitors 36
Angiotensin-receptor blockers 36
Ankle 164, 196
  block 216
  joint 164
    aspiration technique for 197*f*
  pain 164
    management of 164, 166
  sprains 165
  surgery 216
Ankylosing spondylitis 35, 117, 125, 232
Anterior cruciate ligament 156, 208
Antibodies 7
Anticholinergic drugs 55
Anticoagulants 36
Anticonvulsants 16, 45, 55, 59, 82, 99, 113, 122, 217, 261
  agents 102
Anti-cyclic citrullinated peptide 7
Antidepressants 16, 25, 45, 54, 82, 96, 99, 113, 122, 129, 178, 261
Antiepileptics 79
  drugs 177
Antihypertensives 48
  medications 36
Anti-inflammatory
  agents 186
  drugs 178
  effects 247
Anti-inflammatory prophylaxis 106
Antispasmodic 47
  skeletal muscle relaxants 49*t*, 50*t*
Antispastics 47
  skeletal muscle relaxants 49*t*

Anxiety 49, 168
  preoperative 20
Anxiolytics 45
Appetite, loss of 101
Arm sling 136
Arnica montana 244
Aromatherapy 28
Arterial hypotension 49
Arthralgias 169
Arthritis 165
  infectious 157
  juvenile idiopathic 71, 260
  pain, chronic 59
  peripheral 119
Arthroscopic surgery 145, 208
Arthroscopy 140, 158
Artificial intelligence 256, 282
  integration of 283
Ascending pain pathways 3
Ashwagandha 244
Aspiration 141
Aspirin 28, 36
Atrial fibrillation 35
Axillary block 216
Ayurveda 243

B

Back pain 68, 71, 72, 130
  causes of 70
  chronic 15
  diagnosis of 71
  pattern of 69
  postural 69
  psychogenic 126
  psychosomatic 126
  signs of 70
  sports-related 69
  symptoms of 70
Backache 49
  acute low 60
  management of 124
  mechanical 126
Baclofen 45, 47, 59
Barbiturates 50
Bath ankylosing spondylitis disease activity index 119
Behavioral health support 279
Behavioral self-management techniques 86
Behavioral therapy 129

Benzodiazepines 183
Benzydamine 57
Beta-blockers 217
Betamethasone 236
Bier block 45
Bilateral gluteal region 170
Bilateral greater trochanter 170
Bilateral low cervical region 170
Bioelectromagnetics 93
Bioenergetic therapies 243
Biological agents, types of 119
Biomarker development 281
Biopsychosocial model 250, 257
Bisphosphonate 114, 178
   intravenous 114
   oral 114
Bleeding 216
   increased risk of 36
Blood
   pressure 236
   tests 71
   vessels 164
Blurred vision 48
Body mass index 64
Body-based therapies 172
Bone 3, 164
   cysts 207
   infections of 207
   marrow 45
     concentrates 45
     evaluation of 112
   metastases 75
   specific alkaline phosphatase 112
Boswellia serrata 243
Botanical therapies 243
Botulinum toxin 45
Brachial plexus 216
   block 204
   branches of 216
   cord of 216
   division of 216
   injury 140
Bradycardia 52, 216
Brain regions 4
Breast surgery 21
Breastfeeding 50, 52, 234
Budapest criteria 175
Bupivacaine 45, 215
Buprenorphine 41, 43, 44, 92, 221
Burning mouth syndrome 58

Bursae 3
Bursitis 60, 141, 156, 233, 240
Butorphanol 41

C

Calcaneal stress fractures 161
Calcaneus 164
Calcific tendinitis 141
Calcitonin 113
Calcium 114
Capsaicin 58
   patches 45
   topical 101, 133, 173
Capsule soft gel 59
Carbamazepine 32, 45, 59, 88, 177
Cardiac conduction disturbances 50
Cardiovascular disease 104
Cardiovascular risk 76, 108
Cardiovascular system monitoring 119
Carisoprodol 47, 48, 50
Carpal tunnel syndrome 82, 98, 153, 207
   injection 193
     technique for 195*f*
   management of 153
Carpel tunnel release 208
Cartridge-based nucleic acid
   amplification test 128
Causalgia 175, 178
Celecoxib 35, 214, 218
Centers for Disease Control and
   Prevention guidelines 89
Central nervous system 20, 55, 56, 89, 94, 95
   depressants 48, 50
Central neuraxial technique 215
Central sensitization 251
Cerebral palsy 49
Certolizumab pegol 120
Cervical collar 136
Cervical disc replacement 137
Cervical discectomy, anterior 137
Cervical spondylosis 135
   management of 137
   pain management of 135
Cervical traction 136
Chair test 144
Chemotherapy 21
   induced neuropathy 99
Chills 127

Chinese medicine 247
Chlorzoxazone 50
Cholestyramine 32
Chondroitin 133
Chondroprotective agents 133
Chronic inflammatory arthritis 168
Chronic musculoskeletal pain 15, 54, 74, 89
　syndrome 60
Chronic pain 1, 20, 66, 74, 75, 113, 122, 239, 250, 257, 259, 274, 282
　disorders 24
　management 129
Cirrhosis 87
Clonidine 45, 52, 53
Codeine 28, 40, 42, 44, 87
Cognitive-behavioral therapy 5, 8, 11, 17, 28, 129, 172, 212, 243, 246, 251, 258, 262
Colchicine 104, 105
Cold
　extremity, unilateral 177
　therapy 11, 61, 86, 118, 239
Commitment therapy 251, 258
Complementary therapies 12, 262
Complete blood count 7, 128, 170, 182
Complex regional pain syndrome 59, 175
　Budapest diagnostic criteria for 176b
　management of 175
Compression therapy 61
Computed tomography 7, 140, 199, 258
　imaging 200
　scan 71, 118, 128, 135, 157, 166, 200
Connective tissue disorders 170
Conservative management 136, 154, 161, 207
Constipation 44, 48, 50, 54, 76
Conventional radiography 199
Convulsions 48
Coronary artery
　bypass 21
　disease 52
Cortical remapping theory 95
Corticosteroids 24, 36, 45, 102, 104, 105, 122, 158, 186, 223
　injections 123, 145, 150, 162, 198
　intra-articular injections of 45
　oral 233
　parenteral 233

COVID-19 infection 259
C-reactive protein 7, 128, 170
Creatine kinase 170
Cryoablation 201
Cryoanalgesia 45
Cryotherapy 61, 93, 132, 144, 239
　units 28
C-terminal telopeptide 112
Cumulative trauma disorders 207
Cuneiform bones 164
Cyanotic skin 177
Cyclobenzaprine 45, 47, 48, 50, 172
Cyclooxygenase 60, 218
　enzymes 31
　inhibition, effects of 34
　inhibitors 31, 214
Cyclosporine 36
Cytokine 253

D

De Quervain's disease 148, 152
De Quervain's tenosynovitis 82, 148
　management of 149
Degenerative bone 75
Denosumab 114
Depression 20, 50, 168, 177
Dermatomes 177
Desipramine 88
Dexamethasone 45, 52, 217, 218, 236
Dexmedetomidine 45, 52, 53, 218
Dextromethorphan 45
Dextropropoxyphene 40
Diabetes mellitus 98, 104
Diabetic neuropathy 98
Diacetylmorphine 40
Diagnostic sympathetic block 179
Diarrhea 44, 48, 49, 101
Diazepam 49
Diclofenac 35, 57, 58, 119, 218
Digital palpation 170
Digoxin 36
Dihydrocodeine 28
Direct oral anticoagulants 36
Disc herniation 233
Discectomy 130
Discitis 70
Disease-modifying antirheumatic drugs 101, 119, 232
Distal muscles, atrophy of 177

Dizziness 44, 49, 50, 227
Domperidone 33
Doppler imaging 200
Dorsal horn 3
Dorsal root ganglia 95
   stimulation 279
Douleur neuropathique 99
Doxepin 59
Drowsiness 44, 49, 50
Drugs 49, 50, 212
   interaction 36, 48, 55
Dry mouth 44, 48-50, 54
Dual-energy X-ray absorptiometry 112
Duchenne muscular dystrophy 260
Duloxetine 25, 45, 52, 54, 90, 122, 173, 183
Durkan's test 154
Dysesthesias 216
Dystonia 177

E

Edema reduction 240
Education 17, 129
Eichhoff's maneuver 149
Elbow 193
   joint, aspiration technique for 194*f*
   surgery of 216
Electrical muscle stimulation 240
Electrolyte disorders 35
Electromyography 182
   sensors 277, 278
Electrotherapy 239
Eltenac 57
Endoscopic carpal tunnel release 154
Enhanced recovery after surgery 223, 226
   program 225
   protocols 225
Enthesopathy 201
Epicondyle, bilateral lateral 170
Epicondylitis, lateral 143, 201, 208
Epidural blocks 12
Epidural injection 216
Epidural steroid 81
   injections 129, 185, 186, 200, 233
Epilepsy 240
Epinephrine 204
Epiphyseal plates 240
Ergonomics, advantages of 269

Erythrocyte sedimentation rate 7, 118, 128, 170
Esmolol 218
Estimated glomerular filtration rate 89
Etanercept 119
Etoricoxib 35
Euphorbia cactus 62
European League Against Rheumatism 101, 108, 172
Ewing sarcoma 70
Exacerbations, acute 158
Excessive weight bearing 265
Exercise 132, 172, 212, 251
   aerobic 172, 239
   physical 264
   programs 129
   therapy 16, 238, 254
Extensor carpi radialis brevis tendon 143
Extensor pollicis brevis tendons 148
Extensor tendinosis, chronic 59
Extracorporeal shock wave therapy 144, 151, 162

F

Facet joint 125
   blocks 200
   injection 130, 233
Fascia iliaca nerve block 205, 216
Fast-track surgery 225
Fatigue 44, 49, 50, 169
Febuxostat 106
Feeling sick 101
Felbinac 57
Femoral nerve 216
   block 205, 216
Fentanyl 28, 40, 43, 44, 87, 90, 91, 217, 221
Fever 70, 127
Fibromyalgia 15, 54, 55, 60, 168, 171*b*
   classification of 170*b*
   prevalence 168
Finkelstein's test 148
Flexion 128
Fluid disorders 35
Fluoroquinolone antibiotics 48
Fluoxetine 36
Flurbiprofen 57, 58
Food and Drug Administration fetal risk classification system 80*t*

Foot 164
　orthoses 133
　pain 164
　　management of 164, 166
　surgery 216
Forearm, surgery of 216
Fractures 140, 156, 207, 240
　history of 115
　insufficiency 75
　risk 114
　　assessment tool 111

G

Gabapentin 16, 45, 52, 55, 59, 88, 90, 92, 102, 122, 129, 173, 177, 211, 221
Gabapentinoids 28, 52, 53, 88, 173, 211, 212, 221, 227, 229
Gait analysis 7
Gamma-aminobutyric acid 4, 60, 183
　agonists 59
Ganglion cyst 149
Gangrene, ischemic 207
Gastritis 66
Gastrointestinal
　bleeding 108
　disease 236
　disturbances 48
　issues 66, 115
　level 31
　system monitoring 119
　tract 32, 86
Gene therapy 282
Generalized pain 169
GeneXpert 128
Genomic medicine 281
Geriatric musculoskeletal pain 74
Glaucoma 49
Glenohumeral joint 192, 192f, 193
　arthritis 141
Glomerular filtration rate 87, 90
Glomus tumor 207
Glossy skin 177
Glucocorticoids 52, 54, 101, 108, 119, 217
Glucosamine 133
Glucose monitoring 234
Glucose-6-phosphate dehydrogenase deficiency 33
Glutamate 3

Glycine 4
Golfer's elbow 143, 144
　management of 143, 146
Golimumab 120
Gout 157, 232
　acute 106fc, 109
　chronic 104, 106
　treatment of 104
Gouty arthritis 104, 264
Growth factors 253

H

Hair loss 101, 177
Hand
　surgery of 216
　therapy 83
　treatment 82
Hangover effect 49
Headache 44, 49, 50
Heart
　attack 177
　failure 50, 108
Heat therapy 11, 61, 86, 118, 239
Heating pad 60
Heel pain 160
　management of 162
Hematoma 216
　formation 216
Hemolytic anemia 50
Hemorrhage 86
Heparin 36
Hepatic impairment 49
Hepatotoxic medications 33
Hepatotoxicity 48-50
Herbal remedies 93
Herniated discs 59, 70, 98
Heroin 40
Herpes zoster 98
Hip 7
　joint 194
　　aspiration 194, 195, 195f
　pathologies 157
　replacement 208
　surgeries 216
Hirudo medicinalis 60
Hormonal fluctuations 23
Horner's syndrome 216
Human immunodeficiency virus 60
　neuropathy 58

Humeral head degeneration 142
Hyaluronic acid 45, 122, 158
   injections 198
Hydration 105
Hydrocodone 28, 44, 88, 90, 92
Hydrocollator packs 60
Hydromorphone 28, 87, 91
Hydrotherapy 61, 82, 83, 172, 239
Hyperglycemia 236
Hypersensitivity 33, 48, 55
Hypertension 52, 104, 177
Hypertonic dextrose 254
Hyperuricemia, asymptomatic 108
Hypnosis 217, 243, 246
Hypotension 48, 50, 52, 216
Hypothyroidism 172
Hypotonia 48

I

Ibuprofen 35, 42, 57, 58, 65, 66, 119
Ice packs 105
Ileus 217
Immobilization 151, 177
Immunosuppression 236
Indomethacin 35, 57, 58
Infections 70, 98, 151, 155, 240, 241
Infiltration around wound 204
Inflammation
   acute 241
   reduction of 241
Inflammatory pressure ulcers 59
Inflammatory rheumatic diseases 168
Infliximab 119
Infraclavicular block 216
Injury
   ligamentous 156
   traumatic 207
Injury 98, 156, 179
   mechanism of 157
Integrated medicine, role of 243
Intercostal nerve block 12
Intercostal neuralgia 82, 84
Interdisciplinary pain management,
   advantages of 258
Interleukin inhibitors 105, 120
International Association for Study of
   Pain 175, 257
International Olympic Committee 121
Interphalangeal joints 164
Interscalene block 216

Intersection syndrome 149
Interstitial cystitis 168
Interventional pain management 81
Intervertebral disc 7
   degeneration 255
Intra-articular corticosteroids 133, 134
Intra-articular hyaluronic acid 134
Intra-articular injections 132, 133, 158
Intra-articular regenerative therapy 187
Intra-articular steroids 236
Intralesional injectables 123
Intramuscular stimulation 183
Intraoperative analgesic techniques 214
Intraoperative pain management 218
Intrathecal injection 216
Intravascular injection 216
Iontophoresis 151
Ipsilateral phrenic nerve block 216
Irritable bowel syndrome 168
Isoniazid 32
Ixekizumab 120

J

Janus kinase inhibitors 120
Jaundice 50
Joint 3, 164, 235
   complex array of 164
   damage 208
      severe 207
   disorders 141
   effusion 190
   infections of 207
   inflammation 233
   injection 186, 200
      indications 190
      techniques 190
   pain 81, 83
   replacement surgery 208
   surgery 102
Jumper's knee 156

K

Ketamine 45, 52, 53, 59, 214, 217,
   218, 221
Ketoprofen 57, 58
Ketorolac 35
Kidney 50
   disease, chronic 89, 90, 92, 104
Kinesio taping 61

Knee
　arthroplasty 215
　bilateral 170
　joint 196, 196f
　osteoarthritis 7, 58, 201
　pain 156
　　management of 156
　replacement 208
　surgery, posterior 216
Kyphoplasty 114
Kyphosis 70, 207

L

Lactation 49, 50
Laminectomy 130, 208
Lamotrigine 32
Laser
　therapy 61, 239, 241
　　low-level 61
Lateral collateral ligament 156
Lateral epicondylitis 143, 201, 208
　injection for 193
Lateral femoral cutaneous nerve 216
Lateral retropatellar injection technique 196f
Lavage 141
Leech saliva 60
Leeds assessment of neuropathic symptoms and signs scale 99
Lidocaine 183, 204, 221
　nerve block 45
　patches 45, 58, 88
Ligament 3, 164
　repair surgery 208
　skin 177
　sprains 240
Ligamentous tests 157
Light-headedness 50
Lignocaine 204
　infusion 217, 218
Lithium 36
Liver 49, 50
　disease, severe 33
　dysfunction 101
　failure 86, 52
　injury, drug induced 86
　metabolism 86
Local anesthetic 45, 79, 122, 203, 212, 221
　injections 113, 123

Long COVID 169
Lordosis 70
Low back pain 49, 81, 124, 239, 248, 264
Lower limb
　blocks 216
　orthopedic surgery 216t
Lumbar plexus block 205
Lumbar radiculopathy 157
Lumbar sympathetic block 178
Lymphedema 177

M

Machine learning 282
Magnesium 45
Magnetic resonance
　arthrography 140
　imaging 7, 71, 112, 117, 128, 135, 140, 144, 149, 157, 161, 165, 199
　scans 258
Malaise 50
Malignancy 75, 240, 241
Malnutrition 33
Manipulative therapies 245
Manual therapy 16, 150, 238
Massage therapy 61, 238, 245
Medial branch blocks 130
Medial collateral ligament 156
Medial epicondylitis 143
Medical Research Council scale 6
Medications, effects of 78
Medicinal leeches 60
Meditation 243, 245
Meditative movements 172
Meloxicam 35
Membrane stabilizers 53
Meniscal tears 156, 157
Mental health 250
　and musculoskeletal pain 250
　disorders 250
Mental stress 250
Menthol 58
　blocks calcium channels 58
Meperidine 40, 87
Meralgia paresthetica 82, 83
Mesenchymal stem cells 187, 253
Metallic implants 200, 241
Metatarsophalangeal joints 164
Metaxalone 50
Methadone 40, 43, 44, 90, 92
Methocarbamol 47, 50

Methotrexate 33, 36, 119
Methylprednisolone 186, 236
Metoclopramide 33
Migraines 168
Milnacipran 173
Mind-body
  interventions 93, 130
  practices 245
  techniques 17
Mindfulness-based stress reduction 129, 251
Mindset strategies 28
Mini-invasive pharmacological approaches 122
Minimally invasive surgical procedures 276
Mirror therapy 96
Mirror-assisted movement patterns 178
Monitor vital signs 41
Monoamine oxidase 54
  inhibitors 66
Monosodium glutamate 172
Mood swings 23
Morphine 28, 40, 41, 44, 59, 65, 66, 87, 90, 91, 217
  administration 41
  sulfate 41
Mouth, dryness of 50
Mucositis 59
Multidisciplinary pain management, components of 258
Multimodal therapy 241
Multiple sclerosis 49, 98
Muscle 3, 164
  atrophy, prevention of 240
  imbalances 69
  relaxants 11, 45, 47, 48, 51, 129, 261
    role of 47
    types of 47
  skin 177
  spasm 47, 50, 60, 240
    acute 49
    chronic 49
  strains 58, 70, 142
  trauma 216
  weakness 49
Musculoskeletal injuries 175
Musculoskeletal pain 1-4, 6, 7, 9, 32, 46, 47, 63, 81, 93, 120, 199, 207, 214, 240, 247, 248, 250, 260, 262, 268, 270
  assessment of 6, 7
  management 2, 27, 28, 40, 47, 78, 86, 89, 94, 186-188, 203, 232, 238, 247, 252, 260, 262, 268, 281, 283, 284
  preventive strategies for 264
  surgical management of 207
Musculoskeletal tissue engineering 283
Musculoskeletal tumors 142, 207
Music therapy 28, 217
Myalgia 60, 169
Myasthenia gravis 49
Myocardial infarction 35, 54, 108
Myocardial ischemia 141
Myofascial pain syndrome 181
  diagnosis of 182
Myofascial release 245
Myofascial syndrome 181
Myofascial trigger points 183
Myopathy, inflammatory 172

N

Nalbuphine 41
Nalmefene 41
Nalorphine 41
Naloxone 41, 42
Naltrexone 41
Nanoparticle drug delivery systems 282
Naproxen 35, 119
Narcotic analgesics 122
Narrow-angle glaucoma 54
National Center for Complementary and Integrative Health 92
Natural therapies 243
Nausea 44, 48-50, 217, 227
Neck
  musculoskeletal pathology 141
  pain 248
Neer's impingement 140
Nerve 3, 164
  blocks 12, 113, 228
  compression 98
  conduction studies 154
  damage 98
  entrapment 98
  growth factor 100
  injury 140, 151, 155, 216
  root block 233
Neural injuries 175
Neurodermatitis 177
Neurological deficits 127
Neurological disorder muscle spasm 49

Neuromas 165
Neuromodulation 18, 283
  therapies 279
Neuromodulators 101, 102
Neuropathic pain 54, 55, 59, 82, 98, 100, 129, 240, 255
  adjuvants for 88
  chronic 25
  management of 98
  medications 80
Neuropathy 216
Neuropeptides 58
Neuroplastic changes 247
Neurostimulation 93, 279
Neurotransmitter modulation 247
New York criteria, modified 117
Night pain 70
Night splints 154
Nimesulide 58
Nitrates 59
Nitric oxide 59
Nitroglycerine patch 59
N-methyl-D-aspartate 45, 52, 53, 60, 95, 212, 218, 228
  antagonists 217
  blocking agents 59
  receptor
    antagonists 45, 52, 53, 96, 211, 212
    downregulation of 59
Non-low back musculoskeletal injuries 28, 29
Non-narcotic analgesics 122
Nonopioid analgesics 217, 261
Nonpharmacological pain management 118
Nonpharmacological topical analgesia options 61
Nonpharmacological treatment 105, 107, 136, 161, 258
Nonsteroidal anti-inflammatory drugs 11, 13, 16, 27, 28, 31, 34, 36, 38, 42, 45, 46, 58, 60, 66, 76, 79, 80, 82, 87, 91, 95, 101, 102, 104, 113, 118, 121, 122, 129, 133, 136, 141, 144, 150, 154, 158, 161, 173, 178, 183, 203, 210, 212, 217, 218, 220, 227, 229, 235, 261, 281
  adverse effects of 35
  gastrointestinal side effects of 37
  oral 150
  side effects of 38*fc*

systemic use of 56
topical 27, 150
use 37
Nonvertebral fractures, detection of 112
Norepinephrine 60
Nortriptyline 45, 88, 122
Numeric rating scale 6, 8, 261
Nutrition 17, 264
Nutritional deficiencies 99
Nylidrin hydrochloride 180

O

Occupational therapy 17, 118, 261
Omega-3 fatty acids 244
Open carpal tunnel release 154
Open release surgery 145
Open wounds 240, 241
Opioids 11, 16, 25, 27-29, 40, 44, 44*t*, 45*t*, 55, 59, 76, 79, 81, 82, 87, 91, 95, 99, 101, 122, 129, 133, 178, 211, 212, 217, 261
  antagonists 41*b*
  classification of 40*b*
  complex action of 41*b*
  mild 261
  receptors 58
  sparing strategies 43, 46
  synthetic 40
Opium alkaloids, natural 40
Orphenadrine 50
Orthopedic 200
  surgery 84, 217*t*
Orthopedic Trauma Association 27-29
Orthostatic hypotension 177
Orthotics 113, 158, 161
Osteoarthritis 7, 15, 35, 58, 98, 149, 156, 169, 232, 239-241, 248, 255, 264
  advanced 207
  pain management of 132
  severe 208
Osteoarthritis Research Society International guidelines 133
Osteoid osteoma 70
Osteomyelitis 70
  acute 207
  chronic 207
Osteopathic manipulation 245
Osteoporosis 75, 234, 236, 264
  diagnosis of 112

management of 114
severity of 114
Osteoporotic fractures 111
  management of 113
Osteoporotic vertebral fracture 111
Osteosarcoma 207
Osteotomy 158, 208
Oswestry disability index 7
Over thyroid gland 241
Oxycodone 28, 42, 44, 88, 90, 92
Oxygen therapy 42

P

Pacemakers 240
Pain 1, 4, 22, 86, 141, 190, 207
  abdominal 48, 84
  acute 20, 24, 29, 35, 113, 121, 274
  anatomy of 3, 5
  assessment 112
    components of 6
  biopsychosocial model of 250
  burning 177
  characteristics 165
  chronic 1, 20, 66, 74, 75, 113, 122, 239, 250, 257, 259, 274, 282
  clinics 18
  conversion of 20
  education 12, 273
  epicritic 5
  fast 4, 5
  first 5
  flare management 23
  inflammatory 117
  knee 156
  leg 127
  limb 94
  location of 157
  management 1, 74, 82, 84, 89, 90fc, 111, 113, 115, 117, 118, 120, 121, 144, 243, 251, 253-255, 257, 260, 273, 276
  mechanism of 117
  mild 274
  moderate 44, 274
  moderate-to-severe 44
  neuropathic 54, 55, 59, 82, 98, 100, 129, 240, 255
  perception 3, 4
  physiology of 3-5

  reduction 27
  referred 141, 142, 157
  relief 136, 240, 241, 279
    interventional techniques for 185
  second 5
  severe 44, 274
  slow 4, 5
  surgical management of 120
  type 5
Painful diabetic neuropathy 58, 59
Palliative care 260, 274
Palpitation 50
Paracetamol 31-33, 44, 45, 65, 66, 76, 80, 91, 122
  metabolism of 32
Paravertebral blocks 204
Paresthesias, typical 153
Patch 59
Patellar dislocation 156
Patellar tests 157
Patellofemoral pain syndrome 156
Patient-controlled analgesia 221, 228
Patrick's test 128
Pectoral block 12
Pediatric analgesics 65
Pediatric musculoskeletal pain 63
Pelvic pain 84
  pregnancy-related 82
  syndromes 168
Pelvic stabilization, belts for 83
Pentazocine 41, 43
Percutaneous electrical nerve stimulation 279
Periarticular injections 28, 215
Peripheral nerve
  blocks 12, 200, 204, 215, 216t
  stimulation 279
Peripheral nervous system 94, 95
Peripheral nociceptors 3
Peripheral sensory nerve endings 59
Peroneal tendons 164
Persistent nerve compression 207
Personal protective equipment, use of 270
Pethidine 40, 42, 44
Phalen's test 154
Phantom limb pain 94-96
  characteristics of 94
  mechanistic theories of 95

Pharmacotherapy 95, 150
Phenol 45
Phenytoin 32, 59
Pholcodine 40
Phrenic nerve block 216
Physical therapy 5, 11, 16, 64, 84, 86, 100, 113, 118, 136, 141, 144, 146, 150, 158, 162, 212, 235, 238, 261
Physiotherapy 238, 242
  role of 238
Piroxicam 57, 58
Plantar
  fascia 161
  fasciitis 160, 165
    injection for 197, 197f
Platelet-derived growth factor 253
Platelet-rich plasma 18, 187, 282
  injections 145, 162
  therapy 198, 254
Pluronic lecithin organogel 60
Pneumothorax 216
Point-of-care ultrasound 199
Polymyalgia rheumatica 170
Polyneuropathy, chronic peripheral 58
Popliteal fossa block 216
Positron emission tomography 258
Post-COVID-19 169
Posterior cervical decompression 137
Posterior cruciate ligament 156, 208
Postherpetic neuralgia 58, 59
Post-mastectomy pain syndrome 58, 59
Postoperative care 151, 154, 232
Postoperative inflammation 232
Postoperative pain
  control multimodal analgesia approaches 220
  management strategies 220
Post-traumatic dystrophy 175
Postural methods 82
Potent capsaicin analogue 58
Preanesthetic medication 226
Prednisolone 45
Prednisone 36, 235
Preemptive analgesia 210, 212t, 213, 214
  interventions 211
Pregabalin 16, 45, 52, 55, 59, 88, 90, 92, 102, 122, 129, 173, 177, 211, 214, 217, 221
Pregnancy 49, 50, 78-81, 234, 240, 241
Prehabilitation 226

Prerequisites 190, 248
Prilocaine 58
Probenecid 33, 106
Prolotherapy 254
Prostaglandin E receptor 118
Prosthetics 96
Pruritus 217, 227
Pseudogout 157
Psoriasis 58
Psoriatic arthritis 169, 232
Psychiatric disorders 168
Psychological therapy 100, 258, 271
Psychosocial therapy 64

R

Radial styloid tenosynovitis 149
Radial wrist pain 148
Radiation therapy 21
Radiculopathy 207
Radiofrequency 201
  ablation 45, 113, 137, 188
Radiology, role of 199f
Randomized controlled trials 29, 186, 248
Range-of-motion 6, 157, 165
  exercises 150, 151
Rapid inhibitory neurotransmission 183
Rectus sheath block 12
Red flag 70
  indicators 141
  situations 127
Reflex sympathetic dystrophy 175
  Bonica stages of 177t
Regenerative medicine 18, 253, 282
  applications of 255
Regional anesthesia 215
  techniques 45
Regional blocks 92, 228
Regional pain disorders 169
Rehabilitation 113, 123, 145, 151, 154, 166, 283
Relaxation
  techniques 252
  therapy 243, 246
Remifentanil 40
Renal disease, end-stage 89
Renal dysfunction, acute acute 35
Renal excretion 86
Renal failure 89, 120

Renal function 115
Renal impairment 50, 76
  severe 33
Renal system monitoring 119
Respiratory depression 44, 76, 217
Reye's syndrome 66
Rheumatoid arthritis 7, 15, 35, 58, 98,
    157, 169, 187, 207, 232, 241, 264
  management of 101
Rheumatological pain 82
Rib, bilateral second 170
Ribonucleic acid-based therapy 43
Rifampin 32
Romosozumab 115
Rotator cuff tears 140, 141

S

Sacroiliitis 117
Sacroplasty 201
Salicylates 58
Salicylic acid 57
Saphenous nerve 216
Scaffolds 253
Scaphoid fracture 149
Scar management 151
Sciatic nerve 216
  blocks 205, 216
  terminal branches of 216
Sciatica 49
Scoliosis 70, 72, 207
Secukinumab 120
Sedation 44, 48, 54, 227
Seizures 49, 50, 52
  disorders 49
Selective cyclooxygenase inhibitors 122, 210
Selective nerve root blocks 129
Selective serotonin reuptake inhibitors
    36, 43, 52, 54, 55, 92
Semisynthetic opiates 40
Septic arthritis 207
Serotonin syndrome 55
Serotonin-norepinephrine reuptake
    inhibitors 25, 55, 88, 99, 102, 122,
    129, 133, 173, 183, 218
Sertraline 36
Severe acute respiratory syndrome
    coronavirus 2 (SARS-CoV-2)
    infection 169

Sexual dysfunction 54
Shingles 98
Shortwave diathermy 241
Shoulder 191, 216
  girdle 140
  pain 59, 139
    causes of 140
    chronic 141
    management of 139
    traumatic 140
  pathology 139
Shoulder-hand syndrome 175
Six-minute walk test 7
Sjögren syndrome 169
Skeletal muscle
  relaxants 92, 122
  spasm 49
Skin
  edematous 177
  infiltration of 215
Sleep
  disorders 168
  hygiene 17
Smartphone apps 277
Smooth skin 177
Sodium-gated channels, block activity
    of 58
Soft-tissue 7
  injections 236
  injuries 7, 232, 240, 241
  mobilization 150
Soluble epoxide hydrolase inhibitors 43
Somatosensory cortex 4
Somnolence 44, 49
Spasm 177
Spinal blocks 12
Spinal cord 3, 25
  injuries 49
  stimulation 5, 96, 99, 279
Spinal decompression surgery 208
Spinal fusion surgery 208
Spinal injections 236
Spinal injuries 49
Spinal manipulation 238
Spinal stenosis 98, 233
Spondyloarthritis 169, 170
Spondylolisthesis 70
Spondylolysis 70
Spondylosis 49
  cervical 135

Index

Sports injuries 70, 121
  prevention of 266
Sprains 58, 70, 241
Stem cells 253
  therapy 115, 254, 282
Stenosing tenosynovitis 148
Steroids 232, 236, 237
  administration of 233
  injections 154
  role of 11, 232
  types of 235
Straight leg raise 128
Strains 241
Strength testing 6, 165
Strengthening exercises 150, 151, 162, 239
Stress
  fractures 165
  management 18
Stretching exercises 162
Stroke 108
Structural deformities 207
Subacromial corticosteroid injections 141
Subacromial impingement 141
Subtalar joint 164
Success rates 151
Sudeck's dystrophy 175
Sufentanil 40
Suicide 177
Sulfasalazine 119
Supplemental opioid analgesia 229
Suppress inflammation 58
Supraclavicular block 216
Supraspinatus, bilateral 170
Surgery 102, 132, 134, 146
  types of 21
Surgical neuropathic pain 58
Surgical site local infiltration 45
Swelling 148
Sympathetic blocks 96
Sympathetic trunk 180
Symptom severity scale 169
Syncope 50
Systemic autoimmune
  disorders 170
  rheumatic diseases 168
Systemic inflammatory arthropathies 170
Systemic lupus erythematosus 169, 232

T

Tadalafil, oral 178
Talus 164
Tapentadol 28, 40, 43, 44
Tarsometatarsal joints 164
Telerehabilitation 278
Temporomandibular disorders 168
Tender point examination 169
Tenderness 148
Tendinopathies 156, 201, 255
Tendon 3, 164, 235
  instability 152
Tendonitis 233, 240
Tennis elbow 143, 144, 193, 207, 208
  injection technique for 194f
  management of 143, 146
Tenotomy, percutaneous 145
Tension headaches 168
Teriparatide 114
Therapeutic exercises 150, 271
Thermatomes 177
Thermotherapy 60, 132, 239
Thiocolchicoside 47-49, 183
Thoracic outlet syndrome 98
Thoracolumbar interfacial plane 228
Thoracotomy 21
Thrombophlebitis 241
Thrombosis 241
Thumb
  carpometacarpal joint, osteoarthritis of 149
  spica splint 150
Thyroid stimulating hormone 170
Tibialis posterior 164
Tibiotalar joint 164
Timed up and go test 7
Tinel's sign 154
Tissue engineering 254
Tizanidine 45, 47-49, 183
Tolperisone 49
Topical agents 16, 58t, 62, 92, 99, 261
Torticollis 49
Total hip
  arthroplasty 215
  replacement 76
Total knee
  arthroplasty 158
  replacement 76, 215

Tramadol 27-29, 40, 43, 44, 50, 87, 91, 95, 173, 183, 217
Transarterial embolization 201
Transcranial magnetic stimulation 96
Transcutaneous electric nerve stimulation 5, 25, 45, 61, 75, 83, 93, 96, 100, 113, 172, 183, 211, 217, 223, 239, 262, 277
Transcutaneous electrical nerve stimulation, use of 28
Transdermal patches 82, 221
Transduction 4
Transforaminal nerve blocks 200
Transforming growth factor-beta 253
Transient receptor potential vanilloid-1 receptors 58
Transversus abdominis plane block 12
Trapezius
  bilateral 170
  myalgia 201
Trauma 70, 98
  history of 127
Tremor 50, 177
Triamcinolone 186, 236
Tricyclic amines 122
Tricyclic antidepressants 16, 25, 54, 59, 79, 87, 88, 90, 92, 99, 102, 129, 172, 183
Trigeminal neuralgia 58, 59
Trigger point injections 12, 187
Triggers 23
  points 181
Trimeprazine 205, 206
Tropisetron 183
Truncal blocks 12
Tubercular infections 125
Tumors 70, 98
  necrosis factor 89
    inhibitors 119
Tylenol 44
Type 2 complex regional pain syndrome 178

U

Ulcers 66
Ultrasound 7, 140, 144, 149, 157, 161, 166, 199, 200
  therapy 61, 182, 239, 240
Ultrasound-guided interventions
  pain management 200
  types of 200
Upper arm surgery 216
Upper extremity blocks 12
Upper limb
  blocks 216
  orthopedic surgery 216t
Urate-lowering therapy 106
  continuation of 107
Uremic pruritis 58
Urinary retention 217, 227
Urine discoloration 50

V

Valeriana officinalis 244
Vasoconstriction 177
Vasovagal reactions 49
Vastus medialis 216
Vertebral augmentation 201
Vertebral fracture 112
  assessment 112
Vertebroplasty 114
Virtual reality and augmented reality 277
  training 96
Visual analog scale 6, 7, 111, 261
Vitamin
  B 182
  B12 deficiency 99
  C 178
  D 114, 182, 244, 265
    levels 170
  K 265
Vomiting 44, 48-50, 217, 227

W

Warfarin 32, 36
Weakness 49, 52
Wearable pain relief devices 277
Weight
  gain 54
  loss 70, 127, 132
  management 17, 158
  reduction 265
Western Ontario and McMaster universities osteoarthritis index 7

Withania somnifera 244
Workplace injuries, prevention of 266
World Health Organization 13, 27, 28, 46, 89
  pain management ladder 13*fc*, 46*fc*
Worst pain 7
Wound
  care 154
  healing, promotion of 241

X

Xerostomia 49
X-rays 7, 71, 117, 118, 128, 135, 140, 149, 157, 161, 165
Yoga 82, 243, 245

Z

Zingiber officinale 244

EU GSPR Authorised Reprsentative
Logos Europe, 9 rue Nicolas Poussin
1700, La Rochelle, France
Phone: +33 (0) 6 67 93 73 78
E-mail: contact@logoseurope.eu

www.ingramcontent.com/pod-product-compliance
Ingram Content Group UK Ltd.
Pitfield, Milton Keynes, MK11 3LW, UK
UKHW060920270326

469420UK00011B/303